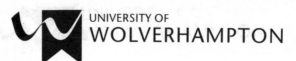
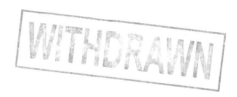

Handbook of

Emotion,

Adult Development,

and Aging

Handbook of

Emotion,

Adult Development,

and Aging

Edited by

Carol Magai
Department of Psychology
Long Island University, Brooklyn, New York

and

Susan H. McFadden
Department of Psychology
University of Wisconsin—Oshkosh, Oshkosh, Wisconsin

ACADEMIC PRESS

San Diego ✦ London ✦ Boston ✦ New York ✦ Sydney ✦ Tokyo ✦ Toronto

This book is printed on acid-free paper. ∞

Academic Press, Inc.
525 B Street, Suite 1900, San Diego, California 92101-4495, USA
http://www.apnet.com

Academic Press Limited
24-28 Oval Road, London NW1 7DX, UK
http://www.hbuk.co.uk/ap/

Library of Congress Cataloging-in-Publication Data

Handbook of emotion, adult development, and aging / edited by Carol
   Magai, Susan H. McFadden.
        p.   cm.
   Includes bibliographical references and index.
   ISBN 0-12-464995-5 (alk. paper)
   1. Emotions. 2. Emotions and cognition. 3. Adulthood. 4. Aging-
-Psychological aspects.   I. Magai, Carol.   II. McFadden, Susan H.
   BF531.H316   1996
   152.4--dc20   96-22522
                                                  CIP

PRINTED IN THE UNITED STATES OF AMERICA
96   97   98   99   00   01   BC   9   8   7   6   5   4   3   2   1

Contents

PART I
Theoretical Perspectives

CHAPTER 1

Emotions and the Aging Brain
Regrets and Remedies
Jaak Panksepp and Anesa Miller

CHAPTER 2

Differential Emotions Theory and Emotional Development in Adulthood and Later Life

Linda M. Dougherty, Jo Ann Abe, and Carroll E. Izard

CHAPTER 3

Ethological Perspectives on Human Development and Aging

Klaus E. Grossman

CHAPTER 4

A Humanistic and Human Science Approach to Emotion
Constance T. Fischer

CHAPTER 5

Psychosocial Perspectives on Emotions
The Role of Identity in the Aging Process
Susan Krauss Whitbourne

PART II

Affect and Cognition

CHAPTER 6

Emotion, Thought, and Gender
Gisela Labouvie-Vief

CHAPTER 7

Emotion and Cognition in Attachment

Victor G. Cicirelli

CHAPTER 8

Emotion and Memory

Kenneth T. Strongman

CHAPTER 9

Emotion and Everyday Problem Solving in Adult Development

Fredda Blanchard-Fields

CHAPTER 18

Quality of Life and Affect in Later Life
M. Powell Lawton

CHAPTER 19

Religion, Emotions, and Health
Susan H. McFadden and Jeffrey S. Levin

PART V

Continuity and Change in Emotion Patterns and Personality

CHAPTER 20

Mood and Personality in Adulthood
Paul T. Costa, Jr. and Robert R. McCrae

CHAPTER 21

Facial Expressions of Emotion and Personality
Dacher Keltner

CHAPTER 22

Personality Change in Adulthood
Dynamic Systems, Emotions, and the Transformed Self
Carol Magai and Barbara Nusbaum

CHAPTER 23

Emotional Episodes and Emotionality through the Life Span
Jennifer M. Jenkins and Keith Oatley

CHAPTER 24

The Story of Your Life

A Process Perspective on Narrative and Emotion in Adult Development

Jefferson A. Singer

Contributors

Numbers in parentheses indicate the pages on which the authors' contributions begin.

Jo Ann Abe (27) Psychology Department, University of Delaware, Newark, Delaware 19711

Paula Smith Avioli (207) Kean College of New Jersey, Union, New Jersey 07083

Victoria Hilkevitch Bedford (207) Behavioral Sciences Department, University of Indianapolis, Indianapolis, Indiana 46227

Fredda Blanchard-Fields (149) Department of Psychology, Georgia Institute of Technology, Atlanta, Georgia 30332

Laura L. Carstensen (227) Department of Psychology, Stanford University, Stanford, California 94305

Victor G. Cicirelli (119) Department of Psychological Sciences, Purdue University, West Lafayette, Indiana 47907

Paul T. Costa, Jr. (369) Gerontology Research Center, National Institute on Aging, National Institutes of Health, Baltimore, Maryland 21224

Brian de Vries (249) School of Family and Nutritional Sciences, University of British Columbia, Vancouver, British Columbia VGT 124, Canada, and Department of Medical Anthropology, University of California, San Francisco, San Francisco, California 94143

Linda M. Dougherty (27) Department of Gerontology, Virginia Commonwealth University, Medical College of Virginia, Richmond, Virginia 23298

Karen L. Fingerman (185) Department of Human Development and Family Studies, Pennsylvania State University, University Park, Pennsylvania 16802

Constance T. Fischer (67) Psychology Department, Duquesne University, Pittsburgh, Pennsylvania 15282

Victor Florian (269) Department of Psychology, Bar-Ilan University, Ramat Gan, Israel

Howard S. Friedman (307) Department of Psychology, University of California, Riverside, Riverside, California 92521

John M. Gottman (227) University of Washington, Seattle, Washington

Jeremy Graff (227) Department of Psychology, Stanford University, Stanford, California 94305

Klaus E. Grossmann (43) Institut für Psychologie, Universität Regensburg, Regensburg, Germany

Carroll E. Izard (27) Psychology Department, University of Delaware, Newark, Delaware 19711

Jennifer M. Jenkins (421) Institute of Child Study, University of Toronto, Toronto M5R 2X2, Canada

Dacher Keltner (385) Department of Psychology, University of Wisconsin—Madison, Madison, Wisconsin 53706

Gisela Labouvie-Vief (101) Department of Psychology, Wayne State University, Detroit, Michigan 48202

M. Powell Lawton (327) Polisher Research Institute, Philadelphia Geriatric Center and Temple University School of Medicine, Philadelphia, Pennsylvania 19141

Richard S. Lazarus (289) University of California, Berkeley, Berkeley, California 94720

Robert Levenson (227) University of California, Berkeley, Berkeley, California 94720

Jeffrey S. Levin (349) Department of Family and Community Medicine, Eastern Virginia Medical School, Norfolk, Virginia 23501

Carol Magai (403) Department of Psychology, Long Island University, Brooklyn, New York 11201

Robert R. McCrae (369) Gerontology Research Center, National Institute on Aging, National Institutes of Health, Baltimore, Maryland 21224

Susan H. McFadden (349) Department of Psychology, University of Wisconsin—Oshkosh, Oshkosh, Wisconsin 54901

Mario Mikulincer (269) Department of Psychology, Bar-Ilan University, Ramat Gan, Israel

Anesa Miller (3) Memorial Foundation for Lost Children, Bowling Green, Ohio 43402

Barbara Nusbaum (403) Department of Psychology, Long Island University, Brooklyn, New York 11201

Keith Oatley (421) Center for Applied Cognitive Science, Ontario Institute for Studies in Education, Toronto, Ontario M5S 1V6, Canada

Jaak Panksepp (3) Department of Psychology, Bowling Green State University, Bowling Green, Ohio 43403

Jan-Erik Ruth (**167**) Department of Social Policy, University of Helsinki, Helsinki, Finland

Jefferson A. Singer (**443**) Department of Psychology, Connecticut College, New London, Connecticut 06320

Kenneth T. Strongman (**133**) Department of Psychology, University of Canterbury, Christchurch, New Zealand

Lillian E. Troll (**185**) Medical Anthropology Department, University of California, San Francisco, San Francisco, California 94143

Joan S. Tucker (**307**) Department of Psychology, Brandeis University, Waltham, Massachusetts 02254

Anni Vilkko (**167**) Department of Social Policy, University of Helsinki, Helsinki, Finland

Susan Krauss Whitbourne (**83**) Department of Psychology, University of Massachusetts at Amherst, Amherst, Massachusetts 01003

Preface

The study of human emotions and feelings has had an uneven history. A first wave of emotions research during the opening decades of this century was followed by a lull of 40 years. During the early 1980s, however, psychology began to renew its interest in the emotions.

The resurgent interest in human emotion and motivation over the past 15 years has had a stimulating effect on many areas of research, bringing new vitality to such topics as cognition, learning, perception, and memory. A recent report by the National Advisory Mental Health Council (1995) indicates that the new wave of research on emotions has had an important impact on federal policy with respect to basic behavioral research, and it is clear that it will continue to do so well into the next century.

This renaissance of research on emotions has similarly enlivened the field of adult development and aging, as is well captured in the 24 chapters in this volume, and it has developed in several interesting ways. For example, in the child developmental literature, attachment research came of age in the 1980s and 1990s, with child development monographs devoted to the topic in 1985, 1989, 1994, and 1995. In the adult developmental literature, there has been a corresponding expansion of work in the area in recent times, as reflected in this volume.

The influence of emotions on health was an early topic for the field of psychosomatic medicine, but because of problems in measurement, this field of research became somewhat marginalized. The old mind–body problem has since been revisited with more sophisticated methods and analyses with the emergence of the field of behavioral medicine. With it comes a resurgent interest in how psychological factors, including stress and emotional reactions, moderate disease processes associated with aging.

Another new trend in the field of adult development and aging that is visible in the present volume is the appearance of the narrative approach to the study of adult psychological processes. Several of the chapters reflect the growing respect for qualitative research and the human science approach within psychology. As psychologists, we find that it is no longer necessary to give up our identity as scientists of behavior to accept a broader approach to the study of emotion, which examines the phenomenology of lived experience. This attention to the contextual framework of everyday life promises to enrich the study of emotion. Moreover, the authors represented in this volume recognize that many different variables (e.g., gender, race, ethnicity, and religion) affect the ways people experience emotion within these life contexts.

In adult developmental work, as within the broader field of psychology, a new rapprochement has emerged with respect to the relation between emotion and cognition. No longer is cognitive research isolated from emotions research and vice versa. It has become obvious that the artificial separation between these two domains of psychological process that existed for so many years no longer represents a viable model for understanding effective human functioning.

All in all, the reconciliation between emotion and cognition, mind and body, and quantitative and qualitative methods heralds a new era in psychology's stance in relation to itself and other disciplines. Linear and nonlinear, multifactorial, and multidimensional conceptualizations of human experience, relationships, and development now live more compatibly with one another, and have been enriched by one another in the process. The field appears to be achieving the kind of integration and maturity that characterizes the postformal cognitive achievements of many older adults—in which opposites can be creatively held in tension, in which ambiguity can be tolerated, and in which there is no "last word."

This volume provides a summary of some of the more important areas of research on emotion that deal specifically with life course issues and aging. Spanning several topical areas, the handbook offers a purview of the exciting and ever-growing body of data on affectivity and aging from a bio-psycho-social perspective. The theoretical perspectives in Part I cover biological, discrete emotions, ethological, humanistic, and psychosocial views. Part II on affect and cognition deals with the crucial role of emotion with respect to issues of memory, everyday problem solving, constructions of self and gender, and internal working models of self and other. Part III covers an expanded treatment of issues of emotion and interpersonal relationships, including relations between parents and their adult children, between siblings, friends, and romantic partners; it also treats the issue of separation and loss. Part IV on health and well-being treats issues of stress and coping, interactions with personality, and religion. Finally, Part V addresses personality over the life span and details issues of continuity and change from a variety of perspectives.

In summary, this volume provides a comprehensive view of some of the most vital work in the field over the past 15 years. Moreover, these chapters suggest many potential avenues for future research. Within this work, readers will detect the sense of excitement and possibility felt by the authors as they suggest a coming agenda in psychology's quest to understand human behavior and experience across the life span. It should be a valuable reference for anyone interested in the new integrated view of human development that has emerged in recent years.

Carol Malatesta Magai
and
Susan H. McFadden

PART I

Theoretical
Perspectives

CHAPTER 1

Emotions and the Aging Brain

Regrets and Remedies

Jaak Panksepp   *and*   Anesa Miller
Department of Psychology   *Memorial Foundation for Lost Children*
Bowling Green State University   *Bowling Green, Ohio*
Bowling Green, Ohio

I. INTRODUCTION

Although there is now abundant evidence that a variety of emotional systems have their basis in the shared heritage of the old mammalian (limbic) brain, quite similar in rats, cats, monkeys, and humans, there is virtually no evidence of how these systems age across the life span of organisms. Much more is known about the early development of these systems. This leaves researchers in the creative position of surmising rather than summarizing scholarly accomplishments in the area. Some information that is emerging from the study of early developmental phases (Panksepp, Knutson, & Pruitt, in press) allows one to anticipate what may be found when psychobiologists eventually focus their empirical tools on the question of how emotional matters change as the brain enters old age. What we can provide here is an overall perspective on the types of brain systems that should be studied in relation to aging, and we will also share some provocative recent work on neurochemical manipulations that can postpone the decay of emotional vitality that reduces the joy of living in old age.

We will focus on the basic emotional systems that are organized within subcortical circuits that are shared by all mammals (MacLean,

1990; Panksepp, 1982, 1985a, 1991, in press). We will use the convention of labeling these systems by simple emotional terms, capitalized to highlight that they do not just designate the garden-varieties of emotional feelings, but also the neurological bases of such feelings. These include neural circuits that mediate separation distress and sorrow (the PANIC system), ones that mediate playfulness and joy (the PLAY system), ones that control sexual desires and pleasures (the LUST systems), and ones for maternal (or parental) nurturance and social bonding (the ACCEPTANCE system). There may be others, such as a system for social DOMINANCE, but because it is debatable whether these are distinct from the others mentioned, we will not discuss them as separate systems.

All of those listed above are based in the extended limbic areas of the brain, as defined by MacLean (1990). In addition, there are the more cold-blooded, reptilian emotional systems of FEAR and RAGE, as well as the ever powerful appetitive motivational system that mediates exploratory drives and foraging behavior (which we have previously called the Expectancy System but will henceforth term the SEEKING system). Some of these, such as FEAR and RAGE, are closely intertwined and mediate, respectively, an organism's defense of bodily integrity and its response to irritations that thwart freedom of action and possession of resources. The extensive and compelling neural evidence on how these psychobehavioral systems function during early development has been extensively discussed elsewhere (Panksepp, in press). In the present chapter we would like to summarize how their sensitivities and responsivities change in old age; because we cannot do so on the basis of available empirical evidence, we shall proceed more on the basis of rational argumentation.

One general factor that complicates any life span analysis of brain emotional systems is that a great deal of learning transpires, and many habits are established, broken, and otherwise changed over time. Because of these fluxes, there is really no way to analyze the changing sensitivities of emotional circuits by using behavioral means alone. One must analyze the changing dynamics of the underlying neural systems using anatomical and electrophysiological approaches, and those analyses have started in earnest but without parallel behavioral data, so it is difficult to relate those findings to psychological issues.

II. EMOTIONAL LEARNING AND THE AGING BRAIN

The brain's intrinsic emotional command systems serve to coordinate instinctual behavioral and affective responses to archetypal survival needs. In addition to generating subjective emotional feelings, they activate changes in behavior, physiological and hormonal balances, and they probably prepare the way for cognitive styles of handling important situations. In addition to coordinating those peripheral effects, the affective feelings that emotional systems generate appear to provide internal value gauges to promote efficient coding of external events in the interest of future behavioral actions (Panksepp, 1991, in press). In other words, the feelings we experience play a key role in various affect-related special-purpose learning and cognitive systems (Barkow, Cosmides, & Tooby, 1995). This is presumably so because the brain has a much easier time retrieving certain types of information if it can resurrect an emotional state with which external information has been linked in memory. For instance, when one is not caught up in the throes of rage, it is difficult to outline dastardly plans of revenge in realistic detail. However, when genuine anger is aroused, all the necessary strategies fill one's mind with ease. When we are young, our emotional systems help establish specific types of behavioral and psychological habits, depending on the success of these behaviors in affecting outcomes in desirable or undesirable ways. However, once behavioral and cognitive habits become ingrained, the role of emotional systems may recede to the background as compared to their centrality in youth.

At this point it may also be worth highlighting the Kennard Principle, which states that young people generally recover from the same types of brain damage more rapidly and effectively than older people (see Kolb & Whishaw, 1990). This is especially evident following cortical damage, for instance, to speech cortex. A massive left hemisphere infarct does not impair a person's language abilities in youth as much as in old age. But behavioral neuroscience has now outlined a host of opposite effects—anti-Kennard effects—whereby the consequences of damage are more severe in youth. These types of damage are typically subcortically situated in the deeper recesses of the basic operating systems of the brain, such as the emotional ones. This suggests that without adequate functions within the operating systems, young organisms cannot develop and thrive normally, whereas older individuals, who have lifelong habits backing up their behavioral strategies, can often cope better. For instance, young rats given lateral hypothalamic lesions in the heart of the SEEKING system, tend to show a permanent failure-to-thrive syndrome, whereas older animals can be coaxed to recover and live on their own abilities again (Almli & Golden, 1974). Similarly, aspiration of the olfactory bulbs (i.e., bulbectomy) and temporal lobe/amygdala can compromise the survival chances of infant rats completely, whereas older animals tolerate such procedures well. Likewise, in sexually mature animals bulbectomy does not modify male sexuality, whereas similar damage in young animals permanently abolishes sexual activity (Wilhelmsson & Larsson, 1973). Apparently, the consequences of earlier learning in such brain-damaged adults help sustain competent behavior. When the basic operating systems of the brain have been allowed to develop to maturity, they have apparently established behavioral subroutines that help promote survival.

As a corollary to this, it seems that a mature organism's cognitive, behavioral, and emotional style has been streamlined to the point that, at least in day-to-day circumstances, powerful emotions are activated less frequently than they were in youth. Does this mean that emotional systems have deteriorated at the physiological level, or does it simply indicate that behavioral habits tend to shape our lives so that emotional arousal is no longer as necessary as it once was for guiding our motivations? One way to describe the situation is to suppose that over a person's lifetime, the experience and expression of various emotions gradually creates a relatively intangible neurodynamic structure composed of individual habits and social responses. The quality of an elderly person's emotional life depends on the successful maintenance of these habits and the reactions they elicit.

Considered in this way, an older person's internally experienced emotions may be more diffused than they were in youth, but at the same time, they may become socially more powerful. For example, in an ideal scenario, over the course of a lifetime devoted to caring for her family, a mother establishes behavioral patterns that express love and nurturance, which in turn produce loving responses. Although the woman's intense feeling of attachment to her babies inevitably undergoes modifications as the children grow and achieve independence, if her pattern of caregiving is successful, then her love becomes established as a social fact, replacing individual intensity with a broader kind of strength that relies on a network of participants.

Similarly, a young person's experience of rage may be intense and even destructive, but ultimately, the same emotion can lead to broader and more powerful results (whether for good or ill) if it is built, over time, into a social movement to counteract the thwarting factors that aroused the rage to begin with. Sadly, neurobehavioral data can tell us little, thus far, about the mechanisms of aging in relation to such changes in emotional experience. Still, as one step toward a greater understanding, we will discuss each of the major emotional systems from a perspective that may prove useful for future inquiry.

III. THE BASIC EMOTIONAL SYSTEMS

A. *The Separation Distress/PANIC System*

It seems logical that certain emotional experiences are crucial to the proper development of young organisms and, therefore, tend to be more acute at an early age than they will become later in life. The PANIC system affords a good example, because cross-species comparison shows that activity in this system can vary as a function of the organism's relative need for care and protection. The neurodynamics of the brain systems that generate separation calls (or distress vocalizations, DVs) vary markedly in species depending on their ecological circumstances and modes of social bonding. For instance, herbivores that are born precocious (at a relatively mature level of motor development), such as guinea pigs, chickens, and ducks, demonstrate separation distress on the first day of life and exhibit a prolonged inverted-U type of trajectory of separation calls that continues until puberty (Panksepp et al., in press; Pettijohn, 1979). Altricial animals, such as most carnivores, including dogs, exhibit similar prolonged patterns of separation distress (Scott, Stewart, & DeGhett, 1973), but they show a delay in exhibiting the emotional response (i.e., till eye opening and some motor competence), because it makes little evolutionary sense to exhibit such noisy behavior as DVs until one is sufficiently mature to have some credible means to get out of harm's way. Thus, although they can obviously generate physical distress calls before their eyes open (for example, when exposed to a cold environment), true social separation DVs—namely those that occur even in a warm, soft, and nondangerous environment—do not begin till about 3 weeks of life (Gurski, Davis, & Scott, 1980). Once developed, these animals exhibit DVs well into puberty.

Human babies tend to follow a similar pattern—the emotional response takes a while to mature, till about 8 months of age, whereupon it is evident for many years. Because humans are one of the most neotenous species on the face of the earth (i.e., we have a remarkably long childhood), we can also understand why strong feelings of loneliness can continue for a lifetime. On the other hand, rats, also born altricial like dogs and humans, exhibit about an 8-day delay in the exhibition of true separation calls, but then only emit them for a short period of a week or two, during which time they also demonstrate a brief period of true attachment to their mothers and nest sites. These patterns presumably reflect the maturation of certain brain systems, such as corticotropin-releasing factor (CRF) systems, which are known to promote this emotional response (Panksepp, Normansell, Herman, Bishop, & Crepeau, 1988).

However, for our purposes, the key question might be, what causes this emotional response to decline in all species as a function of maturation? We can be fairly certain that the most obvious explanation is not applicable to the case: The DV circuitry itself does not degrade, because one can electrically stimulate the diencephalic and mesencephalic trajectories of the system to re-evoke infantile separation calls even when mature animals no longer appear to use this response system in their natural behavioral repertoire (Herman & Panksepp, 1981). One obvious alternative possibility is sexual maturation, and the activation of the pituitary–gonadal system. We have evaluated the role of this factor in guinea pigs (Figure 1), and it does seem that testosterone secretion increases the threshold of this system in males. The age-related decline in DVs was diminished by castration, and testosterone administration has also proven quite effective in speeding the decline in birds (Panksepp, 1985b). Ovariectomy and estrogen administration were not as effective. Thus, it seems that the vigor of this emotional response is controlled to some extent by male hormones and gonadal maturation, both of which presumably promote an asocial form of psychobehavioral independence. On the other hand, females may remain more dependent on social contacts. If this is so, it may explain why adult males tend to be more socially aloof than females, whereas females tend to have stronger social networks and appear more socially interdependent than males. The paradox with this view is that in humans the loss of a spouse has more devastating consequences for a husband than a wife (see Melnechuk, 1988). Of course this may only be a surface paradox, for the greater social networks of a woman may allow her to ride through the grief of loss more effectively than males, whose networks are commonly weaker and often emotionally more superficial. However, we presently know little about the underlying physiological mechanisms, although higher cognitive mechanisms clearly become increasingly important in determining how adult humans respond to loss.

Contrary to earlier beliefs, cortical development is now known to continue well into adulthood (Benes, 1994). The cortex can inhibit, constrain, and channel subcortical processes. Our assumption is that in the mature organism the separation distress system still helps elaborate feelings of loneliness, but that the output is channeled into instrumental behaviors that can help establish social contact. For instance, older organisms, having had many prior experiences with separation, can cognitively buffer the immediate absence of social companions with the confidence that reunion will occur at some fairly predictable future time. As our brains develop into maturity and beyond, cognitive abilities can come to outweigh simple emotional ones. Conversely, changes in higher brain functions in old age may again release subcortical functions, leading once more to the prevalence of certain emotional energies—feelings of frustration, anger, and loss. Of course, such issues need to be experimentally clarified.

B. *PLAY and DOMINANCE Systems*

The development of *PLAY* also exhibits an inverted U-shaped function, whereby the intensity and frequency of rough-and-tumble activities

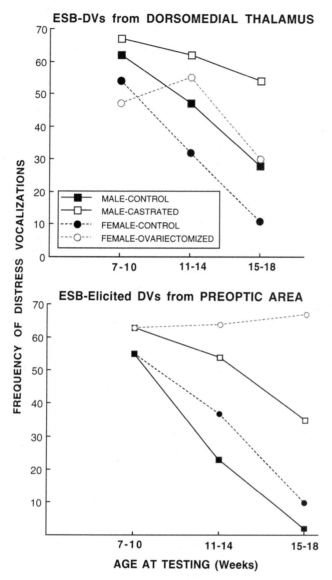

Figure 1. Average brain stimulation elicited distress vocalizations (DVs) in guinea pigs as a function of age and gonadal status from two separate sites within separation distress circuitry (i.e., dorsomedial thalamus and preoptic area). Male and female animals were surgically prepared at least 1 week before testing, and current-intensity curves were run during the three points in early development—late "childhood," (7–10 weeks), late juvenile period (11–14 weeks), and early adulthood (15–18 weeks of age). The data depicted represent results for the highest current level, constant at all ages. Clearly, electrical stimulation of the brain (ESB)-elicited DVs declined as a function of age, and the decline was decreased by gonadectomy in both males and females. These data indicate that the maturation of gonadal hormone systems promotes a decline in the responsivity of the separation distress system of the brain (Sahley & Panksepp, 1983).

diminishes as animals enter late "childhood" and even more as they proceed through puberty (Panksepp, 1993; Panksepp, Siviy, & Normansell, 1984). We do not know what controls this decline, even though, again, testosterone is a participant, because it can reduce juvenile playfulness (Panksepp, 1989). Because we assume that the underlying play circuits are a major source of the joy that organisms experience in social interactions, we have had some interest in seeing whether we might be able to resurrect play in its declining days using neurochemical manipulations. For a synopsis of that work, see section V.

Although there is little empirical evidence on the functions of play, it is likely that this activity exercises the brain systems that mediate various social skills—for instance, how to win or lose gracefully and how to handle oneself in competitive situations. Thus, rough-and-tumble play seems to be a source process for social dominance and submission, which are social issues that do not undergo significant decline as a function of age. Indeed, it is possible that among primates, as an individual grows older, dominance emerges as much from playful, mutually positive and beneficial interchange—from the establishment of friendships and coalitions—as from brute force and intimidation. Indeed, analysis of dominance in primate societies suggests that elevations of brain serotonin can promote dominance (Raleigh, McGuire, Brammer, Pollack, & Yuwiler, 1991) but not simply through an increase in aggression. Rather, the establishment of confident and positive social relationships with other members of the group allows the individuals with pharmacologically elevated serotonin activity to prevail. In rat societies, the animals that have exhibited the highest levels of friendly juvenile play also tend to be dominant. (Adams & Boice, 1989). It seems that juvenile playfulness paves the way to dominance.

In this context, it is also noteworthy that most human societies have provided outlets for the vigorous expressions of playful dominance urges, including medieval jousting and modern sports. The respect that these forms of stylized play enjoy from powerful elderly humans (especially males), including administrators of our universities, not to mention the members of the business community who wrangle to purchase sport franchises, testifies to the importance of play-dominance circuits in human affairs. Even when one's own natural ability to express those urges has markedly diminished, the symbolic value of supporting sport events attests to the continuing powerful role of such motivations in human affairs. We suspect the attraction of those activities throughout the life span, especially in aging males, reflects the fact that the PLAY systems of the brain, which inspire young animals to frolic in youth, are the progenitors of systems and abilities that help mediate dominance in adult social systems. Even when the urge to frolic has diminished, the symbolic power and status urges have not.

C. LUST Systems of the Brain

Male and female brains are organized differently during the fetal period to mediate gender characteristic sexual proclivities (Kinckl, 1990). Robust sexual urges develop at puberty during the activational phase of neurosexual development only if the proper patterns of hormone secretion occur (Crews, 1987; LeVay, 1993). Such erotic urges reflect the maturation of sexually dimorphic LUST systems, which remain partially distinct, and partially overlapping in males and females (Archer & Hansen, 1991). With aging, a hormonally related decline in sexual vigor occurs in all species, but the rate of decline is related to each animal's sexual history and also to the degree of encephalization of each species. For instance, in sexually experienced male rats sexuality declines within several weeks after castration, but in humans who have suffered the same fate, vitality can continue for years (Archer & Hansen, 1991; Crews, 1987). Apparently, thoughts can sustain sexuality when hormones have diminished, but it is possible that these feats of hormone-independent abilities are also due to sustained neural changes of a noncognitive variety. The sustaining effect of past experiences is most evident when hormonal decline is gradual, as in the case of natural aging.

Although sexual habit structures can sustain sexuality in the absence of the hormonal forces that initially drove these energies in earlier years, they will not continue indefinitely in most species without those ancient physiological forces. Since the decline of sex hormones is generally earlier and more precipitous in females than in males in most species, sexual receptivity also declines earlier in females. However, this is not obligatory in humans, where sexuality has been liberated to some extent from immediate sex-hormonal influences by virtue of serving functions other than mere reproduction, such as long-term social bonding, with the resultant sharing of material resources and other defenses against misfortune.

Moreover, in human females, persistent sexual desires are more closely linked to the production of adrenal androgens than in other species (Burger, Hailes, Nelson, & Menelaus, 1987; Morris, Udry, Khan-Dawood, & Dawood, 1987). This suggests quite a different underlying organization for female eroticism in humans than the other mammalian species, whose urges depend on the spontaneously cycling cascades of estrogen and progesterone. Because various neuropeptide circuits of the brain are known to promote sexuality, including vasopressin, oxytocin, and LH-RH (Pedersen, Caldwell, Jirikowski, & Insel, 1992), it will be of great interest to determine how the responsivity of these systems declines and the extent to which they remain resilient in old age.

In any event, the restoration and smooth functioning of the sexual apparatus is greatly enhanced by appropriate hormone supplementation in humans (Burger et al., 1987; Morris et al., 1987). It can also be restored in animals by direct hormone administration into specific parts of the brain: Injections of testosterone into the preoptic area restores male sexuality, and estrogen followed by progesterone into lower brain stem structures restores female urges (Crews, 1987). Recent work has focused on the development of pharmacological aids for restoring sexual ardor in humans as it declines with age (Riley & Wilson, 1994). Animal data suggest the potential utility of dopamine facilitators, for instance monoamine oxidase-B (MAO-B) inhibitors such as deprenyl as discussed in section VI.D.

D. The ACCEPTANCE System(s)

In addition to the brain systems discussed above, the emotion we commonly call love is also closely related to the parental *ACCEPTANCE* systems. In all mammals, nurturance is mediated by distinct brain circuits (Numan, 1988), but it is also remarkably susceptible to the influences of various peripheral hormonal processes and learning (Krasnegor & Bridges, 1990; Winberg & Kjellmer, 1994). How many distinct brain systems should actually be subsumed in this category remains in doubt, but in lower animals the maternal components of nurturant behavior are being well delineated (Krasnegor & Bridges, 1990; Numan, 1988). In laboratory rats nurturant tendency can be monitored simply via measures of "sensitization" or "concaveation." These terms designate the induction of maternal behaviors (nest building, pup retrieval, and hovering over the pups) in virgin rats, both male and female, via prolonged exposure to rat pups. Although males exhibit some nurturance (Brown, 1986), generally, mature females exhibit faster sensitization than males. Likewise, during a brief period of life (perhaps corresponding to the most intense "doll-play phase" of human children), juvenile rats exhibit a high level of nurturance, with no major difference between males and females. However, with the onset of puberty and adulthood, sensitization proceeds more slowly in males than females, although homosexual male rats remain as responsive as females (see Krasnegor & Bridges, 1990; Signoret, Fabre-Nys, & Balthazart, 1994), suggesting that an adaptive value of this phenotype may be to reduce reproduction and facilitate nurturance under stressful circumstances.

Once sensitized, virgin animals exhibit very rapid onset of nurturance on subsequent occasions, indicating the potential power of learning factors. Thus, it is not surprising that females who have already had one litter are better mothers the second time around. Of course, we must be cautious in concluding that this is a mere learning effect, for it remains possible that the previous experiences have modified the arousability of genetic mechanisms, such as the expression of oxytocin-based brain chemistries within nurturant circuits of the brain, an effect that has been observed in various rodent social models (Pedersen et al., 1992). Also, it is known that a single birth can have long-term biochemical consequences on the mothers' physiology, for instance, the levels of certain hormones such as prolactin and dihydroepiandrosterone (Key, Pike, Wang, & Moore, 1990).

In sum, the more experiences an individual has had with nurturance, the more likely these mechanisms are to remain responsive in old age, which probably helps make parents who have had many children excellent grandparents. It will be most interesting to see how the underlying neural systems, such as those that elaborate oxytocin, change as a function of development, and how these changes are modified by various social histories (Insel, 1992).

E. On the Nature of Social Bonding

The developmental nature of social bonding is probably directly related to the responsivity of ACCEPTANCE, LUST, PLAY, and PANIC systems, as discussed elsewhere (Panksepp, in press). Whether there is also a separate social-bonding system independent of the aforementioned neural substrates is not known. No doubt there are several distinct types of social bonding; those that occur in infancy and childhood are neurophysiologically distinct from those that occur in puberty and early adulthood, whereas the friendships of old age can surely be based more on cognitive factors than on elementary affective ones. However, without the continued participation of the affective substrates, it is hard to imagine that such relations could provide adequate satisfaction. Probably the quality of bondings during the earlier phases of life helps determine the responsivity of bonding systems in old age.

Probably the same chemistries that are important in decreasing separation-distress responses and facilitating nurturant responses, namely endogenous brain opioid, oxytocin, and prolactin systems, will be essential ingredients in the construction of social-bonds (Panksepp, 1991). It should be informative to eventually determine, through the use of animal models, whether the underlying neural substrates of the earlier bonding mechanism continue to control attachments in old age. Likewise, some of these systems have been shown to be important in the construction of social memories (Winslow, Hastings, Carter, Harbaugh, & Insel, 1993), and it will be important to determine how such abilities change as a function of age.

F. The SEEKING/EXPECTANCY or "I WANT" System

This brain system, sometimes called an "appetitive motivational" or "behavioral activation" system, mediates certain desires and interests that are especially energized in youth, but the "energies" of which gradually decline through old age. This system promotes active engagement with the world—exploration, investigation, and the anticipation of the rewards to be had in our environments (Panksepp, 1986, 1991). This system is confluent with ascending brain dopamine systems, which course from midbrain zones such as the ventral tegmental area to the basal ganglia and forebrain, in a broad trajectory from which the most vigorous forms of self-stimulation and exploratory arousal are evoked with localized electrical and chemical stimulation of the brain. The fact that this system helps mediate that mysterious process that psychologists call positive reinforcement, in yet unfathomed ways, adds further weight to the thesis that the power of emotional systems in youth can promote learning that lasts a lifetime.

By the mere application of electrical stimulation to this circuit or administration of psychologically addictive drugs such as cocaine and the amphetamines, one can permanently increase the sensitivity of this system (Kalivas & Stewart, 1991). This also occurs in humans, not only because of psychostimulant abuse, but probably because of the incentive sensitizing effects of life stressors and avaricious lifestyles (Robinson & Berridge, 1993). When these systems become sensitized, organisms tend to assume a more chronic craving mode, which makes them more susceptible to the various psychological addictions and materialistic desires whose persistence and increasing prevalence creates much havoc and unhappiness in modern society. Massive overarousal of these systems, in the presence of yet other neuropathologies, may contribute to those strong paranoid tendencies that are diagnosed as adult-onset or functional schizophrenias. Mild overarousal of these systems probably contributes to various types of personality disorders.

Because dopamine is at the heart of this system, serving a command influence, we have an excellent neurochemical marker for the decline of the system with aging. Brain dopamine gradually diminishes in aging rats, and similar patterns are evident in humans (Rogers & Bloom, 1985). The decline in dopamine leads to the general decline in psychomotor arousal as organisms age. The loss of vitality in brain dopamine systems is also responsible for the onset of mild Parkinsonian symptoms in many older adults.

Because this system is vital for the motivational energy of many behavioral acts, it is especially important to find ways to counter its natural decline. This has now been achieved with the sustained administration of deprenyl, and as discussed below, such treatment provides one way to counteract the decline in mental energies as one ages. Because brain dopamine circuits are readily sensitized by chronic exposure to psychostimulants and environmental stressors (Robinson & Berridge, 1993), it will be important to evaluate how the vigor of sensitization changes as a function of aging. When we learn how to reverse such neuroemotional habits of the animal brain, we will have some insight into controlling afflictions that may accumulate with age in humans such as addictive personality and posttraumatic stress disorders (PTSD). On the other hand, perhaps sensitization decreases spontaneously with the aging process, and thereby contributes to the "wisdom" of age. Indeed, we would not be surprised if a decline in sensitization might be promoted by positive social activities and chemistries such as discussed in the previous section, but those possibilities remain to be empirically evaluated.

G. The FEAR System

All mammals have a fundamental FEAR system in the brain, which courses between amygdaloid, medial hypothalamic, and central gray areas of the midbrain (Panksepp, 1991). Manifestations of this system emerge during early human development and have been reasonably well characterized. Human babies are afraid of falling before they are afraid of darkness, and they fear darkness before they fear snakes and other scary animals (Gray, 1987). The ability to cope with fears also probably becomes ever more efficient as organisms grow older, thanks largely to the development of cognitive strategies (i.e., the buffering effect of representations of the past and future). It is possible that older animals' increasing ability to remove themselves from harm's way simply allows for lower activation of the FEAR system as organisms mature. This disuse effect could also be represented in the brain as a gradual weakening of the synaptic connectivities and chemistries of the FEAR system, but that is not an established fact.

Although we know almost nothing about changes in the FEAR system as a function of aging, one important issue to be considered is the ability of this system to also become sensitized as a function of experience. There is suggestive evidence that this occurs, as appears to take place in PTSD. Fear sensitization can be evoked simply by electrically stimulating the headwaters of the FEAR system in the amygdala, which leads to increased permeability of neural pathways to medial hypothalamic components of the FEAR system (Adamec, 1990).

A chronic increase in fearfulness can also be induced by various anxiogenic drugs, especially those "inverse agonists" that promote anxiety by interacting with the benzodiazepine receptor system. These manipulations generate a personality change in experimental animals, whereby formerly friendly animals become chronically hyperdefensive (Adamec, 1990). No one has yet determined whether this increase in "limbic permeability" changes with age, or whether it can be more effectively alleviated at certain phases of development than others. It will be important to address these neuropsychiatric issues in future research because they may have implications for treating anxiety disorders in the elderly.

H. The RAGE System

It is difficult to analyze the status of this basic neural system without direct brain manipulations (Bandler, 1988; Siegel & Pott, 1988). Humans are usually trained to inhibit their anger in public, and there are no good scales to measure the ongoing influence of this system in the daily affairs of humans or animals. However, it is a commonplace observation that humans generally tend to become less volatile as they age, and there are animal data to suggest that high circulating levels of gonadal steroids and hypothalamic releasing factors generally tend to reduce the thresholds of aggression systems (Bermond, Mos, Meelis, van der Poel, & Kruk, 1982; Inselman-Temkin & Flynn, 1973). Thus, in a manner similar to declining hormone-dependent sexual urges, it seems likely that there are age-related declines in the arousability of the RAGE system.

As with the FEAR system, one can sensitize the RAGE system (Adamec, 1990), but the underlying neural mechanisms remain to be clarified. It is possible that despite the decline in the system as one ages, older organisms have more habitual "trigger spots" in such circuits, and if so, it will be especially important to determine how they might be muted with cognitive, affective, pharmacological, and other somatic interventions.

IV. BRAIN CHANGES IN OLD AGE

A. Neuroanatomical Issues

The various forms of neural deterioration that characterize aging are an object of active study. The neuropathologies underlying the most severe age-related mental disorders—Alzheimer's, Parkinson's, and Huntington's disease—have now been well characterized, and there is increasing medical hope for some of them (Parks, Zec, & Wilson, 1993). Each of these disorders entails emotional changes: Alzheimer's is associated with confusional states that can lead to frustration and anger; Parkinson's, with the inability to become actively engaged with world affairs; and Huntington's, with a gradual dissolution of behavioral coherence, so that various emotions can more readily rise to the surface, even though mature people would normally tend to keep their stronger feelings in the background.

There is hope that some of the neural deficits of these disorders, along with the consequence of various forms of cerebral ischemia, can be reduced and prevented with new medicines, although most work along those lines remains in the experimental stages (Ginsberg, 1995). There are strategies for administering neuronal growth factors to delay cell death, and dietary maneuvers that can reduce the influence of free-radical damage to neuronal systems (Mendell, 1995; Russell, 1995). Even surgical procedures, such as fetal tissue grafts and nerve growth factor infusions into the brain have been attempted (Olson et al., 1992). Most importantly though, as described in the next section, there are some neurochemical manipulations that can help preserve the fading vitality of the aging brain.

B. Neurochemical and Neurophysiological Issues

There is abundant evidence that various neurochemical systems decline as a function of age. Probably the best characterized are those related to the diseases mentioned in the previous section: there is loss of prominent basal forebrain cholinergic and cortical somatostatin in Alzheimer's that may be due to specific genetic infirmities (Strittmatter & Roses, 1995); there is basal ganglia dopamine loss in Parkinson's (Wichmann, Vitek, & DeLong, 1995), and loss of all of the interneuron chemistries of the basal ganglia in Huntington's (Young, 1995). The various changes associated with these afflictions are well detailed in many sources.

A characterization of the decline in specific neuropeptide chemistries that mediate specific emotional and motivational tendencies (Panksepp, 1993) remains to be conducted, but it seems likely that most systems lose vitality with age. In general, the aging brain tends to exhibit more slow-wave activity during waking, which reflects a less arousable brain. Similarly, PET scans for glucose metabolism are able to predict the onset of Alzheimer's symptoms by monitoring the early decline of metabolic activity (Kennedy et al., 1995). One of the major lines of future research will be to determine how specific systems can be restored so as to increase the quality of life for aging individuals. As we will see in the next section, important progress is being made.

V. THE NEUROCHEMICAL FOUNTAINS OF YOUTH: SLOWING THE CHANGES OF OLD AGE

The resilience and activity of most neurochemistries decline as a function of age (Rogers & Bloom, 1985). No physician can prescribe the road to a vital and happy old age, but without sufficient joy, energy, health, and sustained good nights' sleep, happiness is difficult to achieve. Quality of life can be enhanced by meaningful activities, close friends and few enemies, but in addition to these self-evident factors, the incommensurate biological declines in different bodily systems can be coaxed in positive directions through the wonders of modern chemistry.

There are now several simple beneficial neurochemical approaches to some of the mood and motivational problems that characterize aging. In addition to generally beneficial metabolic/nutritional manipulations, several neuroendocrine systems can be safely treated to yield general health benefits: brain dopamine (Knoll, 1992), pineal melatonin (Miles, Philbrick, & Thompson, 1989), adrenal dehydoepiandrosterone (Regelson, Loria, & Kalimi, 1988), and other hormone supplements. All three of the above decline gradually during the process of aging. Facilitation of each of these systems can prolong the life span in animals, and there is no evidence that any supplement is harmful if used properly as prophylactic agents.

A. Melatonin and Sleep

Some of the sleep difficulties that accompany aging may result from the decline of melatonin. Recently, this pineal hormone has emerged as a powerful sleep-promoting molecule that can be orally taken, and continues to have reliable effects for extended periods with no significant side effects. Indeed, this molecule offers a great number of positive effects that can promote general health, such as synchronizing bodily rhythms, increasing immune competence, reducing tumor growth, and alleviating psychiatric ailments such as depression, anxiety, and perhaps even some psychotic symptoms (Miles et al., 1989). For those who might not be able to get to sleep because of loneliness, it is worth noting that the molecule is quite effective in reducing separation distress (Nelson, Panksepp & Ikemoto, 1994), and one of the most exciting effects is its ability to increase the life span, which has now been observed under various conditions (Regelson et al., 1988).

B. The Dehydroepinadrosterone Story

Dehydroepinadrosterone (DHEA) manufactured in the body from cholesterol, is the most abundant adrenal hormone in the body that declines dramatically as a function of aging, but its normal physiological function remains uncertain. Some have characterized DHEA as a "buffer hormone" that seems to broadly facilitate the smooth functioning of many bodily systems (Regelson et al., 1988). In the brain, which has an endogenous DHEA system, it promotes memory processes, apparently by a reduction of GABA activity (Flood, Morley, & Roberts, 1992). Oral supplementation with the hormone in aging individuals can have various beneficial effects on the body, ranging from a reduction in cholesterol to a diminished incidence of heart attacks. In the present context, it is noteworthy that a month of oral supplementation markedly increased the overall sense of well-being of middle-aged adults (Morales, Nolan, Nelson, & Yen, 1994). In addition to general health effects, this may partially reflect the ability of this agent to exert a mild antianxiety effect, which has been documented in animal models (Melchior & Ritzmann, 1994).

C. Deprenyl and Sexual and Cognitive Vitality

As mentioned, brain dopamine systems gradually die off as individuals age. The decrease in dopamine is one of the major reasons that active engagement with the world diminishes in old age, ranging from decreased sexual desire to the loss of other lifelong interests. Indeed, animal research shows that one of the predictors of death in male animals is their loss of sexual vigor (Knoll, 1988).

It is known from *in vivo* neurochemical studies that brain dopamine is plentifully released in animals when they are sexually aroused (Pfaus & Phillips, 1991). Thus, it was natural for investigators to ask whether sexual behavior could be restored by restoring brain dopamine activity. Since dopamine is normally destroyed in neurons by the B-variant of the enzyme MAO, an investigator in Hungary decided to determine if inhibition of the enzyme with a drug called deprenyl would restore sexuality in aging male rats (Knoll, 1988). Indeed, long-term administration of low-levels of the drug proved quite effective in maintaining the sexual interests and abilities of older rats. Instead of declining sexual activity at their normal old age, the deprenyl-treated animals continued to copulate for several additional months (the equivalent of several years in human terms). Indeed, deprenyl-treated animals lived longer than expected, and this was not simply due to the fact that they were having more sex.

Apparently deprenyl can protect the metabolic decay of dopamine systems in the brain. Although we do not know for certain, the restored neuropsychic vitality may well be the critical ingredient in sustaining life. Moreover, it should be emphasized that this effect reflected a true increase in the normal life span of the animals. It was not due to more animals simply reaching the maximal extent of their life expectancy: Most individuals were living longer than what would normally be expected. Of course, we do not yet know whether this effect will be evident in humans (there has not yet been time to complete such an experiment), but because the drug is available for other disorders, some are optimistically consuming deprenyl with the assumption that the rats' good fortunes will transfer to the human condition. We do know that deprenyl can prevent the decline of dopamine neuronal death in humans as it does in animals, and hence it is presently used medically to forestall severe Parkinsonian symptoms during the early phases of the disease (Parkinson Study Group, 1989). It also appears to be beneficial in reducing cognitive deficits in Alzheimer-type individuals (Agnoli, Fabbrini, Fioravanti, & Martucci, 1992). There are bound to be many other such prophylactic treatments as the chemical dynamics of the mammalian brain are more fully revealed. However, rather than trying to summarize the details of the many other emerging systems in the limited space available here, let me summarize one general strategy by which our lab has sought to understand—so far without much success—how might one sustain emotional vitality as a function of aging? We have sought neurochemical factors to sustain playfulness.

D. In Search of the Ludic Cocktail—Joy Extension

In our estimation, no other emotional system in the brain can produce as much pure joy as that which elaborates rough-and-tumble play (Panksepp et al., 1984; Panksepp, 1993). This brain system is modulated by opioids, among the most pleasurable molecules in the brain (Panksepp et al., 1985), and by a host of other chemistries, only some of which have been identified (Panksepp, Normansell, Cox, Crepeau, & Sacks, 1987). As discussed above, ludic urges decline as a function of aging, but a substantial degree of playfulness remains in humans and some other neotenous species throughout their lives. Presumably, young children have special brain chemistries that sustain open, childlike attitudes toward existence, but we do not know what they are.

Although our search for that fountain of youth has met with only modest success, let us briefly summarize what we have done. Among the first pharmacological manipulations that we evaluated on play were drugs that affect the major biogenic-amine systems—namely those of serotonin, norepinephrine, and dopamine—as well as those that affect brain opioids. We found that we could marginally increase play with (a) low doses of broadly acting serotonin-receptor antagonists such as methysergide, (b) low doses of apomorphine that reduce brain dopamine activity, and (c) low doses of opiate-receptor agonists such as morphine (Panksepp et al., 1984, 1987). Accordingly, we proceeded to evaluate each of these, as well as all combinations of these agents, to see if we could reinvigorate playfulness when it was declining during late puberty. Unfortunately, none of these agents alone nor in any combination restored playfulness in young adults.

We have not given up the quest. One possibility we are presently evaluating is the recently identified endogenous cannabanoid system of the brain (Childers, Sexton, & Roy, 1993), and we have had some success in restoring playfulness as rats age (Pruitt & Panksepp, 1995). Of course, it remains possible that no neuropharmacological agent shall ever restore full juvenile playfulness. The decline in play may reflect a deterioration of circuits that cannot be resurrected no matter what we do, or it may reflect the decline in the genetic expression of certain play chemistries that cannot be rejuvenated without great advances in our ability to manipulate genetic expression. Of course, we will continue the quest, for it is a worthy journey.

VI.   CLOSING REMARKS

Modern neuroscience is bound to provide aids that can make the natural journey of aging a more positive experience than it has been in the past. The above examples are only the tip of an iceberg of useful knowledge that is being revealed by modern neuroscience. The moral and ethical choices this kind of knowledge will confront us with are many. What should be our choices when we know how to manipulate individual emotions? Will it be a reasonable choice to give people medicines that can turn off discrete types of fear, anger, and loneliness, and those that turn on playfulness, nurturance, and a sense of union with others? What will be our choices when we are eventually able to provoke feelings of love and sorrow independently of the many life events that normally access these natural systems of the brain?

These will be difficult decisions for society to handle. Some will surely say that we should leave the emotional mysteries alone. They are too powerful to tamper with. We should live out our lives in the old ways, in the midst of the joys and frustrations of our families as well as in the midst of the pain and sorrow that old age has always brought. Others will be more enthusiastic for the useful alternatives that science will provide. Hopefully modern cultural and societal thought will continue to mature so as to assure each the right to complete their life journey as peacefully or vibrantly as they wish.

ACKNOWLEDGMENTS

This work was supported in part National Institutes of Health (NIH) grant R15 HD30387, and The Memorial Foundation for Lost Children, Bowling Green, OH 43402.

REFERENCES

Adams, N., & Boice, R. (1989). Development of dominance in domestic rats in laboratory and seminatural environments. *Behavioural Processes, 19,* 127–142.

Adamec, R. E. (1990). Kindling, anxiety and limbic epilepsy: Human and animal perspectives. In J. A. Wada (Ed), *Kindling 4. Advances in behavioral biology* (pp. 329–341). New York: Plenum Press.

Agnoli, A., Fabbrini, G., Fioravanti, M., & Martucci, N. (1992). CBF and cognitive evaluation of Alzheimer type patients before and after MAO-B treatment: A pilot study. *European Neuropsychopharmacology, 2,* 31–35.

Almli, C.R., & Golden, G. T. (1974) Infant rats: Effects of lateral hypothalamic destruction. *Physiology & Behavior, 13,* 81–90.

Archer, T., & Hansen, S. (Eds.) (1991). *Behavioral biology: Neuroendocrine axis.* Hillsdale, NJ: Lawrence Erlbaum Associates.

Bandler, R. (1988). Brain mechanisms of aggression as revealed by electrical and chemical stimulation: Suggestion of a central role for the midbrain periaqueductal grey region. In A. N. Epstein & A. R. Morrison (Eds.), *Progress in psychobiology and physiological psychology* (Vol. 13, pp. 67–154). New York: Academic Press.

Barkow, J. H., Cosmides, L., & Tooby, J. (Eds.) (1995). *The adapted mind: Evolutionary psychology and the generation of culture.* New York: Oxford University Press.

Benes, F. M. (1994). Development of the corticolimbic system. In G. Dawson & K. W. Fisher (Eds.), *Human behavior and the developing brain* (pp. 176–206). New York: The Guilford Press.

Bermond, B., Mos, J., Meelis, W., van der Poel, A. M. & Kruk, M. R. (1982). Aggression induced by stimulation of the hypothalamus: Effects of androgens. *Pharmacology Biochemistry & Behavior, 16,* 41–45.

Brown, R. E. (1986). Paternal behavior in the male Long-Evans rats (*Rattus norvegicus*). *Journal of Comparative Psychology, 43,* 36–42.

Burger, H., Hailes, J., Nelson, J., & Menelaus, M. (1987). Effect of combined implants of estradiol and testosterone on libido in postmenopausal women. *British Medical Journal, 294,* 936–939.

Childers, S. R., Sexton, T., & Roy, M. B. (1993). Effects of anandamide on cannabinoid receptors in rat brain membranes. *Biochemical Pharmacology, 47,* 711–715.

Crews, D. (Ed.). (1987). *Psychobiology of reproductive behavior. An evolutionary perspective.* Englewood Cliffs, NJ: Prentice-Hall, Inc.

Flood, J. F., Morley, J. E., & Roberts, E. (1992). Memory-enhancing effects in male mice of pregnenolone and steroids metabolically derived from it. *Proceeding of the National Academy of Sciences, 89,* 1567–1572.

Ginsberg, M. D. (1995). Neuroprotection in brain ischemia: An update (Part II). *The Neuroscientist, 1,* 164–175.

Gray, J. A. (1987). *The psychobiology of fear and stress* (2nd. ed). Cambridge, UK: Cambridge University Press.

Gurski, J. C., Davis, K., & Scott, J. P. (1980). Interaction of separation discomfort with contact comfort and discomfort in the dog. *Developmental Psychobiology, 13,* 463–467.

Herman, B. H., & Panksepp, J. (1981). Ascending endorphinergic inhibition of distress vocalization. *Science, 211,* 1060–1062.

Insel, T. R. (1992). Oxytocin: A neuropeptide for affiliation-evidence from behavioral, autoradiographic and comparative studies. *Psychoneuroendocrinology, 17,* 3–35.

Inselman-Temkin, B., & Flynn, J. P. (1973). Sex-dependent effects of gonadal and gonadotropic hormones on centrally-elicited attack in cats. *Brain Research, 60,* 393–410.

Kalivas, P., & Stewart, J. (1991). Dopamine transmission in the initiation and expression of drug- and stress-induced sensitization of motor activity. *Brain Research Reviews, 16,* 223–244.

Kennedy, A. M., Frackowiak, R. S. J., Newman, S. K., Bloomfield, B. M., Seaward, J., Roques, P., Lewington, G., Cunningham, V. J. & Rossor, M. N. (1995). Deficits in cerebral glucose metabolism demonstrated by positron emission tomography in individuals at risk of familial Alzheimer's disease. *Neuroscience Letters, 186,* 17–20.

Key, T. J. A., Pike, M. C., Wang, D. Y. & Moore, J. W. (1990). Long term effects of a first preganancy on serum concentrations of dehydroepindrosterone sulfate and dehydroepindrosterone. *Journal of Clinical Endocrinology and Metabolism, 70,* 1651–1653.

Kinckl, F. A. (1990). *Hormone toxicity in the newborn.* Berlin: Springer-Verlag.

Knoll, J., (1988). Extension of lifespan of rats by long-term (−)deprenyl treatment. *Mount Sinai Journal of Medicine, 55,* 67–74.

Knoll, J., (1992). (−)Deprenyl-medication: A strategy to modulate the age-related decline of the striatal dopaminergic system. *Journal of the American Geriatric Society, 40,* 839–847.

Kolb, B., & Whishaw, I. Q. (1990). *Fundamental of human neuropsychology* (3rd ed). New York: W. H. Freeman & Co.

Krasnegor, N. A., & Bridges, R. S. (Eds.). (1990). *Mammalian parenting: Biochemical, neurobiological and behavioral determinants.* New York: Oxford University Press.

LeVay, S. (1993). *The sexual brain.* Cambridge, MA: MIT Press.

MacLean, P. D. (1990). *The triune brain in evolution.* New York: Plenum Press.

Melchior, C. L., & Ritzmann, R. F. (1994). Dehydroepindrosterone is an anxiolytic in mide on the plus maze. *Pharmacology Biochemistry & Behavior, 47,* 437–441.

Melnechuk, T. (1988). Emotions, brain, immunity, and health: A review. In M. Clynes & J. Panksepp (Eds.), *Emotions and psychopathology* (pp. 181–247). New York: Plenum Press.

Mendell, L. M. (1995). Neurotrophic factors and the specification of neural function. *The Neuroscientist, 1,* 26–34.

Miles, A., Philbrick, D. R. S., & Thompson, C. (Eds.). (1989). *Melatonin: Clinical perspectives.* Oxford: Oxford University Press.

Morales, A., Nolan, J. J., Nelson, J. C., & Yen, S. S. C. (1994). Effects of replacement dose of dehydroepindrosterone in men and women of advancing age. *Journal of Clinical Endocrinology and Metabolism, 78,* 1360–1367.

Morris, N., Udry, J., Khan-Dawood, F., & Dawood, M. (1987). Marital sex frequency and midcycle female testerone. *Archives of Sexual Behavior, 16,* 27–37.

Nelson, E., Panksepp, J., & Ikemoto, S. (1994). The effects of melatonin on isolation distress in chickens. *Pharmacology, Biochemistry, & Behavior, 49,* 327–333.

Numan, M. (1988). Maternal behavior. In E. Knobil & J. D. Neill (Eds.), *The physiology of reproduction* (pp. 1569–1645). New York: Raven Press.

Olson, L., Nordberg, A., von Holst, H., Backman, L., Ebendal, T., Alafuzoff, I., Amberia, K., Hartvig, P., Herlitz, A., Lilja, A., Lundqvist, H., Langstrom, B., Meyerson, B., Persson, A., Viitanen, M., Winblad, B., & Seiger, A. (1992). Nerve growth factors affects ^{11}C-nicotine binding, blood flow, EEG, and verbal episodic memory in an Alzheimer patient (Case Report). *Journal of Neural Transmission, 4,* 79–95.

Panksepp, J. (1982). Toward a general psychobiological theory of emotions. *The Behavioral and Brain Sciences, 5,* 407–467.

Panksepp, J. (1985a). Mood changes. In P. J. Vionken, G. W. Bruyn, & H. L. Klawans (Eds.), *Handbook of clinical neurology Vol. 1. (45). Clinical Neuropsychology* (pp. 271–285). Amsterdam: Elsevier Science Publishers.

Panksepp, J. (1985b). *Testosterone promotes the decline of separation-induced distress vocalizations in young domestic chicks.* Unpublished data.

Panksepp, J. (1986). The anatomy of emotions. In R. Plutchik & H. Kellerman (Eds.), *Emotion: Theory, research and experience: Vol. 3, Biological foundations of emotions* (pp. 91–124). San Diego, CA: Academic Press.

Panksepp, J. (1989). *Testosterone promotes the decline in playfulness in juvenile rats.* Unpublished data.

Panksepp, J. (1991). Affective neuroscience: A conceptual framework of the neurobiological study of emotions. In K. T. Strongman (Ed.), *International Review of Studies on Emotion* (*Vol. 1*, pp. 59–99). Chichester, UK: John Wiley.

Panksepp, J. (1993). Rough and tumble play: A fundamental brain process. In K. MacDonald (Ed), *Parent-child play: Descriptions and implications* (pp. 147–184). New York: SUNY Press.

Panksepp, J. (in press) *Affective neuroscience: The foundations of human and animal emotions.* New York: Oxford Univ. Press.

Panksepp, J., Jalowiec, J., DeEskinazi, F. G., & Bishop, P. (1985). Opiates and play dominance in juvenile rats. *Behavioral Neuroscience, 99,* 441–453.

Panksepp, J., Knutson, B., & Pruitt, D. L. (in press). Toward a neuroscience of emotion: The epigenetic foundations of emotional development. In M. F. Mascolo & S. Griffin (Eds.), *What develops in emotional development?* New York: Plenum Press.

Panksepp, J., Normansell, L., Cox, J. F., Crepeau, L. J., & Sacks, D. S. (1987). Psychopharmacology of social play. In B. Olivier, J. Mos, & P. F. Brain (Eds.), *Ethopharmacology of agonistic behaviour in animals and humans* (pp. 132–144). Dordrecht, Holland: Martinus Nijhoff Pubs.

Panksepp, J., Normansell, L., Herman, B., Bishop, P., & Crepeau, L. (1988). Neural and neurochemical control of the separation distress call. In J. D. Newman (Ed.), *The physiological control of mammalian vocalization* (pp. 263–299). New York: Plenum Press.

Panksepp, J., Siviy, S., & Normansell, L. (1984). The psychobiology of play: Theoretical and methodological perspectives. *Neuroscience and Biobehavioral Reviews, 8,* 465–492.

Parkinson Study Group. (1989). Effect of deprenyl on the progression of disability in early Parkinson's disease. *The New England Journal of Medicine, 321,* 1364–1371.

Parks, R. W., Zec, R. F., & Wilson, R. S. (Eds.). (1993). *Neuropsychology of Alzheimer's disease and other dementias.* New York: Oxford University Press.

Pedersen, C. A., Caldwell, J. D., Jirikowski, G., & Insel, T. R. (Eds.). (1992). *Annals of the New York Academy of Sciences. Vol. 652. Oxytocin in maternal, sexual and social behaviors.* New York: New York Academy of Sciences.

Pettijohn, T. F. (1979). Attachment and separation distress in the infant guinea pig. *Developmental Psychobiology, 12,* 73–81.

Pfaus, J., & Phillips, A. (1991). Role of dopamine anticipatory and consummatory aspects of sexual behavior in the male rat. *Behavioral Neuroscience, 105,* 727–943.

Pruitt, D., & Panksepp, J. (1995). *Anandamine and synthetic cannabanoids can increase play in young adult rats.* Unpublished data.

Raleigh, M. J., McGuire, M. T., Brammer, G. L., Pollack, D. B., & Yuwiler, A. T. (1991). Serotonergic mechanisms promote dominance acquisition in adult male vervet monkeys. *Brain Research, 559,* 181–190.

Regelson, W., Loria, R., & Kalimi, M. (1988). Hormonal intervention: "Buffer hormone" or "state dependency." *Annals of New York Academy of Sciences, 521,* 260–273.

Riley, A. J., & Wilson, C. (Eds.). (1994). Sexual pharmacology. New York: Oxford Univ. Press.

Robinson, T., & Berridge, K. (1993). The neural basis of drug craving: An incentive-sensitization theory of addiction. Brain Research Review, 18, 247–291.

Rogers, J., & Bloom, F. E. (1985). Neurotransmitter metabolism and function in the aging central nervous system. In C. E. Finch & E. L. Schneider (Eds.), Handbook of the biology of aging (pp. 645–691). New York: Van Nostrand Reinhold Co.

Russell, D. S. (1995). Neurotrophins: New players, clinical uses? The Neuroscientist, 1, 119–122.

Sahley, T. L., & Panksepp, J. (1983). Effects of castration of prepubertal guinea pigs on brain stimulation induced distress vocalizations. Unpublished data.

Scott, J. P., Stewart, J. M., & DeGhett, V. J. (1973). Separation in infant dogs. In J. P. Scott & E. C. Senay (Eds.), Separation and depression: Clinical and research aspects (Publ. 194). Washington, DC: American Association for the Advancement of Science.

Siegel, A., & Pott, C. B. (1988). Neural substrates of aggression and flight in the cat. Progress in Neurobiology, 32, 261–283.

Signoret, J. P., Fabre-Nys, C., & Balthazart, J. (Eds.). (1994). Hormone, brain and behaviour. [Special Issue] Psychoneuroendocrinology, 19, 403–720.

Strittmatter, W. J., & Roses, A. D. (1995). Apolipoprotein E: Emerging story in the pathogenesis of alzheimer's diseases. The Neuroscientist, 1, 298–306.

Wichmann, T., Vitek, J. L., & DeLong, M. R. (1995). Parkinson's disease and the basal ganglia: Lessons from the laboratory and from neurosurgery. The Neuroscientist, 1, 236–244.

Wilhelmsson, M., & Larsson, K. (1973). The development of sexual behavior in anosmic male rats reared under various social conditions. Physiology & Behavior, 11, 227–232.

Winberg, J., & Kjellmer, I. (Eds.). (1994). The neurobiology of infant-parent interaction in the newborn period. ACTA Paediatrica, 83, [suppl. 397].

Winslow, J. T., Hastings, N., Carter, C. S., Harbaugh, C. R., & Insel, T. R. (1993). A role for central vasopressin in pair bonding in monogamous prairie voles. Nature, 365, 544–548.

Young, A. B. (1995). Huntington's disease: Lessons from and for molecular biology. The Neuroscientist, 1, 51–58.

CHAPTER 2

Differential Emotions Theory and Emotional Development in Adulthood and Later Life

Linda M. Dougherty
Department of Gerontology
Virginia Commonwealth University
Medical College of Virginia
Richmond, Virginia

Jo Ann Abe
Psychology Department
University of Delaware
Newark, Delaware

Carroll E. Izard
Psychology Department
University of Delaware
Newark, Delaware

I. INTRODUCTION

From its inception, differential emotions theory (DET; Izard, 1971) has maintained that emotions are the primary forces in organizing human thought and action (cf. Tomkins, 1962, 1991). DET has also affirmed that it is the emotional component of consciousness and experience that gives richness and meaning to individual life and relationships. Having characterized the emotions in this way, it follows that quality of life in the older adult can best be explained by a principle that affirms the continuity of emotion feelings and emotion expressions across the life span (cf. Barrett & Campos, 1987; Emde, 1980).

This position statement, which sets the tone of this chapter, runs contrary to some earlier views of emotions in adult development. As Malatesta (1981) observed, major theories of emotion have depicted the emotional life of older people as flat, blunted, and impoverished.

It is true that as a result of socialization and cultural rules individuals tend to modulate their expressions of emotions as they age (Malatesta & Izard, 1984). However, this diminished display is not necessarily accompanied by diminished emotional experience. Emotion feelings retain their importance across the life span as an integral component of an individual's life.

Although physiological findings indicate that the aging individual typically takes longer to return to a homeostatic state after high arousal, empirical evidence does not link physiological reactivity with a decrease in the frequency and intensity of discrete emotion feelings or with an increase in negative emotional experience. In fact, Levenson, Carstensen, Friesen, and Ekman (1991) reported that emotion-specific automatic nervous system (ANS) activity is remarkably similar across adulthood.

Over the last decade, evidence has accumulated indicating the continued salience of emotions throughout life (Carstensen, 1992; Labouvie-Vief, DeVoe, & Bulka, 1989; Lawton, Kleban, & Dean, 1993). As a mounting body of evidence suggests a dynamic picture of emotion in late adulthood, there is a growing need for a comprehensive theory of life span emotional development.

The purpose of this chapter is to show how DET may serve as a theoretical framework for emotional development across the life span. Although most investigations using DET as a research paradigm have focused primarily on issues of early development (e.g., Ackerman, Abe, & Izard, in press; Izard & Malatesta, 1987; Malatesta & Haviland, 1982; Weinberg & Tronick, 1994), some efforts to extend research into adulthood were initiated by Malatesta and Izard (1984). Since then, other aspects of DET have been further elaborated, and empirical research has begun to be conducted on emotions in adulthood (e.g., Dougherty & Riggins, 1995; Izard, Libero, Putnam & Haynes, 1993; Malatesta & Izard, 1984).

This chapter consists of five parts. In the first part, we present an overview of DET. In the second part, we discuss key principles of life span emotional development. In the third part, we discuss DET in relation to adult development and aging. In the fourth part, we discuss how DET relates to other models of emotion in adulthood. We conclude by discussing avenues for future research from the perspective of DET.

II. DIFFERENTIAL EMOTIONS THEORY: AN OVERVIEW

As indicated in the opening paragraph of this chapter, the central tenet of DET is that the emotions system is the principal motivational system for human thought and action. A distinctive feature of the theory is that it defines each discrete emotion as a motivational subsystem of personality. Although there are changes in connections between a given emotion and the cognitive and action systems, each emotion retains its unique motivational properties across situations and throughout the life span. For example, the emotion of interest always motivates focused attention, receptivity to information, and learning; fear always motivates protective behavior; and anger drives thought and action toward overcoming a barrier to a goal. Furthermore, a given situation may elicit anger, disgust, and contempt, but in such situations these three emotions remain separate motivational forces (Izard, 1993). They do not blend into the unitary subjective experience of hostility. In terms of affective symptomatology, hostility, as well as anxiety and depression, are convenient but loose labels for a cluster or pattern of discrete emotions, each retaining unique motivational tendencies (Izard, 1971, 1993; Izard & Youngstrom, 1996).

According to DET, a small set of emotions that are fundamental to human motivation constitute independent emotion systems. These emotions include interest, joy, anger, sadness, fear, surprise, and disgust. They emerge early in development and remain a stable part of the repertoire of human emotions. The distinguishing characteristics of the independent emotions are that they are not dependent on cognitive development for their emergence nor on cognitive appraisal processes for their activation (Izard & Malatesta, 1987). Identifying these emotions as independent systems indicates that they can operate independent of the cognitive system. We emphasize this idea as a counterpoint to those theories that assume cognition to be a necessary antecedent of all emotion experiences (e.g., Lazarus, 1991). However, labeling them as independent systems does not mean that they *always* operate independent of cognition. They are frequently activated by cognitive appraisal or interpretation, but they also operate in response to noncognitive activators such as periodic changes in levels of hormones and unanticipated pain.

Each of the fundamental emotions has three aspects: neural-evaluative, expressive, and experiential. The neural-evaluative aspect consists of structures and pathways involved in the process of evaluating sensory data from internal and external stimuli. This component activates processes that lead to the experiential and expressive aspects of emotions. The expressive aspect refers to discrete facial, gestural, and vocalic patterns that have cue value for others in social exchange. This aspect also contributes to the activation and regulation of subjective experience of an emotion through sensory feedback processes. The experiential aspect consists of a quality of consciousness or feeling state that always includes motivation, often includes action tendencies (Bull, 1951) or action readiness (Frijda, 1986), and can activate specific cognitions or a particular type of thought.

Although the neural-evaluative, expressive, and experiential aspects of the independent emotions are highly interconnected and interactive, it is useful to conceptualize these three aspects as distinct functional units because DET proposes that developmental processes may differ among the three aspects, and emotion feeling and emotion expression are dissociable (Izard, 1994). For example, certain facial expressions or component expressive signals are present at birth or soon thereafter, whereas the complete and stable matching of these expressive signals with corresponding feeling states may be dependent on the maturation of the prefrontal cortex during the first few months of life (cf. Kalin, 1993).

Four emotions that we consider fundamental components of human motivation comprise dependent emotion systems. These are contempt, shame, shyness, and guilt. Dependent emotion systems contrast with independent systems in two important ways. Certain cognitive attainments (e.g., self–other differentiation, self-concept) are required before dependent emotion systems can be activated. Additionally, with the possible exception of contempt, dependent emotions do not have universal facial expressions (Ekman & Friesen, 1988; Izard & Haynes, 1988) as have been demonstrated for independent emotions (Ekman, Friesen, & Ellsworth, 1972; Izard, 1971).

III. SOME PRINCIPLES OF LIFE SPAN EMOTIONAL DEVELOPMENT

The central tenets of DET regarding the emotions as the principal motivational system and the stability of the unique motivational properties of each discrete emotion is assumed to hold throughout an individual's lifetime. The broad principles of constancy of emotion feelings and emotion-based aspects of personality have been selected for illustration of the applicability of other DET tenets to life span development.

A. *The Constancy Principle of Emotion Feelings*

DET assumes that the core feeling state of any discrete emotion is constant across the life span (Barrett & Campos, 1987; Emde, 1980; Izard & Malatesta, 1987). Constancy of emotional experience is the foundation of a stable sense of self and personality. Significant developmental changes in the cognitions and actions associated with each discrete emotion feeling are assumed to occur over the course of an individual's life, but these changes occur against a backdrop of constancy in emotion feelings (Ackerman et al., in press). For example, older adults have been found to report similar experiences of emotion and evaluation of change in emotional life but report different elicitors of emotion (Malatesta & Kalnok, 1984).

Constancy of emotion experience is critical for explaining the stability of self-concept and personality traits. Because similar significant events tend to elicit similar emotions across time and over occasions, the individual will have a stable framework for interpreting and responding to life's contingencies. Evidence from investigations in clinical neurology supports the notion that emotion feelings are temporally stable and crucial for the complex task of navigating one's way through the web of interpersonal encounters and relationships. When insult or injury causes a breakdown in the neural substrates of emotion feelings, social skills also break down, and relationships become strained and damaged (Damasio, 1994). This kind of evidence is a dramatic reminder of the essential role of emotions in organizing, motivating, and guiding cognition and social behavior in an orderly, consistent fashion. Such constancy in emotional responses to evocative events and situations, and the resulting stability in self-concept and relationships, would not be possible without constancy in emotion feelings across the life span.

There are several reasons why evolution resulted in emotion feelings that remain unchanged in the context of an ever-changing cognitive system and other developmental processes. First, it is highly adaptive for the individual to have a stable system of subjective experiences amidst myriad changes and a stable framework of motivational forces for responding to environmental contingencies. Constancy of a given emotion feeling guarantees the reliability of the motivational function of that emotion. Thus danger situations will elicit fear, and the fear feeling—always the same—will reliably drive protective behavior. A developmental change in the feeling of fear could result in inappropriate responses to danger.

Second, changes in the feeling state for a particular emotion would alter the status of affective–cognitive structures involving that emotion, and, as discussed later, affective–cognitive structures are the building blocks of personality (Izard et al., 1993). If the quality of the feeling of joy changed substantially, there would be changes in the feeling-thought assemblies involving joy. For an extrovert who enjoys social situations, this could mean that social situations come to elicit a different feeling. This new feeling might not motivate the social behavior that characterizes extroversion, and changes would ensue in this dimension of personality.

Third, relationships depend on the reliable communication of emotion feelings (cf. Hobson, 1993). Such communication is essential to mutual understanding and the development of trust. If the quality of the feeling state that characterizes a particular discrete emotion changed with age and the change was a function of idiosyncratic experience, emotion communication would become unintelligible, and relationships would falter. For example, shared sadness is a basis for empathy, sympathy, and mutual social support. Sadness at the loss of a loved one serves as motivation for strengthening family ties and other social bonds (cf. Averill, 1968). If the feeling of sadness changed with age, it would not serve these critical social functions.

Another great advantage stemming from the constancy of emotion feelings is the ability to learn and generalize from personal experiences. Always having the same feeling (sadness) at the loss of someone or something dear enables us to anticipate and prepare for the emotion that we shall experience in the type of situations that involve such losses. Always feeling fearful in threatening and dangerous situations enables us to anticipate the experience and develop techniques for avoiding unnecessary threats and dangers. None of these adaptive advantages would be accessible if we did not *feel* our emotions. Emotions must achieve consciousness as feeling states in order for us to have some freedom and flexibility in the forming of connections between the motivational power of an emotion and subsequent thoughts and actions (cf. Damasio, 1994).

B. Emotion-Based Aspects of Personality

A key principle of DET that has implications for developmental process in late life is that emotion–cognition relations and affective–cognitive structures are the key components of personality traits. An affective–cognitive structure is a bond or association between a specific emotion feeling and an image or thought stored in memory. In early infancy, an affective–cognitive structure may consist merely of the feeling of enjoyment and an image of the caregiver's face. In later life, the feeling of joy may be associated with the memory of a positive encounter with the loved one.

A number of investigators have shown that emotion-specific affective–cognitive structures are related to personality traits (Izard et al., 1993; Magai, 1995; Malatesta, 1990). For example, the positive emotions of interest and joy are positively correlated with the personality dimension of extroversion, and most discrete negative emotions are related to the dimension of neuroticism. More specific personality traits like achievement may be related primarily to the emotion of interest, and trait aggression mainly to anger, disgust, and contempt.

In DET, emotions provide the motivational component for personality structures. The robust relations among discrete emotions and traits of personality suggest that emotion and traits are overlapping constructs (Magai, 1995). The strength of the emotions associated with a given trait helps to determine its centrality to self-concept and the core personality.

IV. EMOTIONS IN ADULT DEVELOPMENT AND AGING

DET assumes that the most important realm of development in the personality domain is the forming of connections among the emotions, cognition, and action systems. The really important developmental changes are *not* within the emotions system, however. The morphology or basic form of facial expressions of emotion is innately determined and stable over time (Izard et al., 1995). Although there are some age-related changes in the way expressive signals are configured (e.g., full-face to partial or component expressions) (Abe, Takahashi, Putnam, & Izard, 1995; Izard & Malatesta, 1987, Malatesta & Izard, 1984), the signal value of a particular configuration of spontaneous facial muscle expressions remains constant. The core feeling states of the basic emotions are also temporally stable. Significant changes do occur in the formation and continued development of connections and links among personality subsystems, particularly the emotion, cognition, and action systems.

A. Adult Developmental Trends in Emotion–Personality Subsystems

Some emotion–personality subsystem connections are initially activated by early childhood cognitive attainments, reach a plateau in late childhood, and remain stable throughout adulthood. Two such affective–cognitive processes are emotion-expression recognition (identifying the appropriate label for a facial expression from a list of categories) and producing a verbal label for facial expressions of the emotions (Izard, 1971).

Some socioemotional response capabilities that depend on early cognitive attainments and emotion–cognition connections continue to develop over the life span. An example is that of taking into account others' beliefs and desires in anticipating their emotion responses to a particular event. Although children of 5 or 6 years can demonstrate this ability in response to clearly described emotion-specific situations (Cermele, Ackerman, Morris, & Izard, 1995; Harris, 1989), it is reasonable to assume that this affective–cognitive skill increases as long as knowledge of others and their circumstances increases.

It seems probable that this ability to appreciate the beliefs and desires of others and anticipate their emotion responses will continue to develop across the life span. This lifelong process is driven, in part, by continual development of the quality of the social network (Carstensen, 1992). Clearly, the ability to anticipate another's emotion responses facilitates the development and maintenance of friendships and a social support system.

Developmental changes in affective–cognitive structures are hypothesized to continue through the life span by increasing in number and complexity. With increasing age, a specific emotion, like joy, anger, or shame, becomes associated with a virtually limitless number of images and thoughts. Beginning in late childhood and early adolescence, individuals form increasingly complex structures that involve a pattern of emotions and a set of images and thoughts as broad as a value system or personal ideology (cf. Tomkins, 1962, 1991). Because affective–cognitive structures are dependent on cognition, changes resulting from cognitive development will influence the status of these structures and related traits of personality.

There is substantial evidence demonstrating the role of ongoing or prior emotion on cognitive appraisal and subsequent emotion experience. Experimentally induced emotion can directly alter basic perceptual processes (Izard, Nagler, Randall, & Fox, 1965; Neidenthal, Setterland, & Jones, 1994). There is probably general agreement that the affective valence of a specific emotion associated with an image or thought is significantly influenced by the individual's experience and social learning. We hypothesize that situation–emotion relations (i.e., elicitors) of emotion will change with age. As cognitive capabilities increase and differentiate with age, emotion may be activated by multiple sources. For example, an individual may feel the same level of joy watching a sunset as when remembering one.

To summarize, we hypothesize that emotional development is characterized by a blend of stability and continued differentiation and change. Because the basic principles of DET outline a comprehensive model of discrete emotions serving as the primary motivational subsystem of personality, this combination of developmental stability, differentiation, and change is not only expected but anticipated in order to preserve and enhance an individual's adaptation throughout the life course.

B. Emotion Experience and Expression

Research on emotions in adulthood and aging has mainly examined emotion experience and emotion expression. This body of research, although not large, generally supports DET. DET hypothesizes that the frequency and intensity of emotional experience remains stable across the life span, whereas emotional expression exhibits age-related changes.

There appear to be few meaningful age differences in frequency or intensity of emotional experience across the life span. Additionally, empirical evidence supports the view that emotional experience in late life is varied and predominantly positive. Malatesta and Kalnok (1984) found that community-dwelling older adults did not report greater experience of negative affect or less experience of positive affect compared to younger adults. Older adults also did not report greater inhibition of emotion nor did they report that their emotional experience had changed in intensity over their life span.

Subsequent investigations have found similar results. Lawton, Kleban, and Dean (1993) found that older adults reported lower levels of every negative emotion state as well as negative affect factors of depression, anxiety, guilt, hostility, and shyness. Dougherty and Riggins (1995) found that older adults reported their emotional experience to be characterized by more positive emotions than negative. They also reported that profiles of negative and positive emotion experience showed no age differences through middle age and late life.

Levenson, Carstensen, Friesen, and Ekman (1991) did find age differences in emotion experience with respect to frequency. That is, when asked to re-create a given emotion experience, older adults reported experiencing the target emotion less often than young adults. Once the emotion was experienced, however, there were no age differences in rated intensity of the emotion.

DET hypothesizes that the facial display of emotional expression changes over the life span. Beginning in childhood and continuing throughout the life span, facial displays of emotion become characterized by fewer pure, singular emotion expressions and by greater mixed or complex displays. Emotion expression masking, blending, and miniaturization or fragmentation become typical features of adult expressive behavior. This developmental change appears to occur relatively early in the life course and is related to increasing cognitive and social differentiation. Malatesta and Izard (1984) demonstrated that middle-aged and older women showed significantly greater emotion expression masking, blending, and fragmentation compared to young women, but overall amount of facial expressiveness did not differ.

V. OTHER MODELS OF EMOTION IN ADULTHOOD

Most models of emotion focus on emotional development in early life. We have selected three models that consider emotion from a life span perspective to discuss in relation to DET.

Labouvie-Vief and colleagues (Labouvie-Vief, DeVoe, & Bulka, 1989;

Labouvie-Vief, Hakim-Larson, DeVoe, & Schoeberlein, 1989) propose that emotion regulation is related to an individual's cognitive-developmental level. Development and aging are accompanied by changing context for emotional experience, types of emotions experienced, and rules for emotion expression modulation. Their research has indicated that more mature individuals (although not necessarily older) report more differentiated emotion experience as measured by understanding of emotion terms, description of inner and outer emotional experience, monitoring of emotional processes, and reliance on self-generated standards for emotion regulation.

Labouvie-Vief's model builds on Piagetian theory by assuming that the developing cognitive system transforms an individual's repertoire of emotion-related coping skills. The model's focus is on adaptive growth in self-regulatory processes. Labouvie-Vief warns, though, that the increased emotional complexity and abstractness that accompanies development is not always adaptive.

This model of emotional development shares assumptions with DET but differs on several key principles. Both models assert the importance of emotions for adaptation throughout the life span. Labouvie-Vief tends to define development more as a process of cognitive maturity that is related to age, whereas DET emphasizes the importance of developing connections among personality systems. Labouvie-Vief also places emotion in the realm of cognitive development, whereas DET views the emotions system as distinct and as the primary motivational subsystem of personality. Both models hypothesize that with aging comes increased differentiation and change in how emotions are experienced. Again, the key difference occurs in the system responsible; Labouvie-Vief believes the cognitive system organizes and directs differentiation and change, whereas DET points to the emotions system. An additional difference lies in the conceptualization of emotion. DET categorizes discrete emotions into independent and dependent emotion systems, whereas Labouvie-Vief defines emotion in more diffuse terms.

Carstensen's socioemotional selectivity theory (Carstensen, 1992; Carstensen & Turk-Charles, 1994; Fredrickson & Carstensen, 1990) considers emotion experience to be the critical component of social interaction across the adult life span, influencing late-life adaptation. Her theory proposes that individuals select and maintain social interaction to regulate affect and maintain self-identity. This model posits that older adults select interpersonal encounters to enhance positive emotions and diminish negative emotions. Her research provides support for the stability of the frequency and intensity of emotion experience as well as demonstrating the importance of emotional rewards achieved from social interaction.

Carstensen's model considers emotion to be a chief determinant of social interactions. Like Labouvie-Vief's model, this model uses a life span developmental approach to study adaptation in late life. Unlike other models of emotion that focus on the direct effects of emotion, selectivity theory focuses on the linkage of emotions to social processes.

Selectivity theory shares commonalities with DET. Both consider the adaptive role of emotions from a life span developmental approach and both hypothesize consistency in emotion experience across the life span. However, some differences between selectivity theory and DET are particularly salient. Selectivity theory considers emotion in relation to social interaction, whereas DET views the emotions system as the motivational force for the individual and his or her relationships.

Lawton and colleagues (Lawton, Kleban, & Dean, 1993; Lawton, Kleban, Rajagopal, & Dean, 1992; Lawton, Kleban, Dean, Rajagopal, & Parmelee, 1992) have developed a psychometric model of emotion. Their approach uses empirical methods based on confirmatory statistical procedures to identify psychometrically sound measures of emotion that remain invariant across subject groups and dimensions of emotion experience. They attempt to identify the structure and components of affect experience empirically and believe that this information can inform models of emotion.

Lawton's research has confirmed for older adults the two-factor circumplex structure of emotion (Russell & Mehrabian, 1977), consisting of the dimensions of activation and pleasantness or unpleasantness. Although findings provide equivocal support for this circumplex as a measure of emotion across the life span, Lawton and colleagues have provided valuable information about emotional experiences in older adults.

Although the differences between Lawton's approach to the study of emotion and DET are plainly manifest, it is important to note the similarities. Both models attend to the structure of emotion although the methods differ. Where Lawton and colleagues select from existing measures to determine the best statistical model of emotion structure, DET has produced a theory-based measure of emotion experience that is applicable across the life span (Dougherty & Riggins, 1995; Kotsch, Gebring, & Schwartz, 1982).

VI. DIRECTIONS FOR FUTURE RESEARCH

Most research on emotional development across the life span has been conducted cross-sectionally, contributing to our understanding of age differences but leaving unclear the issue of age changes and cohort effects. In order to test the hypotheses suggested in this chapter, longitudinal-sequential research designs need to be employed to disentangle age changes, age differences, and cohort effects. Additionally, the issue of intraindividual change within interindividual variability needs study. Lawton et al. (1992) reported that older adults reported wider variation in the "metaexperience of emotion" (i.e., self-rated patterns of emotions), despite group means showing no age differences in emotion experience.

Another direction for research lies in examining the interdependence of emotions and affective–cognitive structures with adaptive functioning and psychopathology. Consideration of emotion is critical in the assessment, diagnosis, and treatment of psychopathological conditions of older adults. Because signs and signals of psychopathology frequently change with age, awareness of the range of normal emotion experience and expression is essential in order to discern deviations that may be of diagnostic significance. For example, the older depressed patient frequently presents with multiple somatic complaints but few clear affective complaints. Similarly, changes in the emotion systems are frequently an early signal of dementia.

The aging process does not diminish the importance of emotion for the individual. The aging process provides a conduit for emotions system functioning that is affected by, and in turn affects, an individual's life. in this chapter, we have described how DET can serve as a model for emotional development in adult development and aging. The hypotheses we have generated can be used to guide future research efforts on DET and adult development.

REFERENCES

Abe, J. A., Takahashi, M., Putnam, P. H., & Izard, C. E. (1995). *Developmental changes in 13- to 18-month-old infants' expressive behavior and their implications for socioemotional competence in early preschool years.* Unpublished manuscript.

Ackerman, B. P., Abe, J. A., & Izard, C. E. (in press). Differential emotions theory: Mindful of modularity. In M. Mascolo & S. Griffin (Eds.), *What develops in emotional development?* New York: Plenum.

Averill, J. R. (1968). Grief: Its nature and significance. *Psychological Bulletin, 70,* 721–748.

Barrett, K. C., & Campos, J. J. (1987). Perspectives on emotional development II: A functionalist approach to emotions. In J. D. Osofsky (Ed.), *Handbook of infant development* (pp. 555–578). New York: Wiley.

Bull, N. (1951). Experimental investigation of the body-mind continuum in affective states. *Journal of Nervous and Mental Disease, 113,* 512–521.

Carstensen, L. L. (1992). Social and emotional patterns in adulthood: Support for socioemotional selectivity theory. *Psychology and Aging, 7,* 331–338.

Carstensen, L. L., & Turk-Charles, S. (1994). The salience of emotion across the adult life span. *Psychology and Aging, 9,* 259–264.

Cermele, J. A., Ackerman, B. P., Morris, A., & Izard, C. E. (1995). *Children's understanding of the relation between emotion evidence and emotion experiences.* Unpublished manuscript.

Damasio, A. R. (1994). *Descartes' error: Emotion, reason, and the human brain.* New York: Putnam.

Dougherty, L. M., & Riggins, E. C., III. (1995). *Application of the Differential Emotions Scale with an older population.* Unpublished manuscript.

Ekman, P., & Friesen, W. V. (1988). Who knows what about contempt: A reply to Izard and Haynes. *Motivation and Emotion, 12,* 17–22.

Ekman, P., Friesen, W. V., & Ellsworth, P. C. (1972). *Emotion in the human face: Guidelines for research and an integration of findings.* New York: Pergamon Press.

Emde, R. N. (1980). Levels of meaning for infant emotions: A biosocial view. In W. A. Collins (Ed.), *Development of cognition, affect and social relations: Minnesota Symposia on Child Psychology* (Vol. 13, pp. 1–38). Hillsdale, NJ: Erlbaum.

Fredrickson, B. L., & Carstensen, L. L. (1990). Choosing social partners: How old age and anticipated endings make people more selective. *Psychology and Aging, 5,* 335–347.

Frijda, N. H. (1986). *The emotions.* New York: Cambridge University Press.

Harris, P. L. (1989). *Children and emotions: The development of psychological understanding.* Oxford, UK: Basil Blackwell.

Hobson, P. (1993). The emotional origins of social understanding. *Philosophical Psychology, 6,* 227–249.

Izard, C. E. (1971). *The face of emotions.* New York: Appleton-Century-Crofts.

Izard, C. E. (1993). Organizational and motivational functions of discrete emotions. In M. Lewis & J. Haviland (Eds.), *Handbook of emotions* (pp. 631–641). New York: Guilford.

Izard, C. E. (1994). What I should remember from my study of emotions, if I were to return to teaching and practicing psychotherapy. In N. H. Frijda (Ed.), *Proceedings of the VIIIth Conference of the International Society for Research on Emotions* (pp. 149–153). Storrs, CT: ISRE Publications.

Izard, C. E., & Haynes, O. M. (1988). On the form and universality of the contempt expression: A challenge to Ekman and Friesen's claim of discovery. *Motivation and Emotion, 12,* 1–16.

Izard, C. E., & Malatesta, C. Z. (1987). Perspectives on emotional development. I: Differential emotions theory of early emotional development. In J. D. Osofsky (Ed.), *Handbook of infant development* (2nd ed., pp. 494–554). New York: Wiley-Interscience.

Izard, C. E., & Youngstrom, E. A. (1966). The activation and regulation of fear and anxiety. In D. A. Hope (Ed.), *Nebraska Symposium on Motivation: Vol. 43. Perspectives on anxiety, panic, and fear.* Lincoln: University of Nebraska Press.

Izard, C. E., Libero, D. Z., Putnam, P., & Haynes, O. M. (1993). Stability of emotion experiences and their relation to traits of personality. *Journal of Personality and Social Psychology, 64,* 847–860.

Izard, C. E., Nagler, S., Randall, D., & Fox, J. (1965). The effects of affective picture stimuli on learning, perception and the affective values of previously neutral symbols. In S. S. Tomkins & C. E. Izard (Eds.), *Affect, cognition, and personality*. New York: Springer.

Izard, C. E., Fantauzzo, C. A., Castle, J. M., Haynes, O. M., Rayias, M. F., & Putnam, P. H. (1995). The ontogeny and significance of infant facial expressions in the first nine months of life. *Developmental Psychology, 31,* 997–1013.

Kalin, N. H. (1993, May). The neurobiology of fear. *Scientific American,* pp. 94–101.

Kotsch, W. E., Gerbing, D. W., & Schwartz, L. E. (1982). The construct validity of the differential emotions scale as adapted for children and adolescents. In C. E. Izard (Ed.), *Measuring emotion in infants and children* (pp. 251–278). Cambridge, UK: Cambridge University Press.

Labouvie-Vief, G., DeVoe, M. & Bulka D. (1989). Speaking about feelings: Conceptions of emotion across the lifespan. *Psychology and Aging, 4,* 425–437.

Labouvie-Vief, G., Hakim-Larson, J., DeVoe, M., & Schoeberlein, S. (1989). Emotions and self-regulation: A life span view. *Human Development, 32,* 279–299.

Lawton, M. P., Kleban, M. H., & Dean, J. (1993). Affect and age: Cross-sectional comparisons of structure and prevalence. *Psychology and Aging, 8,* 165–175.

Lawton, M. P., Kleban, M. H., Rajagopal, D., & Dean, J. (1992). Dimensions of affective experience in three age groups. *Psychology and Aging, 7,* 171-184.

Lawton, M. P., Kleban, M. H., Dean, J., Rajagopal, D., & Parmelee, P. A. (1992). The factorial generality of brief positive and negative affect measures. *Journal of Gerontology, 47,* P228–P237.

Lazarus, R. S. (1991). Cognition and motivation in emotion. *American Psychologist, 46,* 352–367.

Levenson, R. W., Carstensen, L. L., Friesen, W. V., & Ekman, P. (1991). Emotion, physiology, and expression in old age. *Psychology and Aging, 6,* 28–35.

Magai, C. (1995). Personality theory: Birth, death, and transfiguration. In R. D. Kavanaugh & B. Z. Glick (Eds.), *G. Stanley Hall Lecture Series: Emotion* (pp. 171–201). Hillsdale, NJ: Erlbaum.

Malatesta, C. Z. (1981). Affective development over the lifespan: Involution or growth? *Merrill-Palmer Quarterly, 27,* 145–173.

Malatesta, C. Z. (1990). The role of emotions in the development and organization of personality. In R. Thompson (Ed.), *Nebraska Symposium on Motivation: Socioemotional development* (Vol. 36 (pp. 1–56). Lincoln: University of Nebraska Press.

Malatesta, C. Z. & Haviland, J. M. (1982). Learning display rules: The socialization of emotion expressions in infancy. *Child Development, 53,* 991–1003.

Malatesta, C. Z., & Izard, C. E. (Eds.). (1984). *Emotion in adult development.* Beverly Hill, CA: Sage.

Malatesta, C. Z., & Kalnok, M. (1984). Emotional experience in younger and older adults. *Journal of Gerontology, 39,* 301-308.

Niedenthal, P. M., Setterlund, M. B., & Jones, D. E. (1994). Emotional organization of perceptual memory. In P. M. Niedenthal & S. Kitayama (Eds.), *The heart's eye: Emotional influences in perception and attention* (pp. 87–113). San Diego, CA: Academic Press.

Russell, J. A., Mehrabian, A. (1977). Evidence for a three-factor theory of emotions. *Journal of Research in Personality, 11*, 273–294.

Tomkins, S. S. (1962). *Affect, imagery, consciousness: Vol. 1. The positive affects.* New York: Springer.

Tomkins, S. S. (1991). *Affect, imagery, consciousness: Vol. III.* New York: Springer.

Weinberg, M. K., & Tronick, E. Z. (1994). Beyond the face: An empirical study of infant affective configurations of facial, vocal, gestural, and regulatory behaviors. *Child Development, 65*, 1503–1515.

CHAPTER 3

Ethological Perspectives on Human Development and Aging

Klaus E. Grossmann

Institut für Psychologie
Universität Regensburg
Regensburg, Germany

I. INTRODUCTION

Ethologists began studying species-specific behavior in light of Darwin's theory of evolution around the turn of the century. Their observations were conducted mainly with animals living together in groups. Humans as social and cultural animals were soon included. Sociobiology eventually joined ethology, adding powerful, abstract, predictive models of inclusive fitness for gene survival. Parental investment and kin selection are the prime mechanisms underlying sociobiological models. Observable manifestations of these mechanisms in social animals are the caregiving and protective behavioral systems on the side of parents or elders and the complementary attachment behavioral system on the side of the young. Parental and kin investment is necessary for offspring to continue the line of reproduction. Biological "success" is achieved if the parents' own genes are maximized in future generations. From this perspective, human development beyond the period of reproduction—that is, aging and old age—has been of little interest to ethologists and sociobiologists. I take up the issue in the current chapter.

In the first part I discuss and elaborate upon the fact that in the theory of evolution, principles of natural selection cannot be applied to explain adaptation to old age in humans. Other important factors have to be taken into account. These include aspects of cultural evolution such as approaches to illness, disease, and health that reflect achievements of civilization and medicine. Successful aging largely depends on protection from illness and the curing of diseases. As indicated in the first section, humans have always hoped for a long and productive life and even sought an eternal afterlife. Biologically, however, the best guarantee of successful aging lies in parental investment in children and grandchildren. The concept of parental and kin investment allows one to integrate several theoretical streams of thought—the abstract sociobiological, the group-oriented ethological, and the individually oriented psychological perspectives. In a second section, two historical events are presented to illustrate the effects of parental and kin investment. The Donner Party disaster, and the hardship of the Plymouth Colony, tragedies from early U.S. history, clearly show that especially under extremely life-threatening conditions, human survival greatly depends on kin investment, and especially on parental investment.

In the third part of the chapter we highlight aspects of psychological difference associated with parental investment. The psychological mechanisms behind inclusive fitness are not as yet well understood. However, Bowlby (1982) thought that the emotion system was integral to inclusive fitness. He proposed that not only did emotional responsiveness between social partners foster bonding and mutuality, which is pleasant enough in its own right, but also, and critically, psychological adaptation. However, the capacity for emotional responsiveness and mutuality is a propensity of the human species but not a guarantee. The quality of relatedness that is achieved depends on differential individual and cultural investments in such bonds. These differences will be shown to have consequences for psychological well-being not only in infancy, adolescence, and parenthood, but also in old age.

II. HUMAN LIFE AND CULTURE

Modern developmental psychology is keenly interested in how individuals develop. Crucial to individual adaptation is the development of unique organizational patterns oriented towards ensuring personal well-being. Developmentalists want to understand variations in people's lives, how they develop from early infancy to old age, what they do in coping with other people and with problems of living, how they feel about success and failure, the many ways they strive to adapt to new events and circumstances, and how they cope with threats and challenges to their well-being and health—sometimes even to their lives.

In ethological terms, humans clearly have developed as cultural animals (Lorenz, 1977). Even before birth the human embryo is endowed with brain structures that depend for their development on the investment of other people—mostly parents. Human parents help offspring acquire the cultural aspects of humanness (Trevarthen, 1987), including particular patterns of emotional expression. The emotion system functions as an appraisal system sensitized to various environmental dangers such as falling, darkness, being left alone (Bowlby, 1982), as well as, and perhaps especially, a wide range of desirable and undesirable social conditions. The affect system only guarantees the propensity of infants to form attachments to significant others who then may or may not provide emotional security which, in turn, is critical to the process of becoming a full member of society.

An evolutionary approach to behavioral development is useful "if it integrates diverse facts, if it aids clinical practice, and if it helps us toward a full understanding of human nature" (Hinde, 1991). The individual development of values and emotions engenders an intricate network of human learning propensities (Grossman, 1996) devoted to the acquisition of learning goals worth pursuing, that is, "attachment learning" (Minsky, 1987). Emotional representations of culturally valued domains seem to vary along a continuum of evolutionarily stable dispositions ranging from attachment relations (Bowlby, 1980) to highly individualized dispositions like special giftedness in the arts, literature, or sciences, or even to certain personality characteristics (Plomin & Rende, 1991).

Humans are cultural beings; however, they are nonetheless biological creatures. They are subject to illness, aging, and death. These biological events can be studied both within a life span developmental framework and from the perspective of reproductive strategies (Chisholm, 1993). In terms of modern health psychology, it might even be instructive to inquire why "people often ignore the long-term consequences of behaviors that produce short-term gain" (Hill, 1993, p. 78). What are the implications of an ethological approach for models of aging and life span development? I return to this issue later, after discussing some aspects of the biology of aging.

III. ILLNESS AND DISEASE AS THREATS TO WELL-BEING, HEALTH, AND TO LIFE

Although illness, aging, and death are unavoidable, the meaning of these events has been greatly changed throughout history. In the Western world today, almost all infants who are born in a healthy state are apt to live well into their 70s and 80s, due mainly to an enormously improved health-care system. Even symptoms of bodily aging have been somewhat ameliorated by sophisticated health programs, by knowledge concerning nutrition, exercise, toxic substances, and sleep, as well as the availability of extensive preventative measures. Many individuals, therefore, enjoy their lengthened life span—a most recent gift indeed—as a consequence of cultural and scientific changes, in spite of human's virtually unchanged biological potentials.

Prevention, cure, and amelioration of illness have certainly been the most important factors in extending the life span. Although we may admire certain evolutionary survival strategies, such as fierce protection of infants by high-ranking nonhuman primates, human-made health systems are of an incomparably broader scope. Health as a concept of global well-being may presently be somewhat out of reach for many; yet it still constitutes a useful guide for the future.

Illness is an individual's subjective state of feeling ill. Disease, in contrast, is what medical practitioners have described as morbidity. For example, Jüpner (cited in Schiefenhövel, 1994) found 41 Eipo—natives of the highlands of Papua New Guinea—who had intestinal parasites. The infected people, however, did not feel at all ill. Thomae (1988), in his German longitudinal sample of older people, also found that feeling healthy or ill was more important than being free of disease. As well, in studies conducted in the United States, subjective well-being, independent of various medical diagnosis of disease, was a powerful predictor of "successful aging" (Rowe & Kahn, 1987). On the other hand, the interplay of culture and health is also apparent. Lindeberg and Lund (cited in Schiefenhövel, 1994) found that the systolic blood pressure of the inhabitants of Kitava, one of the Trobriand Islands in the east of Papua New Guinea, remained stable over their life course. It did not show the typical increase of 100-plus-age formula known in Western cultures. Similarly, again based on cross-cultural data, knowledge about the minimum intake of protein becomes questionable when comparing the average protein intake of non-western people (Schiefenhövel, 1994, 220f). Cross-cultural data are necessary and well suited to overcoming the bias of Western views. However, Western bias is bound to become increasingly dominant as Western medical definitions become more pervasive.

It is noteworthy that not all people are affected by health threats in a similar manner. There are wide interindividual differences within our own society in how new cultural insights, some of which are scientifically based, are applied to the maintenance of health. Moreover, traditional peoples across the globe sometimes show an ability to cope with illness more successfully than we do (Schiefenhövel, 1994, p. 226).

In our own society, there are people who are considered incurable by medical experts, but who are nonetheless driven by the hope that a cure may be found outside established medicine. In light of current knowledge about endorphins accompanying placebo effects, such expectations are not entirely unfounded, and improvements or even cures can be expected, and perhaps even have occurred frequently in the past. Modern meta-analyses document the effects of psychological or educational interventions as well as placebo effects on control groups. However, the mediating causal processes through which such effects work—particularly placebo effects—as well as the influence of recipient, provider, and setting characteristics, is considered as the proper agenda for the next generation of treatment effectiveness research (Lipsey & Wilson, 1993, p. 1201). Indeed, psychological data about reactions to diseases and stressors seems to be critical for understanding individual differences in levels of resilience and flexibility in "goal-corrected" behavioral organization (Bowlby, 1988). Our lack of information may, at the same time, force us to be careful in our search for the ethological bases of health and well-being in old age, as well as the general physiological mechanisms that lead to immunological or other physiological changes in our aging bodies.

IV. SENESCENCE: CULTURAL MEANING AND THE BIOLOGY OF AGING

The upper limit on the life span has not changed much during the past few generations, yet more people than ever before reach an age close to the biological limits of the life span—some up to 100 years—in astonishing vitality (Perls, 1995). The chances of surviving life-threatening situations have vastly improved, but our understanding of mechanisms behind aging has scarcely advanced at all. The main goal of today's gerontologists and geriatricians is to continue to improve or maintain the quality of health until the end of life.

Aging and death in our culture are painful and frightening. Jewish and Christian tradition promise a blessed afterlife in paradise without physical decay and infirmities. Although the search for a fountain of youth on earth ("Jungbrunnen," Mittelstrass, 1992) continues as strong as perhaps ever before, the belief in a paradise after death has been relinquished by many people in Western culture. Imhof (1981), a historical demographer, documented the changes in the human life span from the past to the present over the last 300 years. He discusses the fact that without the anticipation of a happy afterlife, our present lives have, in effect, become infinitely shorter than those of our ancestors. No face-lifting or hormonal intervention, or fresh cell injections—the modern fountains of youth—can compensate for a lost eternal life perspective. Such worldly interventions, however, have already become the recourse of many trying to delay or offset the effects of biological aging.

The biological aspect of aging and death has many facets. It is easy to imagine that a world without death would be suffocatingly overcrowded, infinitely more so than it is today. But how would genes "know" this beforehand, and why should they cause their phenotypic expression—our complex bodies—which may have served them well for many years, to invariably wither away? Perhaps our genes have been selected so as to limit the lives of their temporary but worn-out hosts—our bodies—till after they have safely transposed themselves to a new generation of bodies as yet untouched by the ravages of age and overuse (Dawkins, 1976).

Offspring are produced long before old age or senescence. Selection on the basis of inclusive fitness is, according to sociobiology (Voland, 1995; Wilson, 1978), intended to maximize one's own genes in future generations. Forces of selective fitness are restricted to the generative years of sexual reproduction. It is therefore reasonable to expect individuals to live only long enough to produce and successfully raise children until these offspring have children of their own. However, individuals may help in rearing children of close relatives to sexual maturity, as well as assist with parental investment into the subsequent third generation (Crawford, 1989).

Postnatal parental investment in humans, as compared to other animals, is unusually long. Full social maturity is reached only somewhere between 20 and 25 years under conditions of evolutionary adaptedness. At that time the enormous demands of acquiring the necessary and sufficient resources for a competitive existence within one's own culture are established. Sociobiologically, these abilities are relevant for evolution only if they are at least to some degree correlated with genetic endowment. From an evolutionary point of view, one would expect life to last only about 40 years. The difference between 40 years and women's current average life span of well over 80 years (in modern Western cultures), may perhaps be explained by "vitality reserves" necessary for enduring continuous threats to health and well-being throughout the entire life span during the million of years of evolution.

According to Danner and Schröder (1992), there several competing theories of biological aging. Prominent among them are the theories of "aging genes." Other theories explain aging by free radicals that damage the body's cells by programmed deficits—which increase with age—in the body's ability to repair damaged cells by dietary or other deliberate manipulations. In vitro examinations of cell cultures have been performed to help explain known and unknown symptoms of regular, delayed, or premature aging. A distinction is made between longevity genes (longevity assurance genes or longevity determinant genes), which seem to slow down the aging process, and senescence or aging genes, which appear to speed up the aging process (Smith, 1993).

From an evolutionary perspective, a central question emerges: Is aging undesirable because it limits the time of reproduction? Or is aging indifferent to evolution but unavoidable because of costs incurred by the growth and maintenance of our bodies, as seen in such symptoms as age spots, atrophied muscle tissue, bone brittleness, reduction of libido, virility and sperm production, and cancerous tissue growth, all of which may perhaps occur in everyone should they live long enough? Or would the ability to maintain the viability of complex multicellular organisms for longer periods of time (by increasing the upper limits of cell division) simply require a longer evolutionary window of opportunity (Danner & Schröder, 1992)? On the other hand, we must acknowledge that heart muscle cells do not divide and yet they still die! All things considered, the loss of bodily functions, as a consequence of the loss of an efficient genetic repair program, appears to be the mechanism behind the process of aging.

Senescence, as described by anthropologist Kim Hill (1993), "is an age specific increase in age specific mortality even when conditions for survival are ideal" (Hill, 1993, p. 82). The ideal conditions for human longevity up to the nineties and even hundreds are not as yet very clear (Perls, 1995; Smith, 1993). For the human species as a whole, life span theory assumes that "the molecular mechanisms of aging are part of the question rather than the answer to it" (Hill, 1993, p. 82). As mentioned earlier, deleterious effects in old age are hardly under natural selection. "If the same gene that produces a small gain in early fitness leads to the complete collapse of a major organ system late in life, it still may be favored by selection" (Hill, 1993, p. 82). If there is a trade-off between maintenance and reproduction, and if natural selection allocates less energy to maintenance than necessary for eternal survival, then reproduction and subsequent parental investment must eventually lead to death. Hill (1993) cited studies indicating that selection for longevity may even lead to decreased reproductive function. Some studies found that selection for increased fertility correlated with a reduced life span. Still others showed that the act of mating itself may decrease survival, even when not pro-ducing offspring. It is interesting to note that sterilized individuals from species as varied as fruit flies, cats, and humans have longer life spans than sexually intact organisms (Hill, 1993, p. 83). In conclusion, we concur with Schiefenhoevel's evaluation:

> For the end of life, the inexorable effects of mutation and selection have not pro-duced adaptations as meaningful as those for the beginning of life. Favorable bodily, emotional and cognitive features could be transmitted to later generations only if they would exert beneficial effects already at earlier periods in life when they could serve procreation. Properties of life which could help to cope well with old age, and dying itself, are no longer under selection pressure. In other words: The kinds and manners of dying are selectively neutral. This may be the reason why so many people suffer gravely when dying. Since biology and evolutionary psychology are of no help, humans are prone to death anxiety. They must there-fore resort to cultural traditions for consolation. Religious consolations are per-haps the most pervasively found. People must, furthermore, develop new strategies of their own when facing the most threatening event to themselves. (Schiefen-hövel, 1994, p. 238)

V. PARENTAL AND KIN INVESTMENT: TWO HISTORICAL EXAMPLES

Ethological understanding may perhaps help most when we want to understand the strong feelings tied to social relationships, to procre-ation, and to survival. From historical reports we have, unfortunately, al-most no data about how people felt in earlier eras. From the facts, how-ever, one can get the impression that when parents were overwhelmed by too many children, some of them, but by far not all, became negligent, maltreating, abandoning, and even cruel. A purview of European history about 12 to 15 generations ago provides ample evidence for the instabil-ity of even evolutionarily stable systems such as the attachment system; bonds among children, parents, intimate friends, and spouses were se-verely challenged by tremendously traumatic threats to life and unimagin-able economic pressures. At that time, people were selectively wasted rather than conserved (Muhsam in Grossmann, 1995). We shall review two studies from American history that may sharpen our sense of the close interdependence between the human evolutionary endowment and the human response to threatening conditions, especially with reference to age, sex, and relatedness.

The first concerns the famous Donner Party disaster, which occurred in 1846 (Grayson, 1993). The second relates to the Plymouth Colony dur-ing the first crisis year of 1620–1621 (McCullough & Barton, 1991). Both events took a high death toll: 40 out to 87 (45%) in the Donner Party, and 53 of the 103 passengers (51.5%) of the Mayflower in 1620, died during the crises.

A. *The Donner Party (1846–1847)*

The Donner Party "combines powerful American themes" and is "immersed in the romance of the western frontier and the American dream of improving life by taking bold steps," but is also so "awash in death and cannibalisms (that) no Grimm's fairy tale can match it. The . . . Donner Party deaths suggest that the story is even better read as a piece of biology than as a piece of history" (Grayson, 1993, p. 151). Virtually all aspects of the Donner Party mortality can now be explained by our knowledge of the factors that cause differential mortality in human societies. The differential fates of these immigrants show us a natural selection in action (Grayson, 1993). The Donner Party of 87 people trekked along the overland trail to California. In the Wasatch Range of northeastern Utah many strong men depleted their vital resources by cutting a road through dense vegetation in narrow, rugged canyons. After severe losses of cattle in the Great Salt Lake Desert, they were caught in deep snow in the Sierra Nevada mountains, unable to continue or turn back. On November 1, 1846, they had established two camps. Only on April 21, 1847, after many months of grave hardship, the last 47 survivors were rescued.

Who was at risk, and who was protected? Grayson's (1993) analysis revealed that only 23 of the 53 men survived (43.3%), but 24 of the 34 women (70.6%), a ratio of almost 1:2. Survivors were younger than those who died: men averaged 18.2 years, 6.2 years less than those who died; surviving women averaged 15.8 years, 6.1 years less than the nonsurviving women. Finally, even the march of death across the many days of the Donner Party encampment revealed that males not only died in greater numbers, but also sooner. As early as December 15 to January 5, thirteen men died. No deaths occurred within a lull of 18 days between January 6 and 23, but then a fourteenth man died. The oldest men died first, except for 62-year-old George Donner himself, who had a nonhealing hand wound and was intensively cared for by his wife, Tamsen. George Donner survived until March 26, and Tamsen died the very next day (p. 156). Before the lull, men who died averaged 32.4 years—they "could fend for themselves," (i.e., they traveled on their own and had depleted their energies at Wasatch Range and in the Sierra Nevada) but were "doomed by their age and sex" (p. 157). The 13 men who died after the lull—8 of whom were cared for, including George Donner—averaged only 15.4 years. The younger ones died later. The first female died only on February 2, and from then on both men and women died. The somewhat detailed account gives some notion about the events as well as the kind of data that emerged from this experiment in nature.

According to several authors, strong social networks seem to play a decisive role in strengthening energies necessary to fend off health threats to life in our days (Hewlett, 1991) as well as in past times (Imhof, 1984). Within-family assistance was routine among the Donner Party members and the size of the family group had a significant effect on survival. Surviving males traveled with families averaging 8.4 people, nonsurviving males with only 5.7. Family size for females averaged 10.1. Average family size for the men who died early was 5.2, and for those who died later 9.9, almost twice as many. Of the 15 single men between 20 and 40 years, only 3 survived; 9 had already died before the lull in 1846. In men, however, the beneficial effect of family size may have been overridden by the losses of energy during the strenuous tasks they undertook by virtue of their sex role and age.

Grayson's conclusions are the core of our ethological considerations: "Virtually all the deaths that occurred within the Donner Party can now be explained by what we know about general patterns of human mortality: differences between the sexes in resistance to cold and famine, and the role that social networks play in increasing longevity" (p. 158), including the timing of deaths. This example "provides us with a case study of natural selection and action within a human group" (p. 158). It is also interesting to look at the five deaths that had already occurred before the winter camp. One case presumably of tuberculosis, one homicide with subsequent expulsion of the perpetrator from the group, one denial of passage to a 60-year-old man who died soon thereafter, one homicide by fellow travelers, one accidental shooting. "Five deaths, all and typically male: infectious disease, aggression, and violence" (Grayson, 1993, p. 156).

B. The Plymouth Colony (1620–1621)

Whereas Grayson looked at the distribution of risk and protection from an age and gender perspective, McCullough and Barton (1991) studied family relationships and relatedness. Of the 103 passengers of the 1620 voyage of the *Mayflower*, 53 (51.3%) died during the first winter due to malnutrition, disease, and lack of preparedness. In contrast to the Donner Party, there were no differential deaths on the basis of gender or social class. However, children survived more frequently (74.2%) than adults (37.5%). From an ethological perspective, one of the more interesting facts is that all children lived when at least one parent survived the winter. Of the 16 children without at least one surviving parent, 8 died. Somewhat surprisingly, the presence of other relatives had no effect on mortality risk, nor, in this case, did family size. This would have been expected by the sociobiological model of Crawford (1989). However, survivors had a significantly higher mean level of total relatedness than nonsurvivors. Survival was best predicted by level of summed relatedness to survivors, to descendents, and by age.

The special attention to children, as shown in many studies, is typically the province of close relatives (see McCullough & Barton, 1991, p. 204, for further references). Anxiety over the survival of a child may be very intense under certain circumstances. Altruistic care, however, is an expression of profound attachment. Empathy and sadness are responses to the imminent loss of a child or loved one in the context of highly individualized loving investment. It is subjectively represented by the most intense feelings of love, care, anxiety, worry, concern, and rage, anger, and by intensely felt helplessness at the anticipation of death because the integration of emotional organization can no longer be centered around the primary attachment object (Bowlby, 1980; K. Grossmann, 1988; Sroufe, 1990).

There have been times, as already mentioned, when parental readiness to invest in infants and children seemed to have been low. Historical data, however, suggest that at these times, hardship may have been so extreme that they precipitated a disastrous breakdown in caring behavior among many parents. Parts of 17th- and 18th-century Europe were plagued with frequent famine, pestilence, and warfare, constituting extreme challenges to the attachment system (K. E. Grossmann, 1995). In recent times, Egeland, Jacobvitz, and Sroufe's (1988) high-risk Minneapolis sample shows that single parenthood combined with abject poverty constitute profound threats to secure attachment.

The Plymouth survivors do not provide direct data on inclusive fitness—for this the subsequent fertility histories would have to be examined. Several implications for the kin-selection hypothesis of modern sociobiology have nonetheless been drawn: "higher relatedness is associated with higher survival, and surviving parents appear to have adequately protected their offspring. However, children without parents, but having more distant kin, were not protected to the degree commensurate with their level of relatedness" (McCullough & Barton, 1991, p. 204). The authors reflect on this apparent discrepancy by suggesting three possible explanations: that only direct selection, but not kin selection actually worked, or that in small groups relatedness to distant kin is not much greater than to random individuals, or that the payoff to help distant relatives is low in relation to cost of the help. However, the higher survival rates of individuals with large families, such as the case of the Donner Party members, suggest "that kin do, indeed, lend support at least within nuclear families, in complex ways" (McCullough & Barton, 1991, p. 204).

The Plymouth Colony example, although of historical interest and filled with sheer human drama, is perhaps too small and the proportion of variance unexplained too great for adequate sociobiological analysis vis-à-vis the effect of differential relatedness on differential reproductive success over succeeding generations. Nevertheless, both examples—the Donner Party of 1846–47, and the Plymouth Colony of 1620–21—represent well what is known about "the operation of human behavior when faced with a lethal challenge" (McCullough & Barton, 1991, p. 206). Furthermore, data from other parts of the world show that selfish interests of parents favor the protection of those children who have the greatest chance of maximizing their genes. For example, in Krummhörn, North Germany, farmers who married between 1720 and 1750, and who adjusted the distribution of their limited land to their children for maximum survival advantage, had, after 100 years, twice as many offspring as other farmers of their same cohort who did not perform selective parental investment (Voland, 1995).

VI. CONCLUSIONS FROM ETHOLOGICAL AND SOCIOBIOLOGICAL PERSPECTIVES

The ethological data indicate that human parental investment in children and in human relatedness in general function to adaptive advantage when life is endangered. Historical data, however, do not speak to the psychological mechanisms responsible for the differential effects seen in many studies. For a fuller picture on aging we need to understand individual and cultural conditions of individual aging as studied by gerontologists (P. B. Baltes & Mittelstrass, 1992). There is no easy way of resolving individual aging processes—of individuals living today under a multitude of conditions—with that of species-oriented ethological data. However, an ethologically based paradigm such as Bowlby's attachment theory and Ainsworth's attachment research may be of some help in understanding aging in the context of the individual life span. In this last section I shall therefore describe one piece of research on differential psychological relatedness of elderly people and, finally, discuss some of the implications for a theory of psychologically mature aging.

VII. ATTACHMENT RESEARCH ACROSS THE LIFE SPAN

Modern evolutionists assume that our genetic endowment is particularly geared to all those physiological functions that have to do with sexual reproduction. Producing the next generation of individuals who carry half of the parental genes is at the heart of evolutionary selection; this goal is assisted by the biological and cultural products of gender roles, sexual attraction, courtship, reproduction, and the bearing and rearing of children. The most powerful research in developmental psychology today that is concerned with the quality of psychological investment in children is grounded in John Bowlby's attachment theory (Bowlby, 1973, 1980), and Mary Ainsworth's pioneering empirical studies (Ainsworth, 1967; Ainsworth, Blehar, Waters, & Wall, 1978).

Relatedness has been shown to be important for survival. In attachment theory the emphasis is not on survival per se, but on forming secure emotional ties to attachment figures who are ready and willing to help, should assistance be needed. Attachment figures, in addition to providing a secure base for exploration and discovery in infancy and childhood, are also assumed to influence the well-being, the richness or poverty of people's emotional life, and the resilience of personality across childhood, adolescence, and adulthood. An insecure-avoidant attachment, for example, may work against relatedness as a protective factor throughout life. Attachment quality determines an individual's ability to cope with threatening life events on the basis of a goal-corrected partnership in which the individual considers himself or herself worthy of help (Bowlby, 1988). In fact, this may be the decisive link between the sociobiological or ethological advantage of relatedness and its psychological features.

On the other hand, there is no indication in the literature that different attachment qualities, acquired during ontogenesis, influence mate choices or reproductive success. According to Hinde (1991), the attempt of Belsky and colleagues (Belsky, Steinberg, & Draper, 1991) to relate reproductive strategy to insecure attachment experiences is "somewhat tenuous . . . although their thesis does integrate diverse facts about parenting and development" (Hinde, 1991). In any case, differential reproductive success can only be judged, as with Voland's (1995) Krummhörn farmers, after several generations. Nevertheless, the issue of relatedness, the value of attachment relationships, the quality and magnitude of social networks, network resources, and subjective life satisfaction, and the quality of elderly people's perspective of the future are all issues that are well accommodated by attachment theory (Ainsworth, 1985; Bowlby, 1988; Cicchetti, Cummings, Greenberg, & Marvin, 1990; Goldberg, Muir, & Kerr,

1995; Parkes, Stevenson-Hinde, & Marris, 1991; Spangler & Zimmermann, 1995).

In order to understand the role of attachment with respect to the elderly, a brief review of some relevant data is presented. One of the core assumptions of attachment theory is that internal working models of self in relation to others may influence new relationships. This has been longitudinally demonstrated for children (e.g., Sroufe & Fleeson, 1986; Suess, Grossmann, & Sroufe, 1992). We know that mothers' inner working models of attachment, assessed by the Adult Attachment Interview (AAI; M. Main & R. Goldwyn, 1985–1993) correlate closely with the quality of secure base behavior of their one-year-old infants in Ainsworth's strange situation. This was even true when mothers' attachment representations were assessed 5 years later (Main, Kaplan & Cassidy, 1985; Wartner, Grossmann, Fremmer-Bombik, & Suess, 1994), when other methods of analysis were used (K. Grossmann, Fremmer-Bombik, Rudolph & Grossmann, K. E. (1988), or when the AAIs were assessed 1 year before the infants were even born (Fonagy, Steele, & Steele, 1991). However, attachment organization does not appear to simply remain stable over the life course from 12 months to adolescence. Nor is there as yet a satisfying answer to the question of how ethologically preprogrammed attachment behaviors of infants may be transferred into mental attachment representations at later ages in individual development. Zimmermann and Grossmann (1995) demonstrated that in a sample of 44 children, mothers' attachment representations correlated significantly with infants' attachment behavior, as well as predicted these same children's attachment representation as 16-year-old adolescents. But for the children themselves, their strange situation behavior as infants did not correlate significantly with their AAI classifications as adolescents. It appears that a mother's secure attachment representation may have worked towards changing the child's attachment quality from insecure in infancy to a secure representation in adolescence. In contrast, difficult life circumstances, particularly those affecting relatedness such as divorce, separation, grave illnesses, and death, was strongly associated with youngsters' insecure attachment representation independent of his or her infant attachment quality.

How can these discrepancies be resolved? Our hunch is that infants' behavior in the strange situation is but the beginning of a behavior-based, inner workings model of relationships, readily changeable under favorable conditions of caregiver sensitivity (Van den Boom, 1994). Likewise, attachment representations in 16-year-olds are at the beginning of a process of meaning-making, reflection, and self-awareness about attachment relationships as well as about mental exploration and resilient coping with life challenges. This notion is supported by our finding that mothers' attachment representations did indeed significantly correlate with their infants' attachment behaviors as well as predict their youngsters' attachment representations as shown in Q-sorts of transcribed AAIs.

VIII. ATTACHMENT REPRESENTATION AND LIFE SATISFACTION IN ELDERLY PEOPLE

Despite many unresolved questions, we were interested in the adaptive quality of different attachment representation in old age. Though the focus of research on attachment representation in the past has been on relations over time, the issue of attachments in old age had not yet been addressed at the beginning of the study. Direct, ethologically-based observations of elderly people's quality of adjustment and relatedness would have been desirable, but were not within our means at the first assessment. We therefore conducted an interview-based study with 49 grandparents of our Regensburg longitudinal study (K. Grossmann et al., 1988; Sprangler & Grossmann, 1995; Wartner et al., 1994; Wensauer, 1994, 1995; Wensauer & Grossmann, 1995). A questionnaire developed by Yvonne Schütze (1990) assessed the social relationships of this sample. The mean age of the participants was 69 years. Among them, 62 (55%) were still married, 4.2% were divorced, and 33.3% had been widows or widowers for an average of 12 years. About two-thirds considered themselves physically healthy, and 79.2% mentally healthy. Twenty-eight participants (59.6%) claimed that they made life decisions entirely by themselves; for 22 (45.8%) of the grandparents other people or other considerations played influential roles. In the assessment of attachment representation, the grandparents were given the AAI (Main & Goldwyn, 1985–1993). As one of its main features the AAI assesses an individual's ability to reflect upon and cope with emotionally negative memories from childhood, and ability to integrate them coherently into an emotional as well as cognitive understanding of the reasons behind parental behavior, especially when that behavior implied rejection, disregard, and even maltreatment.

In terms of psychological adaptation, attachment theory holds that negative emotions are, in securely attached persons, signals to be utilized in adapting positively to events and circumstances (Grossman & Grossmann 1993). They serve as a guidance system for detecting the causes of negative feelings and for actively coping with them. If emotions are not well integrated in emotional organization, they may grow into maladaptive personality traits (Magai, 1995). Feelings of self-worth and confidence in others are deeply rooted in the emotional appraisal function of inner working models. Without such confidence, feelings of insecurity activate defensive, denying, or devaluing strategies; occasionally, the individual may become so overwhelmed that reflective planning becomes virtually impossible. The best means of learning to integrate negative feelings within a reality-based framework begins in the responsiveness and benevolence of attachment figures; these figures must, of course, be or have been physically available, perceptive, and appropriately responsive—even beyond infancy. Other people besides the biological parents can become attachment figures as well, but this seems to occur less frequently.

The focus of our grandparent study, against the backdrop of attachment theory, was on the relations among social resources, subjective well-being, and attachment representation. We wondered if we would find that optimistic and/or pessimistic life perspectives were anchored in attachment representations in older people with their long, developmentally permeable life histories.

The AAI was conducted according to Main's guidelines, and analyzed according to the Regensburg method (Fremmer-Bombik, Rudolph, Veit, Schwarz, & Schwarzmeier, 1989). Twenty-six of our participants (54%) were classified as having an insecure-repressive attachment representation, two others were insecure-defensive, resulting in 28 participants with an insecure attachment representation. The rest, 20 participants, were secure, 12 because of their fond reminiscences and detailed memories of a tender, loving upbringing ("secure-positive"), or because they had later developed a forgiving understanding attitude towards their mothers or other attachment figures, who, in their memory, were not characterized as very caring or sensitive ("secure-reflexive"; Grossmann, et al., 1988). Many of the participants had suffered frequent and even traumatizing punishments, maltreatments, and separations in their childhood during the 1920s and 1930s (Burkert, 1994). These memories were perhaps comparable to the observations made by Vaughn, Egeland, Sroufe, and Waters (1979) in their Minneapolis high-risk sample in more recent times. In that study of changing, unpredictable, and unstable family relationships, mothers reported various stressful life events that impaired their sensitivity to their children's needs.

In the Regensburg grandparent study, if the participants had secure attachment representations, they were much more well integrated, socially, than their insecure counterparts. They reported more efficiency in using their social network resources if they remembered convincingly caring attachment figures. Regression analyses revealed that apathetic behavior ("resignation") and unresolved mourning contributed significantly to attachment representations. In addition, a most interesting difference emerged with regard to our elderly participants' life satisfaction. Those with secure attachment representations were clearly more contented with their lives than those with insecure representations, as well as physically healthier.

Most of the social network members were relatives (Eben, 1994; Wensauer, 1994), which is not surprising from an ethological perspective or from the Plymouth Colony data. Emotional gratification seems to thrive best in close family relationships. Family members were usually described vividly as individuals, whereas friends and other family persons were mentioned more generally and less often. Despite the fact that all participants had at least one adult child and one grandchild, impressive individual differences in the extent of social integration and relatedness were found to exist.

An efficient use of the social network as a global variable did not directly correlate with the general security versus insecurity of attachment representation, but the particular reported quality of past attachment figure did. Those grandparents who remembered more loving care also more frequently described receiving, as well as giving, help and social support than those who, if they remembered much at all, reported painful rejection by their attachment figures. The former group could easily mobilize support in critical situations, and they could also provide help to others.

The flexible handling of support within family relatedness is one of the ethologically based features we were looking for. Indeed, it was precisely the lack of such resiliency, sympathy, and care within relatedness, combined with some apathy, that is characteristic of insecure-repressive attachment representation. Unfortunately, this combination was also typical, to a certain degree, of secure-reflectives—those individuals' whose attachment classification shifts from insecure to secure (termed "earned security" in Mary Main's system). People who remembered a childhood full of rejection, even if they valued attachments now, in contrast to those with a secure-positive representation from the very beginning, reported fewer helping persons in their networks, fewer persons who assisted in special situations, and a reduced amount of giving and receiving of support. They appeared to be less well adapted to the psychosocial dimension of the aging process (Wensauer, 1995).

Life satisfaction is a well-researched psychological construct. The term implies global satisfaction or well-being, and is grounded not only in life circumstances themselves, but in whether such events have a crippling, depressing effect, or give rise to growth, competence, mastery, and pride. The lesson taught by Glen Elder and his co-workers about age-differentiated effects of the Great Depression in the 1930s (e.g., Elder & Caspi, 1990)—as found in their greatly respected reanalysis of the Berkeley and Oakland Growth studies—has been well received. Psychological security may change for the better or worse under threatening life conditions, but certainly not easily. Security in relatedness seems to be among the most valuable asset a person can have.

IX. CONCLUSIONS FROM SOCIOBIOLOGY, ETHOLOGY, AND ATTACHMENT THEORY

There does not seem to be any direct relation between the classical ethology of the Konrad Lorenz tradition or modern sociobiology and the current psychology of aging. Old age is hardly mentioned in the impressive volumes on comparative ethology and human ethology by Lorenz, nor by his disciple Eibl-Eibesfeldt. Nonetheless, our biological endowment provides us with sufficient vital energy to live beyond the years of reproduction. The ability to live beyond the reproductive years has become available for many by the scientific, technical, and medical advances of modern Western culture. Still, the differential morbidity and mortality of many disadvantaged groups indicates that many do not, or cannot, take advantage of the various medical advances (Imhof, 1984). Moreover, today there are new threats to life, especially among young males, as with the Donner Party members, and there are still enormous differences cross nationally (U.S. Department of Health, 1979). However, these new threats and the tolls they take happen on a small scale relative to the high rates of early mortality in our not too distant past (Imhof, 1981).

The notion of a few highly valued surviving seniors who transmitted vital cultural knowledge to their clans in earlier times was one that was favored by many writers in the 19th century, including Freud. Whether this actually occurred or not is almost irrelevant, because it does not provide a sufficient nor even a necessary working model of old age in our time. Here we emphasize that relatedness has critical survival value as well as a beneficial influence on the qualitative aspects of individual successful aging, though we only have begun to understand the underlying mechanisms.

Likewise, questions about the selective factors in our own past environments promoting evolutionary adaptedness are seldom the focus of developmental psychologists. An important question raised by Hinde and Stevenson-Hinde (1990) bears directly on the issue of attachment and individual well-being: Why are humans so constructed that particular childhood experiences have particular outcomes? The authors suggest a number of cultural and individual desiderata, because "today much behavior is directed toward goals other than the maximization of inclusive fitness" (Hinde & Stevenson-Hinde, 1990, p. 62). They remind us that "natural selection is concerned solely with an individual's reproductive success and that of his or her close relatives devalued by their degree of relatedness," and "from a cultural point of view, behavior is shaped by the norms and values of the society, in which an individual lives, and these may be particularly incompatible with biological desiderata" (p. 70). If psychological well-being is the desired outcome—particularly for the prospects of old age in our culture—then "biological desiderata are less important than cultural or individual ones" (Hinde & Stevenson-Hinde, 1990, p. 70). As in attachment, biological propensities, of course, do affect the cultural desiderata. However, they do so differentially in different cultural epochs (K. E. Grossmann, 1995), and under different life circumstances (Elder & Caspi, 1990).

The circumstances in which individuals develop psychological well-being are, after all, cultural products made by humans. Secure attachment, as an ideal in human relatedness, is a prime example. Security in human attachments is almost universally desired, though obviously not always fulfilled. For aging individuals, the battle to prevent organ breakdown at the ever-increasing costs of energy expenditure may never be won. The trade-off between reproduction and self-maintenance, however, can become somewhat more balanced in the future with cultural development. Attachment is a compelling case in point. The progression in cultural evolution may lead to "secure" relatedness with all the associated benefits throughout life "from the cradle to the grave" (Bowlby, 1988), whereas detachment remains a path towards withdrawal, resentment and hostility, emotional emptiness, joylessness, and isolation. The options are clearly between our present Western culture's striving for human preservation, as contrasted to cultures or epochs of human wastage. A whole gamut of other lifestyles is encapsulated between these two extremes. New ideas and their realization must be created at the service of our individual well-being in old age, and at the service of society's attempt to accommodate the increasing number of their senior members. Culture, as a human product, unfolding in the course of evolution, is challenged to invent new responses to the process of aging. It is now challenged anew by the prospect of an unprecedented population bulge at the upper end of the life span. Our personal investments in successful aging, however, must not be developed at the expense of young parents' investment in infants and children. Withholding resources from our children would indeed be clearly shortsighted. It would signal the imminence of a truly impoverished and selfish culture of aging in the future, in addition to a poorer life for future generations.

There is yet a telling lesson from ethology. Evolutionary pressures have resulted in two basic developmental lines: interpersonal relatedness and self-definition. Successful aging is autonomy within a context of re-latedness, but not autonomy versus dependency, as conceived by Baltes and Silverberg (1994). Recognition of the dialectical nature of interaction between autonomy or individuality and relatedness is fairly new to Western psychology, but bears important "implications for social policy and for facilitating more balanced development of both dimensions in all members of society" (Guisinger & Blatt, 1994 p. 104). The psychological well-being and life satisfaction of aging individuals would seem to depend largely on their fondness and concern for the well-being of the younger generation.

ACKNOWLEDGMENTS

Thanks to E. Voland who provided me with his seminar outline on sociobiology of humans, to Karin Grossman, as always, for critical feedback, and to the editors of the present book for turning my chapter into readable English.

The research in section IX, Attachment Representation and Life Satisfaction in Elderly People, was supported by Deutsche Forschungsgemeinschaft (German Research Council) Gr 299/23.

REFERENCES

Ainsworth, M. D. S. (1967). *Infancy in Uganda*. Baltimore: The Johns Hopkins Press.
Ainsworth, M. D. S. (1985). Attachment across the life span. *Bulletin of the New York Academy of Medicine, 61,* 792–811.
Ainsworth, M. D. S., Blehar, M., Waters, E., & Wall, S. (1978). *Patterns of attachment.* Hillsdale, NJ: Erlbaum.
Baltes, M. M., & Silverberg, S. B. (1994). The dynamics between dependence and autonomy: Illustrations across the life span. In D. L. Featherman, R. M. Lerner, & M. Perlmutter (Eds.), *Life-span development and behavior* (Vol. 12, pp. 41–90) Hillsdale, NJ: Erlbaum.
Baltes, P. B., & Mittelstrass, J. (Eds.). (1992). *Zukunft des Alterns und gesellschaftliche Entwicklung* [Future of aging and societal development]. Berlin: Walter de Gruyter.
Belsky, J., Steinberg, L., & Draper, P. (1991). Childhood experience, interpersonal development, and reproductive strategy: an evolutionary theory of socialization. *Child Development, 62,* 697–670.
Bowlby, John (1973). *Attachment and loss, Vol. II: Separation, anxiety and anger.* London: The Hogarth Press.
Bowlby, John (1980). *Attachment and loss, Vol. III: Loss, sadness and depression.* London: The Hogarth Press.

Bowlby, John (1982). *Attachment and loss, Vol. I: Attachment* (2nd ed.). London: The Hogarth Press.

Bowlby, J. (1988). Developmental psychiatry comes of age. *American Journal of Psychiatry, 145,* 1–10.

Burkert, E. (1994). *Beschreibung internaler Arbeitsmodelle älterer Menschen: soziohistorische Einflüsse und Wege der Tradierung* [Description of internal working models of older people: socio-historical influences and pathways of tradition]. Unpublished Diplom-Thesis, Universität Regensburg, Germany.

Chisholm, J. S. (1993). Death, hope, and sex. Life-history theory and the development of reproductive strategies. *Current Anthropology, 34,* 1–24.

Cicchetti, D., Cummings, M., Greenberg, M., & Marvin, R. (1990). An organizational perspective on attachment beyond infancy: implications for theory, measurement, and research. In M. T. Greenberg, D. Cicchetti, & M. Cummings (Eds.), *Attachment during the preschool years* (pp. 3–49). Chicago: University of Chicago Press.

Crawford, C. B. (1989). The theory of evolution: Of what value to psychology? *Journal of Comparative Psychology, 103,* 4–22.

Danner, D. B., & Schröder, H. C. (1992). Biologie des Alterns (Ontogenese und Evolution) [Biology of aging (ontogenesis and evolution)]. In P. B. Baltes & J. Mittelstrass (Eds.), *Zukunft des Alterns und gesellschaftliche Entwicklung* (pp. 95–123). [Future of aging and societal development]. Berlin: Walter de Gruyter.

Dawkins, R. (1976). *The selfish gene.* Oxford: Oxford University Press.

Eben, M. (1994). Strukturelle und funktionale Analyse sozialer Netzwerke älterer Menschen [Structural and functional analysis of older people's social networks]. Unpublished Diplom-Thesis, Universität Regensburg, Germany.

Egeland, B., Jacobvitz, D. & Sroufe, L. A. (1988). Breaking the cycle of abuse. *Child Development, 59,* 1080–1088.

Eibl-Eibelfeldt, I. (1995). *Die Biologie des menschlichen Verhaltens* [The biology of human behavior]. München: Piper.

Elder, G. H., & Caspi, A. (1990). Studying lives in a changing society: sociological and personological exploration. In A. I. Rabin, R. A. Zucker, & S. Frank (Eds.), *Studying persons and lives* (pp. 201–245). New York: Springer.

Fonagy, P., Steele, H., & Steele, M. (1991). Maternal representations of attachment during pregnancy predict the organization of infant–mother attachment at one year of age. *Child Development, 62,* 891–905.

Fremmer-Bombik, E., Rudolph J., Veit, B., & Schwarzmeier, I. (1989). *The Regensburg Method of Analyzing the Adult Attachment Interview.* Unpublished manuscript. University of Regensburg, Regensburg, Germany.

Goldberg, S., Muir, R., & Kerr, J. (Eds.). (1995). *Attachment theory: Social, developmental and clinical perspectives.* Hillsdale, NJ: The Analytic Press.

Grayson, D. K. (1993). Differential mortality and the Donner Party disaster. *Evolutionary Anthropology, 2,* 151–159.

Grossmann, K. (1988). Trauerarbeit nach Verlust des Kindes—Biologie und Psychologie der Trauer um ein Un- oder Neugeborenes und ärztliche Hilfen für die verwaisten Eltern [Mourning after loss of a child—Biology and psychology of mourning for an unborn or newborn child and physicians' help for the parents]. In H.-J. Prill, M. Stauber & A. Teichmann (Eds.), *Psychosomatische Gynäkologie und Geburtshilfe 1987* (pp. 32–47). Berlin: Springer Verlag.

Grossmann, K., Fremmer-Bombik, E., Rudolph, J., & Grossmann, K. E. (1988). Maternal attachment representations as related to patterns of infant–mother attachment and maternal care during the first year. In R. A. Hinde & J. Stevenson-Hinde (Eds.), *Relationships within families* (pp. 241–260). Oxford Science Publications.

Grossmann, K. E. (1978). Das Tier als Modell: Biologische und Psychologische Verhaltensforschung [Animals as models: biological and psychological behavior research]. In A. Stamm & H. Zeier (Eds.), *Lorenz und die Folgen. Die Psychologie des 20. Jahrhunderts* (pp. 505–527). Zürich: Kindler.

Grossmann, K. E. (1995). The evolution and history of attachment research and theory. In S. Goldberg, R. Muir, J. Kerr, (Eds.), *Attachment theory: Social, developmental and clinical perspectives* (pp. 85–121). Hillsdale, NJ: The Analytic Press.

Grossmann, K. E. (1996). Lerndispositionen des Menschen [Learning dispositions in man]. In J. Hoffmann & W. Kintsch (Eds.), *Lernen. Enzyklopädie der Psychologie* (pp. 131–178). Göttingen: Hogrefe.

Grossmann, K. E., & Grossmann, K. (1993). Emotional organization and concentration on reality from an attachment theory perspective. *International Journal of Educational Research, 19,* 541–554.

Guisinger, S., & Blatt, S. J. (1994). Individuality and relatedness. Evolution of a fundamental dialectic. *American Psychologist, 49,* 104–111.

Hewlett, S. A. (1991). *When the bough breaks. The cost of neglecting our children.* New York: Basic Books.

Hill, K. (1993). Life history theory and evolutionary anthropology. *Evolutionary Anthropology, 2,* 78–88.

Hinde, R. A. (1991). When is a evolutionary approach useful? *Child Development, 62,* 671–675.

Hinde, R. A., & Stevenson-Hinde, J. (1990). Attachment: Biological, cultural and individual desiderata. *Human Development, 33,* 62–72.

Imhof, A. E. (1984). Wandel der Säuglingssterblichkeit vom 18. bis 20. Jahrhundert [Changes in infant mortality from the 18th to the 20th century]. In H. Schaefer, H. Schipperges, & G. Wagner (Eds.), *Gesundheitspolitik. Historische und zeitkritische Analyse* [Health policy. Historical and epochal analyses] (pp. 1–35). Köln: Deutscher Ärzte-Verlag.

Imhof, A. E. (1981). *Die gewonnenen Jahre. Von der Zunahme unserer Lebensspanne seit dreihundert Jahren oder von der Notwendigkeit einer neuen Einstellung zum Leben und zum Sterben. Ein historisches Essay.* [The gained years. About the increase of our life span since three hundred years, and about the necessity of a new attitude to life and death. An historical essay]. München: Beck Verlag.

Lipsey, M. W., & Wilson, D. B. (1993). The efficacy of psychological, educational, and behavioral treatment. Confirmation from meta-analysis. *American Psychologist, 48,* 1181–1209.

Lorenz, K. (1977). *Behind the mirror. A search for a natural history of human knowledge.* New York: Harcourt Brace Jovanovich.

Magai, C. (1995). Bindung, Emotionen und Persönlichkeitsentwicklung [Attachment, emotions, and personality development]. In G. Spangler & P. Zimmermann (Eds.), *Die Bindungstheorie. Grundlagen, Forschung und Anwendung* [Attachment theory. Foundations, research and application] (pp. 122–130). Stuttgart: Klett-Cotta.

Main, M., & Goldwyn, R. (1985–1993). Interview based adult attachment classifications: Related to infant-mother and infant-father attachment. Unpublished manuscripts.

Main, M., Kaplan, N., & Cassidy, J. (1985). Security in infancy, childhood, and adulthood: A move to the level of representation. In I. Bretherton & E. Waters (Eds.), Growing points in attachment theory and research. *Monographs of the Society for Research in Child Development, 50,* 66–106.

McCullough, J. M., & Barton, E. Y. (1991). Relatedness and mortality risk during a crisis year: Plymouth Colony, 1620–1621. *Ethology and Sociobiology, 12,* 195–209.

Minsky, M. (1987). *The society of mind.* London: Heinemann (Pan Books, Picador Edition, 1987).

Mittelstrass, J. (1992). Zeitformen des Lebens: Philosophische Unterscheidungen [Time patterns of life: Philosophical differentiations]. In P. B. Baltes & J. Mittelstrass (Eds.), *Zukunft des Alterns und Gesellschaftliche Entwicklung* [Future of aging and societal development.] (pp. 386–407). Berlin: Walter de Gruyter.

Parkes, C. M., Stevenson-Hinde, J., & Marris, P. (Eds.). (1991). *Attachment across the life cycle.* London and New York: Tavistock/Routledge.

Perls, T. T. (1995). Vitale Hochbetagte [Vital elderly]. *Spektrum der Wissenschaft,* March, 72–77.

Plomin, R., & Rende, R. (1991). Human behavioral genetics. *Annual Review of Psychology, 42,* 161–190.

Rowe, J. W., & Kahn, R. L. (1987). Human aging: Usual and successful. *Science, 237,* 143–149.

Schiefenhövel, W. (1994). Krankheit, Altern, Tod [Illness, aging, death]. In W. Schiefenhövel, C. Vogel, G. Vollmer, & U. Opolka (Eds.), *Zwischen Natur und Kultur* [Between nature and culture] (pp. 217–224). Stuttgart: Georg Thieme Verlag.

Schütze, Y. (1990). Fragebogen "Soziale Beziehungen" ["Social relationships"]. Berlin: Max-Planck-Institut für Bildungforschung. Unpublished manuscript.

Smith, D. W. E. (1993). *Human longevity.* New York: Oxford University Press.

Spangler, G., & Grossmann, K. (1995). Zwanzig Jahre Bindungsforschung in Bielefeld und Regensburg [Twenty years of attachment research in Bielefeld and Regensburg]. In G. Spangler & P. Zimmermann (Eds.), *Die Bindungstheorie. Grundlagen, Forschung und Anwendung* [Attachment theory. Foundation, research, and application.] (pp. 50–63). Stuttgart: Klett-Cotta.

Spangler, G., & Zimmermann, P. (Eds.). (1995). *Die Bindungstheorie. Grundlagen, Forschung und Anwendung.* [Attachment theory: Foundations, Research and Application]. Stuttgart: Klett-Cotta.

Sroufe, L. A. (1990). The organizational perspective of the self. In D. Cicchetti & M. Beeghly (Eds.), *The self in transition* (pp. 231–307). Chicago: University of Chicago Press.

Sroufe, L. A., & Fleeson, J. (1986). Attachment and the construction of relationships. In W. Hartup & Z. Rubin (Eds.), *Relationships and development* (p. 27–47). Hillsdale, NJ: Erlbaum.

Suess, G., Grossmann, K. E., & Sroufe, L. A. (1992). Effects of infant attachment to mother and father on quality of adaptation in preschool: From dyadic to individual organisation of self. *International Journal of Behavioral Development, 15,* 43–65.

Thomae, H. (1988). *Das Individuum und seine Welt. Eine Persönlichkeitpsychologie* [The individual and his/her world. A personality theory]. Göttingen: Verlag für Psychologie.

Trevarthen, C. (1987). Brain development. In R. L. Gregory (Ed.), *The Oxford companion to the mind* (pp. 101–110). Oxford: Oxford University Press.

U.S. Department of Health, Education, and Welfare (1979). *Healthy people.* (Publication No. 79-55071). Washington, D.C.: Public Health Service.

Van den Boom, D. C. (1994). The influence of temperament and mothering on attachment and exploration: An experimental manipulation of sensitive responsiveness among lower-class mothers with irritable infants. *Child Development, 65,* 1457–1477.

Vaughn, B., Egeland, B., Sroufe, L. A., & Waters, E. (1979). Individual differences in infant-mother attachment at twelve and eighteen months: Stability and change in families under stress. *Child Development, 50,* 971–975.

Voland, E. (1995, June). Kalkül der Elternliebe—ein soziobiologischer Musterfall [Calculating parental love—a sociobiological prototype]. *Spektrum der Wissenschaft,* 10–17.

Wartner, U., Grossmann, K., Fremmer-Bombik, E., & Suess, G. (1994). Attachment patterns at age six in south Germany: Predictability from infancy and implications for preschool behavior. *Child Development, 65,* 1014–1027.

Wensauer, M. (1994). *Die Bedeutung internaler Arbeitsmodelle für erfolgreicher Altern.* [*The meaning of inner working models for successful aging*]. Unpublished doctoral dissertation, Universität Regensburg, Germany.

Wensauer, M. (1995). Bindung, soziale Unterstützung und Zufriedenheit im höheren Erwachsenenalter [Attachment, social support, and life satisfaction in high adult age]. In G. Spangler & P. Zimmerman (Eds.), *Die Bindungstheorie. [Attachment theory. Foundations, research, and application] Grundlagen, Forschung und Anwendung* (pp. 232–248). Stuttgart: Klett-Cotta.

Wensauer, M., & Grossmann, K. E. (1995). Qualität der Bindungsrepräsentation, soziale Integration und Umgang mit Netzwerkressourcen im höheren Erwachsenenalter [Quality of attachment representation, social integration and use of network resources in old age]. *Zeitschrift für Gerontologie und Geriatrie, 28,* 444–456.

Wilson, E. O. (1978). *On human nature.* Cambridge, MA: Harvard University Press.

Zimmermann, P., & Grossmann, K. E. (1995, March/April). *Attachment and adaptation in adolescence.* Poster presented at the biennial meeting of the Society for Research in Child Development, Indianapolis, IN.

CHAPTER 4

A Humanistic and Human Science Approach to Emotion

Constance T. Fischer

Psychology Department
Duquesne University
Pittsburgh, Pennsylvania

I. INTRODUCTION

Rather than summarizing what philosophers who are associated with human science psychology have said about emotion and development, and rather than reviewing several dozen qualitative studies of diverse emotions, this chapter presents my own humanistic and human science approach to adult emotion. I hope that this strategy will provide the reader with a coherent journey through territory that is still unfamiliar to many social scientists. My work, of course, has drawn heavily on historical and contemporary kindred authors. Although more and more researchers are working within this general human science framework, a body of systematic investigation into emotion is only beginning.

This chapter first characterizes humanistic and human science psychology and related approaches to understanding human affairs. A qualitative research method then is introduced, followed by the major section of this chapter, a human science analysis of one emotion, anger. With that background, a human science understanding of emotion is then presented. A brief speculative section first addresses the relation of Erikson's

(1959) stages of development to what adults become emotional about, and then relates a human science conception of emotion to well-being. The chapter's final section addresses the question, So what difference does a humanistic, human-science approach make?

II. HUMANISTIC AND HUMAN SCIENCE PSYCHOLOGY

From a 20th- and 21st-century perspective, *humanism* is a philosophy of human nature that regards humans as neither basically divinely transcendental nor as basically the material stuff addressed by natural sciences. Rather, humans are distinguished by our capacity for linguistic expression, self-reflection, and choice—all involving personal meaning, individuality, and cultural context. From a humanist perspective, these characteristics cannot be reduced to the subject matters of theology nor of natural science, even though humans certainly are both material and capable of spirituality.

Historically, the 14th-century Renaissance is regarded as the major humanist accomplishment—a turning away from the dominating concerns with Church doctrine and afterlife to a search for inspiration in the classics of ancient Greece and Rome. We are familiar with the fantastic *human* achievement of that age in art and architecture, as creative people looked to their own secular as well as spiritual experience to guide their explorations into what is possible. We are perhaps less familiar with humanism's looking to the classics' renditions of lives for guidance in living moral lives. In addition, the Enlightenment (late 17th and 18th centuries) also is regarded in part as humanist in its emphasis on human reason and in its openness to discovery through observation. However, by the 19th century some philosophers criticized the growing notion that the study of humans should follow the assumptions and the particular methods of observation and discovery of the new natural sciences. Dilthey (1977/1894), for example, argued that the *Geisteswissenshaften* (sciences of spirit, of mind; human studies) were their own legitimate realm and should be studied with methods appropriate to human nature. Uniquely human phenomena do not lend themselves to study by the methods of the natural sciences, which were designed to study objects.

But Descartes's (and others') emphasis on reason, and on a separation of mind and body, encouraged simplistic, mechanical views of human functioning. In North America, psychology eventually designated itself as the study of behavior, pretty much seen as determined by assorted measurable variables—quite suitable to laboratory models of investigation. By the 1960s, many authors had begun protesting the concomitant and subsequent demeaning of humans. The natural science model meant that experience was ignored (if you can't count it, it doesn't count), and that study was focused on deviation from statistical norms. Hence our literature emphasized decrement, disease, deficiency, disorder, and so on. The other psychological movement of the day, psychoanalysis, was also deterministic and deviation-oriented. The psychologists who argued for a corrective emphasis on positive potential, growth, experience, the individual and his or her differences, and on choice and responsibility, came to be known as *humanistic psychologists*. This appellation became popular after the founders of the movement established a publication (1961) titled, *The Journal of Humanistic Psychology*. That title won out over options such as "person psychology," "self psychology," and "orthopsychology" (Greening, 1985; Sutich, 1962).

Up to this point, the humanist tradition had not been evoked in relation to what was to become known as the humanistic psychology movement. In the past two decades, the influence of each has been enhanced through recognition that both have emphasized human possibility, discovery, creativity, and respect for the individual. From my perspective, the major thrust of humanistic psychology has not been so much a philosophical or theoretical system as it is a corrective, in outlook and practice, to psychology's positivist, determinist value system. Maslow (1962) and Rogers (1951) are perhaps the best-known early contributors to this corrective. Please note that this force in psychology is not the popular counter-culture movement of the 1960s, although they share an underlying critique of the mainstream, and many psychologists did engage in the popular movement's feel-good, here-and-now excesses (cf. Smith, 1990). By now, "humanistic" refers broadly to approaches that sustain humanist values, including concerns for well-being and about interpersonal morality. These approaches range from William James's (1902/1985) through those of human science, existential, and transpersonal psychology. The history and current contributions of humanistic psychology have been published, as part of the American Psychological Association's centennial, by its Division of Humanistic Psychology (*The Humanistic Movement: Recovering the Person in Psychology*, Wertz, 1994).

In the 1960s and 1970s, other psychologists, also discontented with mainstream psychology's restrictive emulation of natural sciences, turned to Dilthey's work and to the related work of phenomenological philosophers such as Heidegger (1927/1962), phenomenological psychologists such as Merleau-Ponty (1945/1962), and the Dutch phenomenological psychologists such as Strasser (1974).

Phenomenology can be said to be a philosophy of being and knowledge that advocates putting aside explanatory theories, as best as we can for the moment, in order to learn more about how the world appears to us before we see it in terms of those theories. Phenomenology is the study of (ology) those appearances (phenomena) to reveal how humans constitute our world.

At Duquesne University in the 1960s, the psychology department founded its approach to psychology conceived as a *human science,* grounded in phenomenological and existential philosophies [see Giorgi's (1970) seminal text]. Human science psychologists regard physical, cultural, and social environments as well as neurobiology as providing limits and possibilities for human meaning-making and action. Meaning-making and related action are the province of human science psychology's research, which will be characterized briefly in the next section. In the meantime, I hope I have intimated that contemporary social scientists may identify simultaneously with human science, hermeneutic, and narrative orientations simultaneously, while emphasizing one or another. These orientations share a general epistemology: that human knowledge can indeed be only human—necessarily developed in contexts, such as cultural, historical, or professional. All data are produced and examined from perspectives; humans cannot escape functioning in terms of meaning—interpretations related to our ongoing sense of and accounts of whatever is going on. Indeed over roughly the past decade, psychology's broadening accounts of both emotion and human development have reflected a new openness to exploring life holistically, to recognizing the importance of personal meaning as well as its physical contexts.

III. EMPIRICAL PHENOMENOLOGICAL RESEARCH METHOD: DESCRIBING WHAT A PHENOMENON IS

In the meantime, for thirty-some years at Duquesne University we have been developing and using an empirical method for describing how people approach, take up, and move through various kinds of situations. During that pursuit, we have not yet conducted research that includes the subject matters of neurology, sociology, and so on, but instead have asked a preliminary question: What *is* this phenomenon as it is lived in ongoing life? For example, we ask *what is* being anxious, waiting for one's biopsy report, deciding whether to have an abortion, being criminally victimized? *Then* we can take our findings to other researchers and theorists for all of us to develop a more comprehensive understanding of the phenomenon.

There are many variations in the following description of research procedure, which I present here in greatly simplified form. In general we have undertaken our research by first studying what scholars and researchers have said about a topic, in order to become sensitized to its depth, complexity, and relation to other phenomena. Then after gathering a range of discovered and requested descriptions of actual (empirical) instances of, say, being angry, the researcher zeroes in on a particular phase, setting, population, and so on, for example, adolescents' angry outbursts at their parents. Observers' accounts (e.g., parents') as well as first person accounts (e.g., angry adolescents') may be collected. Typically, research participants are asked to write a description of the event, starting before it began, going through it, and saying what happened as the event was over.

The researcher then interviews each participant, asking for clarification and elaboration. The initial description together with the interview becomes the text for analysis. The researcher breaks the text into numbered units at natural breaks in order to have manageable chunks to reflect on. He or she then puts aside theories, and asks the following kinds of questions of each unit (while bearing in mind the textual context): What is being said here about where the person is on the way to?; how is he or she attending to self, world, and others?; and what about that attending is essential to the phenomenon that I'm studying? To maintain fidelity to the wholeness of the initial description, the researcher usually then rewrites the participant's account, in temporal format, preserving concrete detail essential to the phenomenon (e.g., "John had been planning to take the family car that night") but dropping nonessential details (e.g., make of the car, the day of the week).

After formulating a set of these edited descriptions, the researcher then drafts a "general structure" of the phenomenon, which is of course more abstract; but it eschews constructs and presents a temporal weaving of themes that were present in every description. In developing this structure, the researcher also asks what the edited descriptions imply about being human that a particular theme emerged. For example, in the research below, the crime victims' being jarred out of routine reminds us that we normally go through our days on the ground of an assured orderliness. In that all themes are essential for the phenomenon to be what it is, no one of them is regarded as explaining the others, although some one theme may be useful for a particular purpose.

Validity of edited descriptions and of a general structure is *not* pursued in terms of procedural precision nor of the logic of deductions and extrapolations. Rather, rigor is pursued procedurally by making available to others the full descriptions as well as the text units that illustrate each theme, so that others can judge whether all material has been taken into account and whether they would agree with the researcher's characterizations. The rigor of reflection and evocative formulation is tested through readers' recognition of, or disparate experience of, the phenomenon as they have lived it or have encountered it in reports (Fischer, 1994). Even upon publication, findings are regarded as communal work in progress, with readers being expected to offer more felicitous wording, qualifications, corrections, or challenging examples.

The structure presents a holistic, coherent comprehension of the phenomenon, in which no one aspect is explained in terms of (i.e., reduced to) another. These structural descriptions can be formulated with varying length, detail, and abstraction, depending on the literatures, issues, and audiences one hopes to address. For example, a 400-word descriptive structure of being criminally victimized begins as follows:

> *Being criminally victimized is a disruption of daily routine. It is a disruption that compels one, despite personal resistance, to face one's fellow as predator and oneself as prey, even though all the while anticipating consequences, planning, acting, and looking to others for assistance. These efforts to little avail, one experiences vulnerability, separateness, and helplessness in the face of the callous, insensitive, often anonymous enemy. Shock and disbelief give way to puzzlement, strangeness, and then to a sense of the crime as perverse, unfair, undeserved. Whether or not expressed immediately, the victim experiences a general inner protest, anger or rage, and a readiness for retaliation, for revenge against the violator. (Fischer & Wertz, 1979, p. 149)*

A 21-page variation unfolds the experience at length and inserts illustrative quotations from victims (Fischer, 1984). The most compact of five versions of the results reads in full:

> *Criminal victimization is a violation by one's fellow, an outrageous assault upon one's assumptions about social order as well as upon explicit social covenants. Safety, freedom, sanctity, future are all thrown into question. Existence stands out as uncertain and problematic as one lives the tensions of being simultaneously object and agent, dependent and responsible, same and different, together and separate. Whether the person balances these tensions toward a sense of mutuality with others or falls into alienation [among others experienced as "them"] depends upon the extent to which he [or she] becomes actively involved with what he [or she] experiences as responsive community. (Fischer & Wertz, 1979, p. 150)*

In the last two sections of this chapter, I will discuss what difference all this emphasis on whatness and human science makes for our understanding of adult emotion and development. For now I want to mention that there are numerous other qualitative research approaches that also have arisen in efforts to go beyond natural science methods when studying phenomena unique to humans. Examples are ethnomethodology, ethnography, grounded theory, discourse analysis, and feminist standpoint research [see Denzin & Lincoln's (1994) *Handbook of Qualitative Re-*

search.] Further discussion of empirical phenomenological research may be found in Giorgi (1985) and Valle and Halling (1989). Examples of growing openness to qualitative research within gerontology are the volumes by Reinharz and Rowles (1988) and Thomas (1989).

IV. BEING ANGRY: AN EMPIRICAL PHENOMENOLOGICAL STUDY

A. Examples (Unelaborated)

The following are examples of angry outbursts or of wanting to burst out. They can be distinguished from "displays of anger" that are calculated to intimidate, from a chronically angry style, from the quickly evaporated "Damn!" from annoyance, and from anger at wrongs against society. I have opted to sacrifice inclusion of diverse emotions, including celebratory emotion, in order to discuss one emotion, anger, in some detail.

1. Observation: Tommy, about 2½, is "playing" with his blocks. Twice he has built a tower nearly two feet high, which, because it was lopsided, collapsed as he attempted to place the next block. At the first collapse, he looked startled and hurt or disappointed, but confidently started over. Upon the second collapse, he looked anguished and became teary, but again started over, determinedly stacking the blocks. As the third tower wavered, Tommy's shoulders sagged and his face fell; then he pulled himself tall, his face flushed, and he energetically kicked the base of the tower, destroying his work before it could collapse on its own.

2. Marge (27 years) reports to her therapist: "I mean, there I was, racing around all weekend doing things by myself, things that are important, that both of us believe in, presumably. We both had done our assigned chores, but he just stayed on the couch reading his stupid magazines. By myself I put in a new flower bed, and I got 16 signatures on a petition for recycling, and he just laid there the whole time. I was so mad I could have exploded. I wished I could have blown *him* up."

3. An account provided by John (46 years), a friend: "I was looking forward to presenting my fund-raising ideas. And if I say so myself, my handout and accompanying arguments were persuasive. But Sally (the Committee Chair) interrupted the beginning discussion to say that we could all think about my proposal and discuss it another time, that there were more urgent items on the agenda. I just got quiet. Then as I watched her joke and direct everything the way she wanted it, I got madder and madder. At some point I made a cutting remark that I guess I meant to be

clever, but as the meeting went on, I was in turmoil: I was even angrier at her but also feeling pretty transparent and small about my dumb remark."

B. The Structure of Anger

The following working version of the structure of being angry was developed from formal unit analyses as described above, through implicit dialogue with prevailing theories, and through refinements as I have encountered instances of anger in the news media, from psychotherapy clients, literature, and examples provided by colleagues and from my own life:

In the midst of going about activities, one finds him- or herself thrown back, progress blocked. Initially one tries again and/or quickly estimates availability of alternative means. A sense of being thwarted enlarges and becomes focal against a horizon of vague reminders of past failures and nemeses. Up to this point one has been perturbed *at* the disruption.

As one becomes increasingly attuned to the personal importance of the activity—to its centrality for who one sees him- or herself to be, being thwarted becomes construed as being endangered. Whether fleetingly or remarkably, one's body pulls in (intake and holding of breath, tightened abdomen and throat, trunk and head drawn back). Attention likewise is pulled in, scanning less and less beyond the immediate scene.

At a later moment, it may become peripherally or focally apparent to self or others that the personal meaning of being stopped was that of being made to be helpless to continue one's course, and of being demeaned (made to feel unable, shamed, unsure, awkward, unimportant, discounted, dumb, etc.). The blocked course is not just the one of building, planting, convincing, and the like, but is also one of being some special aspect of oneself, as well as being on the way toward being a competent, appreciated, valued person in general. Implicitly one becomes angry *about* being lessened as a person through being derailed from his or her previously taken-for-granted project of being a particular kind of worthy person.

Now an angry protest arises *toward* the offender, who becomes the center of one's attention. Even when the obstacle is a material thing, one perceives it as villainous, as intentionally or witlessly getting in the way of one's obviously rightful course. Resentments at past wrongs become salient, even if subconsciously. One turns away from any glimpses of one's own role in these situations, instead sustaining or escalating the protest by self-righteously recounting the offender's arbitrary, unfair, unjustified intrusion.

Promoting one's own rage, he or she feels charged, pumped up, explosive, powerful. Nostrils flare, eyes widen; posture stiffens; jaw and hands clench. At the same time, one quickly scans the situation, both to check on the reality and intransigence of the threat and to identify any further risk. This pause may allow one to restrain aggressive desire, to deescalate, to back away, and to regroup. Or one may give way to outward protests aimed at annihilating the obstacle in a defiant, seemingly sudden and powerful protest that conveys, "You can't do this to me!!" The protest may be verbal (expletives, commands, argument), behavioral (hitting, stomping out, breaking something), or it may be a perceivably strained restraint of such impulses.

Following the explosive protest, one may feel vindicated, and remain proudly and vigilantly ready to reassert the protest. Or, in the aftermath of tiredness he or she may catch clearer glimpses of what the protest was *about* (the meaning for one's sense of self and one's progress), beyond what it was *at* (the incident that blocked one's way), and beyond *toward* whom the protest was felt or expressed. One may then feel abashed, embarrassed, defeated, or enlightened, depending on one's sense of being able to revise the earlier course and still be one's self.

C. Comments

Although being angry may serve to ward off continued or repeated thwartings, for the most part it is a self-deceptive and self-defeating defense against acknowledging one's relativity and vulnerability. The protest is self-deceptive in that it vociferously denies what one has already construed as the other's having made one helpless and demeaned. Through anger one actually diminishes one's self as a person so far as he or she is unable to empathize with and relate to others in their own rights. This anger is also self-defeating in that rather than enabling one to change events, it disallows attending to the larger situation, and continuing one's course in creative ways. After all, realizing that one has just been thwarted does not inevitably lead to anger. One may pause to ask whether he or she has truly been rendered helpless, whether the obstacle is culpable, and whether he or she can cope rather than defend. (See Fischer, in press, for a discussion of the implications of the above comprehension of anger for personal growth, community, and physical health.)

The above brief structural representation of being angry echoes the work of other researchers who also have focused on life-world events, for example: deRivera's (1976) characterization of emotions as being between the person and his or her life space rather than being within the person, as well as his drawing out of the "ought" dimension of emotion;

Sarbin's (1989) description of the passions as dramatistic rhetorical acts performed in the interest of maintaining or enhancing one's moral identity; Sartre's (1962) emphasis on the magical intent of emotions; and Stevick's (1971) identification of the angry person's having been made to feel unable, and his or her depersonalizing of the other person.

How does the above representation of anger differ from other approaches to emotion? It is grounded in descriptions of *what* anger is as it is lived and immediately observed. The description and representation are structural: All aspects are essential for the phenomenon to be anger; no one aspect is more critical for the phenomenon to be anger; and if any aspect is transformed, then the state is no longer anger. Note that even the present abstract characterization remains in the life world rather than superimposing constructs such as drives, motives, biological necessity, and so on. The presented structure of anger allows us to see anger as other than a thing, force, or motive, to see it instead as a complex *relationship* among a person, his or her projects, and the situation.

These characteristics of an empirical-phenomenological representation allow us to see touch points with the contributions of such diverse perspectives as those of Darwin, psychoanalysis, and cognitive-behavioral psychology. Each perspective affords a cogent and useful articulation of a particular dimension of anger. The contribution of an empirical-phenomenological account is that it attempts to remain faithful to the holistic complexity of phenomena, recognizing that, for example, anger is at once an interpersonal relation, a self-appraisal, a protest, and a self-deceptive defense, all with societal and moral implications.

V. WHAT IS EMOTION?

Through reflection on qualitative human science research, such as the above representation of being angry, I have thus far developed the following understanding of what we call *emotion*. Consistent with implicit current practice, I use the term emotion to indicate the bodily and psychological arousal from which we infer that an event has personally affected someone. It seems to me that what has been affected is the individual's course toward being a particular kind of person (safe, honest, mothering, powerful, etc.). In that we are always maintaining or becoming ourselves, we also are always potentially emotional. Our *mood* is our unfocused sense of how the passage is going in general. *Emotion* has to do with our response to shift in course. I differentiate three subterms under the collective term, emotion. These falsely clear but useful distinctions became evident to me through my understanding of humans as beings who pursue goals, for whom all events have personal meaning, and who make choices (albeit within very limited frames), and through my reading of phenomenological studies of being emotional.

The first subterm is *feeling.* Feeling is the experience of signs through which we recognize that we have been affected by a change in course. Feeling includes experiencing body sensations, such as palpitations, shallow breathing, sighs, tensions, teariness, grimaces, queasiness, release and relief, and so on, as well as subtler named and unnamed states. The latter include inclinations, such as desires for escape, for reorientation, and for reaching particular objectives. Reports of how one "feels" are personal readings of how one has been affected. When we ask, "How would you feel about that?" we are asking how the issue would affect the person.

The second subterm is, then, *being affected*—being struck by the implications of a situation for one's projects (immediate tasks, focal and subliminal projected life course, the person one is trying to be both focally and subliminally). One may find him- or herself saddened, dejected, relieved, pleased, bewildered, disgusted, and so on.

The third subterm is the *stance* one takes toward how he or she has been affected. One may accept being affected, resign oneself to it, celebrate it, work to override it, turn away from it, deny it, or protest it. I rejoin most psychologists and the public in using *emotion* not only as an umbrella term but also as a subterm referring to the stance. However, I think that most often we imply that emoting is a strong reaction (anger, joy, crying). Through recognizing the stance aspect of emotional phenomena, we can see that although some emotions are bold and disruptive, others are quiet and unobtrusive. The phase distinctions allow us to be mindful of the difference between finding oneself affected and how one takes up that circumstance.

For example, one finds oneself worried and anxious (affected) about a pet being ill. One's ensuing emotional stances will vary in accordance with unfolding broader meanings. If the pet's illness, pain, and possible demise put one in touch with the downside of caring, then the worry and anxiety might come to be accompanied by a sad stance of acknowledgment. If one takes up the pet's condition as another instance of unfair personal anguish, the emotional stance might be one of angry protest. If the situation is understood in terms of impossibility of ever maintaining affectionate companionship, the stance might be that of desolate giving in. The latter two stances may partially override worry and anxiety. Note that stances vacillate as the person comes in touch with different meanings.

The distinctions (feeling, being affected, taking an emotional stance) help us to track the temporal moments through which how being affected (e.g., being impatient) can become an emotional stance (such as irritability, or anger at delay).

A useful feature of the distinction between being affected and being emotional is that it recognizes the following possibility: having found one-self affected, one can reassess the situation and one's projects and options, and can actively shift course rather than remaining passively affected or reacting with an unreflective emotional stance.

Note that the above characterization of emotion purposely has not placed it in a separate realm from, say, cognition, personality, or inter-personal relations. We theorists impose false order and clarity when we speak as though these aspects are separate just because we can make reflective distinctions. Indeed, having offered the above subterms, I nev-ertheless caution that the formulations are artificially precise. Life's dy-namic complexity does not hold still to fit our categories and linear ways of thinking and speaking. Still, the distinctions help us to grasp our situ-ations and to better maneuver through them.

Unfortunately, we often lose part of what we know implicitly in our everyday lives when we turn to our scientific frameworks. Note that the Latin origins of *emotion* are *to move* and *to remove,* which are consistent with my understanding of stance. Note also that *to be affected* is passive, whereas *to emote* is active, which again is consistent with my understanding of the double moments of emotional phenomena.

VI. DEVELOPMENTAL CONSIDERATIONS

A. *Life Cycle and Emotion*

My research and reflections on emotion seem to be generally conso-nant with Magai and Hunziker's (1993) analysis of the role of emotion in the life cycle. I would add three speculations:

1. The structure of named emotions seems to remain fairly consis-tent across the life cycle. Note that we recognize our own adult anger not only in Marge's and John's instances, but in that of 2½ year-old Tommy.

2. The prevalence of different emotional stances may change across the life cycle. One example: I noted while reading the centenarian De-lany (1993) sisters' stories of their lives that although they remain feisty and involved, these Eriksonian eighth-stagers (wisdom) reported no in-stances of anger in their last decades.

3. A less speculative impression: What I differentiated as the "toward which/at which/about which" aspects of emotion vary with developmen-tal stages and life circumstances. The people and things around us vary with our age and situations, and hence so do the targets *toward which,* for

example, we angrily protest. Perhaps in infancy and senility the toward which is amorphous; in early childhood it is toys, household objects, siblings, and parenting figures; in later childhood the "toward which" includes neighborhood and school people and assignments; by teenhood, the toward which includes society, cliques, boy- or girlfriends, adults in general; and so on. Similarly, the *at which* of angry protest varies with stage and circumstance. In infancy the protest is at being wet, cold, hungry; in toddlerhood it is at being thwarted in one's newfound mobility and independence; skipping, for the sake of brevity, to adulthood, the at which shifts to a wider range: being jilted, losing a promotion to a suck-up, being cheated by the repairman, one's child being needlessly hurt, losing one's spouse to early death, and so on.

One's course and projects inevitably involve stage-appropriate and epigenetically residual tasks, of both general Eriksonian sorts and personal sorts. For all of us, as individuals and as therapists or researchers, for any developmental stage, exploring an affect's or emotion's *about which* can afford access to developmental and personal meanings. Marge, for example, seemed to have been living through a stage-appropriate task of achieving intimacy and solidarity as she continued to pursue fidelity to her earlier environmental ideologies. The "about which" of Marge's angry stance toward her husband turned out to be that his couch-reclining/declining were experienced by Marge as rendering her helpless to continue her course toward shared ideals and mutual effort.

B. Well-Being

This human science investigation of emotion offers implications for our conceptions of positive societal as well as individual development. At the individual level, eruptive emotions need not be seen as states that happen to us, that we merely undergo at the time ("I couldn't help it—I was angry"). Instead, when we find ourselves affected we can then reflect on the situation and consider which stances are viable for our goals, sense of self, and so on. Occasional angry stances may serve positively to put others on notice, and upon reflection to self-inform. We are usually better off curtailing repetitious anger, thereby foregoing self-righteousness and negative totalizing of the other person. Bypassing a self-deceptive angry stance allows for self-consistency, circumspection, openness to others, agency, creative solutions, and continuity toward overall life goals. For example, during Marge's psychotherapy session, she heard herself as she castigated her couch-embedded husband, and after a while spontaneously reflected on her assumptions that he had to share her activities to affirm them, or even that he had to affirm her social activism to affirm her and the marriage. She gradually saw that her husband's disinterest in helping may indeed be a sign of danger to their earlier relationship, but that it did not have to inhibit her beliefs, activities, or sense of self. Nor did the couch behavior impede her from addressing the course of the marriage. Later, Marge learned to identify surges of initial protest as signs to pause before allowing herself to indulge in being angry. She then could move beyond experiencing herself as being blocked. In contrast, the self-help presentations that teach that anger is a force to be channeled or managed, and that emoting "gets it out of the system," discourage responsible reflection on the overall situation, on personal meanings and goals, and on constructive options.

At a societal level, we again can see that emotion is not some*thing* inside us, but is instead a relationship between oneself and other people or events. The interpersonal aspect of emotion is also a moral one involving values and choices that hold implications for the development of society. For example, to the extent that a biologically reductive conception of emotion sanctions angry stances, we condone object-ifying other people and we undercut the development of empathy, which is essential for both personal and societal growth and well-being.

VII. WHAT DIFFERENCE DOES A HUMAN SCIENCE APPROACH MAKE?

The premise of human science psychology is that the nature of being human is not adequately addressed through traditional natural science methods alone. A human science approach, in this case to emotional phenomena, takes as its starting point that in our daily lives and our lives as researchers we perceive and act in terms of lived meanings—holistic engagement in our situations. Working consistently within a human science frame allows us to be mindful of the importance of human language, reflexivity, culture, and creativity, thereby resisting slippage into neater, simpler, but life-less explanatory systems.

Yes, efforts to be faithful to the human order require us to describe *what* events are within that order, rather than to explain in terms of putatively separate variables. And yes, those descriptions are forever unfinished because of their openness to perspective, to inherent ambiguity, and to the evocative possibilities of language. Holistic, structural description nevertheless is a cohesive account of the particular human phenomenon. But yes, from a human science perspective, the empirical phenomenological descriptions of the sort presented here also are not adequate by themselves. The challenge for researchers entering the 21st century is to respect human nature as belonging at once to mutually influencible human, biological, and physical orders.

In the meantime, I hope that this chapter has suggested the viability of qualitative research within a human science framework. Attending to firsthand observations and reports, we found that emotion can be seen as phasic, moving through finding oneself affected, into taking an emotional stance toward that happening. We found that across developmental stages we can distinguish a toward which, at which, and about which of emotional stances, and that the latter has to do with implications for one's meaningful life course. This account suggests revisions of reductive notions of emotion. The difference that a human science approach makes is that it allows us all to integrate our daily life humanistic values with our professional work, and it allows that work to elucidate those limited cross-points where choice is possible.

REFERENCES

Delany, S., & Delany, A. E. (1993). *Having our say: The Delany sisters' First 100 years.* New York: Kodansha International.

Denzin, N. K., & Lincoln, Y. S. (Eds.). (1994). *Handbook of qualitative research.* Thousand Oaks, CA: Sage.

deRivera, J. (1976). *Field theory as human-science: Contributions of Lewin's Berlin Group.* New York: Gardner Press.

Dilthey, W. (1977). *Descriptive psychology and historical understanding* (R. Zaner & K. Heiges, Trans.). The Hague: Niijhoff. (Original work published 1894).

Erikson, E. H. (1959). Identity and the life cycle [Monograph]. *Psychological Issues, 1,* 1–171.

Fischer, C. T. (1984). Being criminally victimized: An illustrated structure. *American Behavioral Scientist, 27,* 723–738.

Fischer, C. T. (1994). Rigor in qualitative research: Reflexive and presentational. *Methods: A Journal for Human Science,* (annual edition), 21–27.

Fischer, C. T. (in press). An empirical-phenomenological analysis of the angry outburst. In R. Valle (Ed.), *Phenomenological inquiry in psychology: Existential and transpersonal dimensions.* New York: Plenum.

Fischer, C. T., & Wertz, F. J. (1979). Empirical phenomenological analyses of being criminally victimized. In A. Giorgi, R. Knowles, & D. L. Smith (Eds.), *Duquesne studies in phenomenological psychology* (*Vol. III,* pp. 135–158). Pittsburgh: Duquesne University Press.

Giorgi, A. (1970). *Psychology as a human science: A phenomenologically based approach.* New York: Harper & Row.

Giorgi, A. (Ed.). (1985). *Phenomenology and psychological research.* Pittsburgh: Duquesne University Press.

Greening, T. (1985). The origins of the *Journal of Humanistic Psychology* and the Association of Humanistic Psychology. *Journal of Humanistic Psychology, 25,* 7–11.

Heidegger, M. (1962). *Being and time* (J. Macquarrie & E. Robinson, Trans.). New York: Harper & Row. (Original work published 1927).

James, William (1985). *The varieties of religious experience.* Cambridge, MA: Harvard University Press. (Original work published 1902).

Magai, C., & Hunziker, J. (1993). Tolstoy and the riddle of developmental transformation: A lifespan analysis of the role of emotions in personality development. In M. Lewis & J. M. Haviland (Eds.), *Handbook of emotions* (pp. 247–260). New York: Guilford.

Maslow, A. H. (1962). *Toward a psychology of being.* New York: Van Nostrand Reinhold.

Merleau-Ponty, M. (1962). *Phenomenology of perception.* (C. Smith, Trans.). London: Routledge & Kegan Paul. (Original work published 1945).

Rogers, C. R. (1951). *Client-centered therapy: Its current practice, theory and implication.* Boston: Houghton-Mifflin.

Rienharz, S., & Rowles, G. D. (Eds.). (1988). *Qualitative gerontology.* New York: Springer.

Sarbin, T. R. (1989). Emotions as narrative emplotments. In M. J. Packer & R. B. Addison (Eds.), *Entering the circle: Hermeneutic investigation in psychology* (pp. 185–201). Albany: State University of New York Press.

Sartre, J. P. (1962). *Sketch for a theory of emotions.* London: Meuthen.

Smith, M. B. (1990). Humanistic psychology. *Journal of Humanistic Psychology, 30,* 6–21.

Stevick, E. L. (1971). An empirical investigation of the experience of anger. In A. Giorgi, W. F. Fischer, & R. Von Eckartsberg (Eds.), *Duquesne studies in phenomenological psychology (Vol. I)* (pp. 132–148). Pittsburgh: Duquesne University Press.

Strasser, S. (1974). *Phenomenology and the human sciences: A contribution to a new scientific ideal.* Pittsburgh: Duquesne University Press.

Sutich, A. (1962). American Association for Humanistic Psychology: Articles of association. *Journal of Humanistic Psychology, 2,* 96–97.

Thomas, L. E. (Ed.) (1989). *Research on adulthood and aging: The human science approach.* Albany: State University of New York Press.

Valle, R. S., & Halling, S. (Eds.) (1989). *Existential-phenomenological perspectives in psychology: Exploring the breadth of human experience.* New York: Plenum.

Wertz, F. J. (Ed.). (1994). *The humanistic movement: Recovering the person in psychology.* Lakeworth, FL: Gardner Press.

CHAPTER 5

Psychosocial Perspectives on Emotions

The Role of Identity in the Aging Process

Susan Krauss Whitbourne
Department of Psychology
University of Massachusetts at Amherst
Amherst, Massachusetts

I. INTRODUCTION

Within the traditional framework of Erikson's life span psycho-social development theory, emotions are viewed as both the stimulus for movement from one crisis transition to the next, and as the products of successful crisis negotiations. Although multiple sets of changes are theorized to move the individual along the epigenetic trajectory, the maturation of new emotions or the ability to take a more mature perspective on affectively laden experiences can propel the individual into a new set of psychosocial issues. The successful resolution of a psychosocial crisis, in turn, can have an emotional component that accompanies the emergence of greater differentiation within the ego (Magai & Hunziker, 1994). Conceptualizations of emotions within the Eriksonian framework, however, are not given in-depth elaboration, as the primary focus of this perspective is on the emergence of values and ego functions. Nevertheless, the psychosocial perspective can offer important insights into the functions of emotions throughout the adult years and particularly in old age.

II. CONCEPTUAL BACKGROUND

A. Erikson's Psychosocial Theory

Erikson proposed that after adolescence, with its often tumultuous search for identity, adults pass through three psychosocial crisis stages. The stages corresponding to the early and middle adult years focus on the establishment of close interpersonal relationships (intimacy vs. isolation), and the passing on to the future of one's creative products (generativity vs. stagnation). In the final stage (ego integrity vs. despair) the individual must resolve conflicted feelings about the past, adapt to the changes associated with the aging process, and come to grips with the inevitability of death. Erikson's ideas, although difficult to operationalize, have provided a major intellectual inspiration to workers in the field of personality development in adulthood and old age.

In Erikson's model, each psychosocial crisis is theorized to offer an opportunity for the development of a new function or facet of the ego. However, the crisis involving identity has special significance as it establishes the most important functions of the ego: self-definition and self-awareness. Following the development of identity, according to Erikson, additional functions of the ego evolve, including love, care, and wisdom. In old age, according to Erikson (Erikson, Erikson, & Kivnick, 1986), the individual engages in a process of reviewing past experiences and incorporating those into a cohesive and positive identity. The sense of identity that emerges from this process, which Erikson called "existential" identity, plays an important role in adaptation to the changes experienced in later life and the ability to meet death without fear. For some elderly individuals, this process might involve a reassessment of their goals and expectations to meet future needs and for others it might mean taking time to examine their sense of self and to conform their identity to the life that they have actually lived.

In addition to the development of an existential identity in later adulthood, Erikson proposed that the end of life brings with it concerns regarding ego integrity—the achievement of a sense of wholeness and completion in one's life and self. According to Erikson, positive emotions in later life are associated with a state of ego integrity in which the individual can look at the past without regrets and the future without fear. Such an individual has a positive attitude toward life, accepts life for what it was.

a sense of accomplishment, and a feeling that if life could be lived over again, it would be done so without major changes. This sense of accomplishment and completion allows the individual to face death and not see it as a premature ending or even to be dreaded. By contrast, older adults who feel that they did not fulfill their potential or who have a weak and fragmented sense of self are in a state of despair. Such individuals constantly regret past decisions and wish they could live their lives over again. They fear death because it will occur before they have corrected their past errors. Erikson's choice of the term *despair* implies an emotional reaction that engulfs the self in dread of the future, despondency over the past, and a landscape of psychic pain in the present.

B. Identity: Contents and Processes

The concept of identity incorporates affective and cognitive processes in the adaptation of the individual to the aging process and to the events associated with life tasks in the social role involvements of adulthood. Attributions of emotional qualities can be seen as forming an integral part of the individual's psychological sense of self. Furthermore, the interactions of the individual's identity with the environment have affective consequences that operate in a cyclical manner to influence identity processes and the way that subsequent events are approached and interpreted.

The construct of identity has been used in the area of adult development and aging to refer to the individual's sense of self over time. It is conceptualized as incorporating various content areas, including physical functioning, cognition, social relationships, and experiences in the world. In this model (Whitbourne, 1996), identity is theorized to form an organizing schema through which the individual's experiences are interpreted. The affective content of identity, for psychologically healthy adults, takes the positive self-referential form encapsulated in the expression, "I am a competent, loving, and good person"; that is, competent at work, loving in family life, and good in the sense of being morally and ethically righteous. In this model, such self-attributions are seen as contributing to the individual's emotional well-being. The developmental imperative for normal, nondepressed adults to regard themselves as having these qualities may be seen as providing a driving force in development in the adult years.

The individual's experiences, both past and present, are postulated to relate to identity through processes of assimilation and accommodation. The process of identity assimilation is defined as the interpretation of life events relevant to the self in terms of the cognitive and affective

Susan Krauss Whitbourne

schemas that are incorporated in identity. The events and experiences to which the assimilation function applies can include major life events, cumulative interactions with the environment over time, or minor incidents that can have a potential impact on identity. Each type of experience can have a different meaning across individuals depending on the nature of their current self-conceptualizations in identity. The process of identity accommodation, by contrast, involves changes in the self in response to these identity-relevant experiences. Positive and negative affective states may be seen, within the identity model, as emerging from congruence between one's identity and experiences within these domains of adult identity. The processes of identity assimilation and identity accommodation modulate the interaction between identity and experiences with the goal of maximizing the individual's favorable emotional states.

In previous work on identity assimilation and accommodation, the underlying assumption has been that events or experiences serve as stimuli in relation to identity over single points in time. An event that reflects unfavorably on one's identity is likely to be processed first through assimilation, and only after such efforts prove unsatisfactory will identity accommodation follow (Brandtstadter & Renner, 1990).

As a general principle, it is theorized that a healthy state of emotional adaptation involves a balance or equilibrium between the two identity processes so that the individual maintains a sense of consistency over time but is able to change in response to the experience of large or continuous discrepancies between the self and experiences (Kiecolt, 1994). In keeping with the notion of a dynamic equilibrium or balance, it is expected that individuals who use one identity process to the virtual exclusion of the other will be more likely to experience interactions with the environment that lead to dysphoric affect. In part, such negative emotional states emerge from an increasing mismatch between the subjective experience of the self and the nature of the self as experienced by others. Furthermore, there may be objective negative consequences of failing to maintain an identity that is congruent with the environment. For example, the individual whose memory is failing but who refuses to acknowledge (through assimilation) the loss of cognitive abilities is likely to suffer problems in completing the tasks of everyday life, as well as to be exposed to criticism from others.

The processes of identity assimilation and accommodation were translated into operational terms in an interview study of adults 24–60 years (Whitbourne, 1986). Moving from the level of qualitative analysis of transcripts, scales developed to test the relationships between identity assimilation and accommodation and emotional well-being on a broader scale are currently being tested on a larger cross-sectional sample of adults.

The Identity and Experiences Scale-General (IES-G) assesses the individual's use of identity assimilation and accommodation in a generic sense, with subscales developed on the basis of response categories that emerged from the semistructured interviews. Examples of identity assimilation items and the interview categories from which they are derived are "Try not to think about things that make me feel bad about myself" (self-justification); "Find myself blaming others when something bad happens to me" (identity projection); "Feel that I am pretty secure in my way of life and don't seek to change it (defensive rigidity); and "Spend little time wondering why I do things" (lack of insight). Identity accommodation is measured by items such as "Have many doubts and questions about myself" (self-doubts); "Depend heavily on others for advice and feedback" (responsivity to external influences); and "Have thought about other lifestyles that may be better for me" (looking at alternatives). The concept of balance or equilibrium is measured by items derived from the former "favorable change" category of identity accommodation: "Feel that the bad things I've experienced were worth the pain." Respondents are also asked to choose a significant recent change that has occurred to them (older adults are asked specifically to describe an age-related physical or cognitive change) and then to complete assimilation and accommodation ratings with regard to this particular change. An example of an assimilation item is "It doesn't change the way I think about myself," and an accommodation item is "I see myself very differently as a result of this."

In subsequent research, the IES will be used to assess how assimilation, accommodation, and balanced identity processes within the realm of physical identity predict affective consequences. The availability of this instrument will also make it possible to test the identity model across a broader range of ages and domains than is possible with the interview. Relationships to outcome measures such as depression, anxiety, and well-being will also be tested to determine the impact of imbalanced identity processes on psychological adaptation.

The aging process presents a particular challenge to the maintenance of a stable sense of identity over time. Events caused by physical aging, cognitive changes, and the alterations of relations with significant others and within the social context are qualitatively different from other experiences in adulthood that are of a more transitory or fleeting nature. An unpleasant encounter in a chance meeting with a stranger that reflects unfavorably upon one's social identity may be dismissed through identity assimilation as lacking direct personal relevance. If this encounter is of a one-time nature, its potential significance to identity will fade with time. Aging, however, is a process that does not fade with time. The changes that occur as a result of the aging process remain a constant challenge as the individual must find ways to integrate them into identity throughout adulthood.

C. A Multiple Threshold Model

A related theoretical concept that can inform the understanding of identity in later life is the multiple threshold model. According to this model, individuals approach changes in physical and cognitive functioning associated with the aging process as a function of their own unique identities. Central to the identity of each individual is a set of physical and psychological attributes that are of particular importance to that individual. For example, the person for whom playing tennis forms a central focus of identity either as a professional endeavor or a valued leisure time activity values the combination of physical agility and mental judgment demanded by the game. The artist values visual and fine motor skills, the gardener relies on being able to dig in the dirt, and the word-game fanatic cherishes the functions of memory and language. In the emotional domain, individuals have views of themselves as being able to control their emotions. Fear of the effects of the possible ravages of aging on cognitive functions may threaten the individual's sense of being able to maintain a sense of dignity when faced with emotionally challenging situations.

For each individual, a particular set of age-related changes will have relevance to this central feature of identity. Although the aging process brings with it many changes in physical and psychological functioning, changes in central functions are the ones that will have maximum salience and impact for the individual (Pelham, 1991). According to the multiple threshold model, individuals monitor age-related changes in each of these functions. Social context affects these expectations, as individuals' lay theories about the effects of aging, and their beliefs in the ability to control aging changes further interact with their own conceptualizations of these possible changes (Heckhausen & Baltes, 1991).

Emotions form part of the content of adult identity, according to this model, but may also be seen as consequences of the quality of identity processes used in relation to age-related experiences. Thus, individuals who have characteristically used identity assimilation and have found themselves able to adapt to life changes without needing to examine the deeper implications of these changes to identity may find that assimilation becomes less effective over the years as new changes require greater adaptive flexibility. Conversely, individuals who have relied upon identity accommodation as their primary mode of interacting with experiences may find that they become demoralized and hopeless when they begin to notice changes in valued aspects of functioning. It is assumed within this model that for nondepressed adults, the desire to view oneself in a positive light forms a basic framework for approaching new experiences. However, if this view of the self is built on a shaky or insecure foundation, aging will become the source of dysphoric affect not as yet equalled in the individual's lifetime.

D. Physical Identity and Aging

The substantive content of identity incorporates the domains of physical, psychological, and social functioning. Within the domain of physical functioning are the attributes of appearance, competence, and health (Whitbourne & Primus, 1996). Physical identity may be regarded as one of the fundamental, yet overlooked, areas of personality within psychological gerontology. Yet, implications of the aging of the body for the individual's psychological well-being, however, are manifest.

The emotional outcome of changes in valued aspects of physical identity may be seen as a function of whether individuals rely on identity assimilation, identity accommodation, or balanced identity processes. Theoretically, individuals who use identity assimilation would be expected to deny the importance of age-related changes in valued aspects of physical functioning. Changes in functioning related to age are not acknowledged as a result of the aging process, but instead are attributed to transitory states of health or health-related behaviors. This type of denial occurs as an effort, both conscious and unconscious, to preserve and protect the individual's sense of the self as competent and consistent over time. As long as denial can be effectively maintained, the individual will feel a subjective sense of well-being; there is evidence that individuals are capable of such assimilation for many years and in the face of objectively defined declining health (Heidrich & Ryff, 1993).

Those older adults who rely more or less exclusively on identity accommodation overreact to small events or experiences and draw overly broad and sweeping conclusions from one instance or situation. With regard to aging, they would be expected to overreact even to small age-related changes, prematurely concluding that they are "over the hill" and failing to take preventative actions (Woodward & Wallston, 1987). The individual may start to "feel old" as soon as these external changes begin to occur. It is likely that individuals who rely on accommodation begin to adopt the self-image of being too weak or feeble to continue to maintain their participation in activities that were formerly rewarding to them (Janelli, 1993). They will become unduly depressed and hopeless (Parmelee, Katz, & Lawton, 1991), and their negative evaluations of the self, world, and future may begin to take the form of the traditional cognitive triad of depression (Beck, Rush, Shaw, & Emery, 1975). The experience of pain may also contribute to depressive affect, particularly when this results in the restriction of activities (Williamson & Schulz, 1992).

A balanced approach to adapting to age-related changes in valued aspects of physical functioning involves taking precautions and attempting to preserve functions for as long as possible, and adapting to losses when they occur by finding ways to compensate for them. One may reach a compromise between assimilation and accommodation by recognizing that aging is taking place but not letting this knowledge interfere with daily functioning or future plans. Although there may be emotional costs involved in the recognition of impending losses, individuals who maintain a balanced approach rebound from setbacks with renewed vigor and optimism (Ryff, 1989).

E. The Interaction of Coping and Identity

The processes of identity assimilation and accommodation add a needed dimension in examining the impact of physical changes on identity and well-being in adulthood and old age. However, the concept of coping must also be factored into this model to predict behavioral and affective outcomes from the interface between identity and age-related experiences. Two major categories of coping strategies have been identified in the stress literature: emotion-focused and problem-focused coping (Lazarus & Folkman, 1984). In emotion-focused coping, the individual attempts to change the way he or she thinks about or appraises a stressful situation rather than changing the situation itself. Problem-focused coping involves attempts to reduce stress by changing the stressful situation.

As a general statement, it appears that individuals who use problem-focused coping strategies are more likely to maintain higher activity levels (Preston & Mansfield, 1984; Speake, 1987). These individuals view aging as a challenge to which they apply the coping strategies found to be effective in other life domains (Die, Seelbach, & Sherman, 1987). They are better able to meet their perceived physical needs and tailor their expectations and behavior to fit the changes in their physical identity (Hennessy, 1989). Active involvement in sports or exercise not only promotes physical functioning but can serve as an important coping mechanism (O'Brien & Conger, 1991). Coping style also seems to be related to reactions to a variety of physical health problems (Berkman, Millar, Holmes, & Bonander, 1991). Training in problem-focused coping methods has proven helpful in facilitating pain management and reducing anxiety (Fry & Wong, 1991). Similarly, problem-focused coping may enable individuals to take advantage of rehabilitative methods that can assist in their recovery and decrease the incidence of depressive symptoms following physical trauma, such as hip fractures (Roberto, 1992).

The relationship between coping and health can be seen as cyclical. Individuals who successfully use coping strategies to manage stress may actually experience improved physical functioning. Active efforts to reduce stress through seeking social support or physical exercise can have physiological advantages in terms of improved immune system functioning (McNaughton, Smith, Patterson, & Grant, 1990). A more competent immune system in turn can lower the elderly individual's risk of certain forms of cancer and influenza (Miller, 1993).

In contrast to the positive effects of problem-focused coping is evidence of the deleterious effect of emotion-focused coping on psychological and physical health outcomes. Individuals who use avoidance are also likely to report higher levels of physical and psychological symptoms and depression (Bombardier, D'Amico, & Jordan, 1990), even continuing for months after the stressful situation has subsided (Smith, Patterson, & Grant, 1990). However, emotion-focused coping can have positive adaptive value if the situation is completely out of one's control, or if excessive rumination is harmful to improvement. As long as the individual follows prescribed treatment, the outcome may still be positive and in some cases denial may actually be adaptive (Pearlin & Schooler, 1978). The use of denial as a coping mechanism becomes maladaptive if it prevents the individual from taking action that is beneficial to recovery.

In existing research on coping, the amount of variance accounted for leaves considerable room for the input of variables related to identity and the self. As a way of gaining a more comprehensive prediction of variations in response to challenges to physical identity associated with the aging process, it may be helpful to combine coping types with identity processes. Such an approach produces a fourfold matrix to account for adaptation to the physical aging process. Specific behavioral and adaptive predictions can be made for individuals within each of the four cells created by this matrix.

Individuals who use identity assimilation and emotion-focused coping are likely to deny the relevance of aging to their identities and, at the same time, engage in few behaviors intended to offset or compensate for aging changes. Adverse health, emotional, and behavioral consequences are more likely to occur for aging individuals who take an assimilative approach to age- or disease-related bodily changes and use emotion-focused coping. They may find it more comfortable not to think about the diagnosis or problem and instead go on with life as usual, not changing their identities in response to the knowledge that they are suffering a major change in health or functioning or even have a potentially terminal illness. Consequently, they will not take active efforts to protect and promote their body's ability to fight the condition or disease. Those who use identity assimilation and problem-focused coping, by contrast, would actively become involved in behavioral controls that could serve a preventative or compensatory function. However, they would not integrate into their identities the knowledge that their body has changed in fundamental ways or faces severe health threats. Thus, at the behavioral level, the individual is engaging in appropriate health maintenance and rehabilitative strategies, and is able to take advantage of these strategies in terms of improvements in physical health. However, the individual has chosen not to give particular thought or emphasis to the implications for identity of the problem or disorder. Such an approach may not have negative emotional consequences, and in fact may have a protective emotional function.

Identity accommodation may also occur in conjunction with either problem- or emotion-focused coping. Individuals who tend to use accommodation to the point that they overreact to a diagnosis or physical disorder may suffer the same adverse consequences as those who deny through assimilation the significance of physical changes or illness. Such individuals believe that what they do in reaction to these changes or diseases will make no difference, and through the emotion-focused strategies of distancing, denial, or avoidance, fail to take the necessary steps to maximize their functioning. Their emotions are likely to be highly dysphoric, and they feel a loss of the ability to control or predict the future course of their physical development or changes in health condition. Individuals who use accommodation but also take steps to confront the changes in physical status through problem-focused coping may be likely to take extremely active steps to help reduce their symptoms. It is probable that such individuals feel that they are able to control the events in their lives, leading them to be less likely to use palliative coping strategies in favor of ones that address the situation (Blanchard-Fields & Irion, 1989). These individuals would react to disease or physical changes by harnessing their available resources, and they would actively seek further medical treatment as well as less proven alternate treatments. They might become preoccupied with their bodies, but at the same time they would use every opportunity to talk to others and get help, using coping strategies such as confrontation, seeking social support, and planful problem solving. The risk of this type of coping in combination with identity accommodation is that although the individual adjusts well to the physical identity stressor by taking active steps, he or she may ruminate excessively about the disease and experience periods of extreme depression when unable to use direct action coping strategies.

Healthy adaptation within this fourfold model involves a balance between assimilation and accommodation in terms of the impact of age changes or disease on identity and flexibility of coping style. When problems arise, such individuals can focus on the physical identity stressor and are open to seeking help from others, but they avoid being preoccupied with the illness when necessary in order to focus on other concerns, such as family or work involvements. This ability to adapt to the challenges of aging reflects what once was described as characteristic of "successful" aging (Clark & Anderson, 1967) and, more recently, has been identified as a protective factor against depression in later adulthood (Brandtstadter & Rothermund, 1994).

In this discussion of identity and coping, it is important to emphasize that the individual's use of these processes is not fixed across the span of the aging years. Individuals may use a variety of coping strategies that complement or offset their identity style. Furthermore, given the emphasis in the coping literature on the variable nature of coping processes (Folkman & Lazarus, 1980; Folkman, Lazarus, Gruen, & DeLongis, 1986), it may be more reasonable to propose that the identity processes are used within the same individual on different occasions, or even within the same individual on the same occasion (Brandtstadter & Renner, 1990). As is true for coping strategies, individuals may use one, then another, of the identity processes in their attempts to adapt to changes in the body's appearance, functioning, and health.

Further research is needed to establish the extent to which these related concepts overlap with the proposed mechanisms described here. Interestingly, the prospect that individual differences in identity processes mediate the relationship between age and personal control beliefs may help to explain the lack of consistency in the literature on age differences in sense of control (Lachman, 1986). More recent work on the concept of primary and secondary control (Heckhausen & Schulz, 1995) seems to be particularly relevant to the proposed interaction between identity and coping methods, and is worthy of exploration.

III. EMPIRICAL INVESTIGATIONS OF IDENTITY AND EMOTIONS

Initial investigations of the adult identity processes of assimilation and accommodation provided evidence of emotional ramifications of the ways that adults incorporate experiences into identity (Whitbourne, 1986). Interview data on adults in the middle years provided initial glimpses into the nature of the identity processes within content areas of work, family, and values. Although not a specific focus of the study, emotional states of a generic positive or negative quality were clearly evident in relation to identity themes and issues within each of the particular domains.

In the case of the family domain, respondents derived emotional gratification from the opportunities to establish close, companionate relationships characterized by high levels of intimacy. Similar findings were observed in a study of young and middle-aged married couples, for whom intimacy and companionship served not only as sources of pleasurable interactions, but also as verification for the individual's identity as a "loving" spouse (Whitbourne & Ebmeyer, 1990). Even more central, perhaps, within the realm of relationships were statements made by respondents concerning their identity as parents. Feelings of personal fulfillment along with, at a simpler level, the emotions of pride, enjoyment, and security, were associated with the parent identity. Subsequent research on the parent identity in particular has shown, further, that identity accommodation in the context of relationships with growing children can stimulate increasingly complex emotions, both positive and negative, particularly as they move into the adolescent years (Tolman & Whitbourne, in press). Furthermore, as children move into adulthood, their accomplishments reflect on the parent's identity in ways that can engender considerable emotional ambivalence (Ryff, Lee, Essex, & Schmutte, 1994).

In the domain of work, positive affective states related to feelings of competence, autonomy, positive regard by others, the ability to see results, and intellectual stimulation result from interactions between identity and experiences. Job-related stress can also be seen, at least in part, as a function of the individual's interpretation of challenges and pressures present in the workplace that are relevant to identity; work-related experiences tap into a fundamental sense within identity of the self as competent and respected by others.

IV. CONCLUDING COMMENTS: IDENTITY AND EMOTIONS IN OLD AGE

In this chapter, I have outlined several broad areas in relation to identity and aging, highlighting the role of emotions within identity and as the outcome of interactions between self and experiences. The general assumption has been that favorable emotional states, such as happiness, life satisfaction, subjective well-being, and positive morale occur when identity and experiences are in synchrony and neither identity assimilation nor accommodation has become a dominant force. This position is consistent with themes in the gerontological literature that emphasize the flexibility shown by adapted elders in coping with the challenges and threats presented by the aging process (Aldwin, 1991; Brandtstadter & Rothermund, 1994).

It is also important to recognize, however, that the lens of gerontological researchers may at times become clouded by the selective nature of the sample we study. The elders available for our scrutiny are, after all, the ones who have survived death in youth, middle age, and beyond due to illness, high-risk behavior, or exposure to accidents, disasters, and war. To make generalizations from the available populations to the "aging process" and, even further, to "successful" aging, runs the risk of becoming tautological. The nonsuccessful agers are no longer represented in the population. Thus, the observation that successful elders have managed to learn to titrate their emotional experiences (Carstensen, 1993) or coping mechanisms (McCrae, 1989) may say less about the aging process than about the nature of people who are survivors and have been for their entire lives.

Furthermore, it is important to maintain a clear sense of what is meant by "positive" emotions or "favorable" adjustment. In this chapter, as in much of the literature on coping with the aging process, there is an implicit assumption that the best one can hope for in old age is to "adapt" or, in the sense of the identity model, to "accommodate" to the trials and tribulations of aging. Within this research, elders who cope well are seen as reactive rather than proactive—able to match wits with the vagaries of the aging process and not lose ground until the very end. However, one must also keep in mind the possibility that aging can bring with it emotional satisfaction from the pursuit of new goals and challenges (Rapkin & Fischer, 1992). The terms *assimilation* and *accommodation* do not give credit to this creative element of the self, in which experiences are sought because they elaborate one's identity rather than being adapted to in a passive manner. Future research on identity, coping, and the emotions should address the creative capacities of the elderly, and the unique perspective offered by their lifetime of experiences in both seeking and adjusting to change.

In returning to the themes of a psychosocial perspective on emotions and aging, it is clear from the concepts and data presented in this chapter that it is essential to view the emotional life of the older adult as a reflection of previous developmental transitions. In particular, the individual's sense of identity as it has evolved over the adult years plays a vital role in influencing the older adult's daily moods and overall sense of well-being. On the other hand, although Erikson's theory has provided a comprehensive and useful framework for understanding the psychosocial development of the individual, it requires considerable elaboration beyond its original propositions. By examining more specifically the components of the psychosocial crisis elements, particularly those applicable to the adult years and beyond, it may be possible to link contemporary work on emotions in later life with a developmental approach that provides insight into the antecedents of the individual's range and level of emotional expression and experiences.

REFERENCES

Aldwin, C. M. (1991). Does age affect the stress and coping process? Implications of age differences in perceived control. *Journal of Gerontology: Psychological Sciences, 46*, P174–180.

Beck, A. T., Rush, A. J., Shaw, B. F., & Emery, G. (1975). *Cognitive therapy of depression.* New York: Guilford.

Berkman, B., Millar, S., Holmes, W., & Bonander, E. (1991). Predicting elderly cardiac patients at risk for readmission. Special Issue: Applied social work research in health and social work. *Social Work in Health Care, 16*, 21–38.

Blanchard-Fields, F., & Irion, J. (1989). Coping strategies from the perspective of two developmental markers: Age and social reasoning. *Journal of Genetic Psychology, 149*, 141–151.

Bombardier, C., D'Amico, C., & Jordan, J. (1990). The relationship of appraisal and coping to chronic illness adjustment. *Behavior Research and Therapy, 28*, 297–304.

Brandtstadter, J., & Renner, G. (1990). Tenacious goal pursuit and flexible goal adjustment: Explication and age-related analysis of assimilative and accommodative strategies in coping. *Psychology and Aging, 5*, 58–67.

Brandstadter, J., & Rothermund, K. (1994). Self-percepts of control in middle and later adulthood: Buffering losses by rescaling goals. *Psychology and Aging, 9*, 265–273.

Carstensen, L. L. (1993). Motivation for social contact across the life span: A theory of socioemotional selectivity. In J. Jacobs (Ed.), *Nebraska Symposium on Motivation* (Vol. 40, pp. 209–254). Lincoln: University of Nebraska Press.

Clark, M., & Anderson, B. (1967). *Culture and aging: An anthropological study of older Americans.* Springfield, IL: Charles C. Thomas.

Die, A. H., Seelbach, W. C., & Sherman, G. D. (1987). Achievement motivation, achieving styles, and morale in the elderly. *Psychology and Aging, 2*, 407–408.

Erikson, E. H., Erikson, J., & Kivnick, H. Q. (1986). *Vital involvement in old age.* New York: W. W. Norton.

Folkman, S., & Lazarus, R. S. (1980). An analysis of coping in a middle-aged community sample *Journal of Health and Social Behavior, 21*, 219–239.

Folkman, S., Lazarus, R. S., Gruen, R., & DeLongis, A. (1986). Appraisal, coping, health status, and psychological symptoms. *Journal of Personality and Social Psychology, 50*, 571–579.

Fry, P. S., & Wong, P. T. (1991). Pain management training in the elderly: Matching interventions with subjects' coping styles. *Stress Medicine, 7,* 93–98.

Heckhausen, J., & Baltes, P. B. (1991). Perceived controllability of expected psychological change across adulthood and old age. *Journal of Gerontology: Psychological Sciences, 46,* 165–173.

Heckhausen, J., & Schulz, R. (1995). A life-span theory of control. *Psychological Review, 102,* 284-304.

Heidrich, S. M., & Ryff, C. D. (1993). Physical and mental health in later life: The self-system as mediator. *Psychology and Aging, 8,* 327–338.

Hennessy, C. H. (1989). Culture in the use, care, and control of the aging body. *Journal of Aging Studies, 3,* 39–54.

Janelli, L. M. (1993). Are there body image differences between older men and women? *Western Journal of Nursing Research, 15,* 327–339.

Kiecolt, K. J. (1994). Stress and the decision to change oneself: A theoretical model. *Social Psychology Quarterly, 57,* 49–63.

Lachman, M. E. (1986). Locus of control in aging research. *Psychology and Aging, 1,* 34–40.

Lazarus, R. S., & Folkman, S. (1984). *Stress, appraisal, and coping.* New York: Springer.

Magai, C., & Hunziker, J. (1994). Tolstoy and the riddle of developmental transformation: A lifespan analysis of the role of emotions in personality development. In M. Lewis & J. Haveland (Eds.), *Handbook of emotions* (pp. 247–259). New York: Guilford.

McCrae, R. R. (1989). Age differences and changes in the use of coping mechanisms. *Journal of Gerontology: Psychological Sciences, 44,* P161–169.

McNaughton, M. E., Smith, L. W., Patterson, T. L., & Grant, I. (1990). Stress, social support, coping resources, and immune status in elderly women. *Journal of Nervous and Mental Disease, 178,* 460–461.

Miller, R. A. (1993). Aging and cancer—Another perspective. *Journal of Gerontology: Biological Sciences, 48,* B8–9.

O'Brien, S. J., & Conger, P. R. (1991). No time to look back: Approaching the finish line of life's course. *International Journal of Aging and Human Development, 33,* 75–87.

Parmelee, P. A., Katz, I. R., & Lawton, M. P. (1991). The relation of pain to depression among institutionalized aged. *Journal of Gerontology: Psychological Sciences, 46,* P15–21.

Pearlin, L., & Schooler, C. (1978). The structure of coping. *Journal of Health and Social Behavior, 19,* 2–21.

Pelham, B. W. (1991). On confidence and consequence: The certainty and importance of self-knowledge. *Journal of Personality and Social Psychology, 60,* 518–530.

Preston, D. B., & Mansfield, P. K. (1984). An exploration of stressful life events, illness, and coping among the rural elderly. *Gerontologist, 24,* 490–494.

Rapkin, B. D., & Fischer, K. (1992). Framing the construct of life satisfaction in terms of older adults' personal goals. *Psychology and Aging, 7,* 138–149.

Roberto, K. (1992). Coping strategies of older women with hip fractures:

Resources and outcomes. *Journal of Gerontology: Psychological Sciences, 47,* P21–26.

Ryff, C. D. (1989). In the eye of the beholder: Views of psychological well-being among middle-aged and older adults. *Psychology and Aging, 4,* 195–210.

Ryff, C. D., Lee, Y. H., Essex, M. J., & Schmutte, P. S. (1994). My children and me: Midlife evaluations of grown children and self. *Psychology and Aging, 9,* 195–205.

Smith, L. W., Patterson, T. L., & Grant, I. (1990). Avoidant coping predicts psychological disturbance in the elderly. *Journal of Nervous and Mental Disease, 178,* 525–530.

Speake, D. L. (1987). Health promotion activities and the well elderly. *Health Values: Achieving High Level Wellness, 11,* 25–30.

Tolman, A., & Whitbourne, S. K. (1996). *Remothering the self: The impact of adolescent children on women's sense of identity.* Unpublished manuscript.

Whitbourne, S. K. (1986). *The me I know: A study of adult identity.* New York: Springer Verlag.

Whitbourne, S. K. (1996). *The aging individual: Physical and psychological perspectives.* New York: Springer.

Whitbourne, S. K., & Ebmeyer, J. B. (1990). *Identity and intimacy in marriage: A study of couples.* New York: Springer-Verlag.

Whitbourne, S. K., & Primus, L. A. (1996). Physical identity in later adulthood. In J. E. Birren (Ed.), *Encyclopedia of aging.* San Diego, CA: Academic Press.

Williamson, G. M., & Schulz, R. (1992). Pain, activity restriction, and symptoms of depression among community-residing adults. *Journal of Gerontology: Psychological Sciences, 47,* P367–372.

Woodward, N. J., & Wallston, B. S. (1987). Age and health care beliefs: Self-efficacy as a mediator of low desire for control. *Psychology and Aging, 3–8.*

PART II

Affect and
Cognition

CHAPTER 6

Emotion, Thought, and Gender

Gisela Labouvie-Vief
Department of Psychology
Wayne State University
Detroit, Michigan

I. INTRODUCTION

Many theories of thought and its development are based on a polarity of modes of functioning (e.g., Bruner, 1986; Epstein, 1990; Labouvie-Vief, 1994). One mode is associated with rational thought, conscious decision making, and the ability to think in terms of decontextualized principles. The other mode appears more inherently tied to holistic and contextualized principles, and often links thinking to the emotions and to basic organismic schemata through the use of metaphor, image, and other figurative symbols, and through narrative and psychological rather than scientific constructions of reality. This differentiation of thought into two modes also has provided a model within which to represent more and less mature ways of thinking: traditionally, mature thought has been described as the ascent of the former mode over the latter.

However, in contrast to this hierarchical view, many recent views suggest that figurative and narrative forms of thought (and emotional schemata on which they are based) themselves are important modes of thinking that continue to interact with and enrich development throughout the course of life (for review, see Labouvie-Vief, 1994). These forms of thinking give direction to patterns of development by relating them to core emotion-relevant experiences, such as those relating to birth, death, sexuality, love, and generational succession. They provide a basis of rich concrete texture and emotional associations, forming a medium through which abstractions are removed from the realm of the impersonal and grounded and rendered personally meaningful through rich networks of self-relevant associations. Thus, many recent theories have begun to examine how more rational and more figurative forms are integrated, and what are the conditions under which they become fragmented or dissociated.

In this chapter, I discuss this linkage to two modes of thinking from the perspective of gender. One particularly important dimension of the differentiation of modes of thought is that it is based upon an elaborate imagery and narrative structure of gendered personifications (e.g., Labouvie-Vief, 1994; Lloyd, 1984; Neumann, 1973; Schott, 1988). Thus the rational mode is often associated with the masculine, the emotive with the feminine. This pervasive imagery has influenced the ability of men and women to emotionally integrate into their self a sense of self as thinker and effective agent in the world, as opposed to a sense of self as passive recipient of others' agency. Thus, the area of thought and gender becomes a particularly rich domain within which to discuss the linkages of more rational and conscious and more emotive and intuitive forms of knowing.

II. EMOTIONS AND THOUGHT

The emancipation of the emotions from a somewhat devalued position has begun to sweep psychology and other disciplines. That movement was united by a wide-ranging critique of the cognitivism and objectivism prevalent in the past grand theories of behavior, foremost the psychoanalytic movement launched by Freud and the cognitive-developmentalism fathered by Piaget. These theories provided a standard of adult thinking that was based on classical models of reason with their emphasis on conscious-rational processes of integration. Instead of the prevalent cognitivism inherent in these theories, what began to emerge is a view of adult thought in which rationality is but one component that must be integrated into a broader self structure, which itself is characterized by multiplicity, contextual (cultural, historical, and interpersonal) situatedness, and the primacy of biological-emotional forms of regulation (see e.g., Commons, Richards, & Armon, 1984; Fischer, Shaver, & Carnochan, 1990; Gilligan, 1982; Labouvie-Vief, 1994). This gradual reevaluation and reconstruction of a traditional model of maturity has made the study of emotions and its linkages with cognition a mainstream endeavor.

While Freud and Piaget in some sense continued important assumptions of rationalism, in another sense they also began significant breaks with rationalist theories (see Labouvie-Vief, 1994). Thus Freud argued that all of human behavior, including advanced forms of rationality, ultimately are to be placed in the context of important emotional systems. For Freud (e.g., Freud, 1911/1957), thought no longer was defined by reason alone, but rather was based on the tension and balance between two modes of being and of defining reality. One is primary process, an organic mode in which an inner world of desires and wishes prevails. The other is secondary process, a conceptual mode no longer directed by the inner reality of wish fulfillment and fantasy. Rather, this mode strives to find out what is objectively true, what holds in the outer world.

Piaget's theory, too, began with a dialectic of two modes of thinking. On the one hand, there were figurative forms of thinking that were tied to the inner (physiological, emotional, experiential) states of the organism; on the other, there were operative forms, governed by abstractive reflection and the ability to dissociate form from content. Paradoxically, however, neither theorist carried that notion of a dialectic of two forms of thinking to its logical conclusion. Freud's theory, for example, is less aimed at a harmonious balance between inner and outer reality, but more at a fairly complete victory of the secondary process over the primary process principle. Indeed, the former is called *reality principle,* whereas the latter is termed *pleasure principle.* Thus, Freud defines education "as an incitement to the conquest of the pleasure principle, and to its replacement by the reality-principle" (Freud, 1911/1957, pp. 43–44). Similarly, the ideal of the adapted individual is the scientist who "comes nearest to this conquest" (Freud, 1911/1957, p. 43). The result of this differential valuation of the two basic modes of thinking was a view of maturity as the triumph of ego control over biology and instincts. In a similar fashion, for Piaget (e.g., 1955) development became equated with the ascent of operative thought over figurative forms.

Many recent writings on the interface between reason and emotion instead reflect the view that emotions themselves may constitute an important and irreducible form of processing (e.g., Labouvie-Vief, Hakim-Larson, DeVoe, & Schoeberlein, 1989; Lazarus, 1991). That view was, in fact, anticipated by Jung (see Whitmont, 1969). Jung's famous break from Freud was motivated out of his belief that Freud, though in one sense liberating primary process from taboo, in another sense had continued to imprison it in a rationalist perspective. For Jung, the broad organismic heritage expressed in story, myth, and visual symbol was not merely a primitive mode of processing displaced by the ascent of reason, but potentially was a rich and highly advanced mode of processing and thinking in its own right. Beyond the capacities of reason, it revealed a larger context that constrains reason, a context of universal biological heritage consisting of the enduring emotional patterns relating to birth, death, sexuality and love, and generational succession.

Jung's work anticipated the recent (see Bruner, 1986; Epstein, 1990; Labouvie-Vief, 1994) tendency to think of the mind in terms of two modes of thought. As was true of Freud, he assumed that these two modes always were interlinked, limiting and constraining each other. However, unlike Freud, Jung suggested that this interlinkage changed in important ways during the process of development. Early, in the process of forming a primary adaptation based on conscious ego control, the individual disowns many emotional experiences that are not congruent with the ideals of culture. Nevertheless, these aspects of the rejected self strive for expression in distorted ways, as in processes of dissociation and splitting. Jung believed that the unique potential of mature development consisted of working on overcoming these splits and forming a more integrated structure. In that process, there is also a reevaluation of the role of rational processes, with the realization that they are undergirded by these powerful emotional prototypes—the *archetypes*.

However, when emotions entered the study of thinking, they did so through the vehicle of a prevalent cognitivism (also fostered by the Schachter and Singer position that it was cognitive classification that gave emotions their specific quality). For example, following Piaget (1981), many studies examined how cognition and its development restructures the emotional and self systems across the life span. This research, represented by such authors as Damon and Hart (1988), Kegan (1982), Labouvie-Vief (1994), Noam (1988), and Selman (1980), has taken its impetus from Kohlberg (e.g., 1984) and Loevinger (1993) and suggests that changes in cognitive complexity across the life span also have a bearing on how individuals regulate their emotions. For example, our own research (e.g., Labouvie-Vief et al., 1989; Labouvie-Vief, Chiodo, Goguen, & Orwoll, 1995) has demonstrated that younger individuals described emotions in terms of outer appearance, conventional standards, relatively static impulse monitoring, and an emphasis on control and the ideal. In contrast, those older or of higher ego level conveyed a more vivid sense of differentiation of self from norms, of an individuality that is distinct, historically formed, and subject to change and transformation, and of complex psychological transactions both within the self and between self and others.

However, more recent positions have pointed out that such cognitively based views of emotions and their development do not go far enough in accounting for the basic nature of the emotions as core organizing systems in development (e.g., Fischer et al., 1990). There is increasing recognition that thinking must be placed, first and foremost, within the context of human selves who are embodied and subject to powerful organismic systems providing constraints on so-called objective forms of thinking. Thus, much recent attention has focused on the ways in which the self is constructed not only through means that are primarily rational, but rather that have to do with narration and imagination (Bruner, 1986; Gergen, 1994; Hermans & Kempen, 1993), and that reflect the operation of powerful emotional schemata related to the vicissitudes of human relationships.

The relationship system whose implications for theories of the mind has been studied most carefully thus far is the attachment system, especially as it is mediated through early parent–child relationships. Although more rationally based theories such as Piaget's have examined the development of the ability to represent persons as a simple parallel to the development of impersonal concepts, this work (see e.g., Case, 1991; Fischer et al., 1990; Labouvie-Vief, 1994; Stern, 1985) has suggested that the ability to develop integrated concepts of self and others depends not just on the level of conceptual complexity; it also is a function of interpersonal embedding experiences. Depending whether or not primary others in development respond to the developing self in a coherent and supportive way or in an incoherent and narcissistic way, individuals will be able to form representations of self and others that emphasize a sense of continuity and coherence of diverse emotional states, or else may give evidence of fragmentation of self and other representations.

Such processes of fragmentation are greatly influenced by relatively pathological variations of the attachment process, such as those found in abuse and neglect. However, a certain degree of fragmentation is also part and parcel of a more normal developmental course. In growing up, the individual needs to learn to define reality in large part by the conventions of culture (as mediated first by direct attachment figures later by more abstract institutions such as those related to education, work, and government). In this process the individual remains dependent on others for a definition of reality, and as a result he or she may be forced to sacrifice a sense of organismic selfhood in the interest of survival and of accommodation to communal settings (see Labouvie-Vief, 1994). The resulting forms of dissociation can be found in the case of another important emotional system—sexuality—which will be the focus of the remainder of this chapter.

III. THOUGHT AND GENDER

Traditional beliefs in the independence of reason from emotion and other figurative forms are belied by the rich systems of metaphors and images that underlie concepts of mind (e.g., Labouvie-Vief, 1994; Lakoff, 1987; Schott, 1988). When we speak of "being in the dark" or of "seeing the light," of "giving birth" to an idea, of "defending" an argument or "being defeated" in one, we translate activities of thinking into an emotional and interpersonal field and thus give evidence that notions of reason actually are undergirded by an elaborate structure of metaphors, images, and stories. These images and stories speak of the nature of reason in terms of emotion-salient symbols: height versus depth, rise versus fall, victory versus defeat, light versus dark, birth versus death, activity versus passivity all are images that evoke powerful emotional associations. All of those associations indicate our tendency to think of the mind in terms of two layers of rather different value.

Such a hierarchical view was first articulated by Plato (see Labouvie-Vief, 1994; Simon, 1978), who evolved a two-layered conception of the individual. A layer of mind, abstract thought, soul, spirit, or ideals was opposed to a layer of body, matter, and enslavement to concrete sensory and organismic happenings. These layers were arranged hierarchically, with mind-spirit forming the superior pole, and body and senses forming the inferior one. Gaining maturity was represented as a heroic journey from the lower, darker, passive layer to the higher, lighter, active one.

That hierarchical worldview also became associated with gender. Thus in the *Symposium* Plato argued that the spiritual love between men who create ideas is more valuable than the physical and material love with women—love that results in bodily procreation rather than the creation of universal ideas (Labouvie-Vief, 1994). This association of masculinity and femininity with different forms of creating was relatively implicit in Plato's work, but became much more explicit in that of his student Aristotle (see Lerner, 1986). For example, Aristotle (*De Generatione Animalium*) argued that different forms of creativity were evident in processes of sexual reproduction. He theorized that the woman contributed the more primitive material principle to the embryo, but denied that the man's contribution also was of a material sort. Instead, he held that the masculine contribution was more spiritual and divine. This superiority of the masculine principle was derived from the belief that the male principle is active, the female principle passive.

A similar association between qualities of the mind and gender has persisted, with some variations, throughout the ages, and is still evident in contemporary theoretical discourse. Thus, the tendency to frame models of the mind as a single pole of which the second pole is merely a degradation ultimately is built upon an imagery of forms of sexual relations. As Lacqueur (1990) has argued, correlated with such models is a one-sex view of gender, which pervades the conceptualization of desire right down to notions of sexual anatomy. Thus, female anatomy is conceived as a hollow, negative space, characterized by passivity, and simply receiving (male) life force. In contrast, male anatomy is viewed as positive, active, creative, and truly generative. More generally, these metaphors have been adopted directly or indirectly by many psychological theorists who have used them to describe gender as a psychological construct. Thus masculinity is seen as active and intrusive, but femininity as passive and receptive (e.g., Erikson, 1951; Freud, 1925/1963).

Significantly, this dualism is extended to notions of mind and self, as well. Thus the male is viewed as the desiring subject, the representor who represents the woman as an object of his desire. Femaleness, in turn, is constituted out of its being the object to masculine desire: the woman is the one gazed upon and acted upon, the one represented, the other to the desiring and willful self (Benjamin, 1988; deBeauvior, 1952; Lloyd, 1984). Thus Freud proposed that women's lack of phallic sexuality made their sexual and psychological orientations more passive and masochistic (Freud, 1925/1963); others taught that the anatomy of women's brains made them less capable of conscious, rational thought and of extraordinary creativity or achievement (Bem, 1993; Labouvie-Vief, 1994). Even in this century, the notion became popularized by Simone deBeauvior (1952), who argued that woman is closer to nature because physiology makes her so. Her mode of creating is by submitting to a natural bodily function, by remaining enslaved to her biological fate, whereas the man creates by "acts that transcend his animal nature" (p. 71). By creating culture, the man is thought to be involved with a new, freer form of creation, one that transcends what is organismically given and shapes the future.

The notion of the masculine as identified with mind, spirit, and transcendence is even more pervasive in mythology and religion, literature and art—disciplines that were friendly to the emotion-relevant imagery that underlies our notion of the nature of the mind. In all of those, one polarity of human functioning tends to be idealized and even inflated as 'masculine': it is based on an imagery of rise, light, and sun, and it symbolizes such psychological qualities as leadership, rational self-control, self-assertiveness, and individuality and willfulness. The other polarity, in turn, is degraded and devalued: its imagery is based on falling, being conquered and surrendering, and of engulfment in dark spaces, and it symbolizes suffering, powerlessness, and entrapment in unconscious processes. In mythology and religion, such imagery often occurs as the theme of the overthrow of original female divine figures by the male godheads or heros who came to be the original creators, creating the world not organically but conceptually, by pronouncing a word (Lerner, 1986). Another example of this process of the replacement of the feminine principle is offered by the great Greek tragedies by Aeschylus and Euripides, centering around the myths of Agamemnon and Orestes, in which fatherhood is said to have replaced motherhood as a principle of creation (Labouvie-Vief, 1994).

How universal is this equation? Much recent writing has suggested that such patriarchal ideologies in actuality came to replace more women-focused ones of previous times. Originally proposed by Bachofen in 1861 (Duby & Perrot, 1992/93), this "matriarchy" thesis holds that there must have been, in prehistoric times and before the rise of the major patriarchal societies, the reign of a maternal principle. One hypothesis holds that the patriarchal principle came into ascendancy with the rise of complex social structures that also brought abstract systems of thought and writing. However, the historical accuracy of this thesis has recently been questioned. True, there may have been *some* early societies in which gender was less polarized than it came to be, quite universally, with the rise of major patriarchies. Still, most historical and anthropological evidence (Duby & Perrot, 1992/93; Ortner & Whitehead, 1981; Rosaldo & Lamphere, 1974) does not support the view that earlier and/or less civilized societies granted women more power *universally*.

Moreover, strong patriarchal systems in which women are devalued along a nature–culture dimension exist world-wide in preliterate societies. Often such societies also have myths of early matriarchies that eventually were superseded by the rule of man. However, such matriarchy myths can be part of an ideology that devalues women (Rosaldo & Lamphere, 1974). Around the world, such myths often tell of the past bad behavior and evil of women that eventually was ended when men overturned the power of women and took control. In this way, matriarchy myths can be used to justify the masculine order. They form part of a cultural code distinguishing men from women in terms of morality and authority; they incorporate the values that grant men more power in social life. Thus even though they talk about a time before the current social order, they fix that order as legitimate and invariant. The myths constantly reiterate that women are not capable of handling power, that they represent the rule of chaos and trickery.

Such claims as to the capacities and characteristics of women mirror, of course, those of more modern writers, among them Freud, who have held that women by nature are made to be intellectually inferior to men. However, several more recent writers have suggested that the very vehemence with which women's abilities are denigrated points to powerful systems of defense against the power of women—defenses that lead to the wide-spread normalization of female inferiority.

Bettelheim (1962) pointed to these defenses when suggesting that the distortion of female competencies is the result of male envy of those competencies. Unlike Freud, who had assumed that gender envy was a feminine problem, Bettelheim suggests that male envy of the attributes of women is, in fact, an extremely pervasive phenomenon. He notes that "men stand in awe of the procreative power of women, that they wish to participate in it" (p. 10), and he goes on to suggest that evidence of such envy of female procreative powers can be found widely in many societies, although on the whole, it may be severely repressed. In less highly civilized cultures, these attitudes are freely expressed, though in highly symbolic form. This is evident worldwide in male initiation rites; such rites typically involve some symbolic wounding in which the initiate is made to bleed in imitation of female menstruation, or even has part of his genitalia altered to mimic female anatomy. Often, these aspects of bodily mutiliations are followed by systematic instruction in sacred and secret teachings, in which the male initiate is instructed into the realm of spirit and mind, a realm considered as differentiated from female, material ways of being. Such practices appear to be aimed at defining the unique nature of the "masculine" as a way of creation unique to men and "better" than the "feminine." Yet in this attempt there is usually a defensive inversion in which the feminine is considered a lesser version of the masculine. Such a process of inversion appears to be basic to how gender is constructed in many cultures.

In a related fashion, Chodorow (1978) has suggested that masculine development requires that the boy push away from the mother, defining his identity in opposition to the feminine. Adopting a similar argument, Stoller (1985) also maintains that, contrary to the classical assumption of the primacy of the "masculine" realm, femininity in actuality constitutes a primary state in human development. This state of "protofemininity" results from the mother's pervasive role in early development, because it is the mother who defines an early core of identity. Says Stoller,

> *I suspect that the problem boys have with creating their masculinity from the protofemininity leaves behind a "structure," a vigilance, a fear of the pull of the symbiosis—that is, a conflict between the urge to return to the peace of the symbiosis and the opposing urge to separate out as an individual, as a male, as masculine. Much of what we see as masculinity is, I think, the effect of that struggle. For much of masculinity, as is well known, consists of struggling not to be seen by*

oneself or others as having feminine attributes, physical or psychologic. One must maintain one's distance from women or be irreparably infected with femininity. (Stoller, 1985, p. 18)

Complementary to the definition of manhood, womanhood in many cultures is defined by practices by which women are made into sexual and psychological objects to the action of men. Such practices can range from direct genital mutilation as a way of subordinating female desire (and ultimately, female fertility) to that of men, to isolating her from participation in public life through exclusion from education and high status work (deBeauvoir, 1952; Labouvie-Vief, 1994; Ortner & Whitehead, 1981).

IV. THOUGHT AND GENDER IN DEVELOPMENT

Cultural definitions of masculine and feminine aspects of the mind have deeply influenced men's and women's identification with aspects of the mind. Whereas masculinity has been associated with increases in abstract thought and rational decision making, femininity has been tied to context sensitivity and field dependence. At the same time, the cultural idealization of rational domains of mind, with their associated symbols of heavenly heights and golden light, and their equation with masculinity has allowed men to claim so-called masculine attributes with a sense of pride and self-confidence. However, these domains were not so valued in women—as Kant had it, women who know Greek or mathematics "might as well even have a beard" (Kant, quoted in Battersby, 1989, p. 77): Knowledge makes them grotesque, freakish, even "loathsome." At the same time, so-called feminine domains of thought were devalued and did not provide an important alternative source of self-worth. As a result, masculine development often has been associated with increases in individuality, agency, and independence, whereas women often have experienced their development as renunciation, surrender, and victimization—a loss of voice, a process of silencing (Bem, 1993; Brown & Gilligan, 1992; Labouvie-Vief, 1994).

The silencing of women is a historical reality, because women have left few direct records of their experience (Brown & Gilligan, 1992; Duby & Perrot, 1992/93). This silence of women has often been taken as evidence of their biological limits (see Gould, 1981), but with the rise of feminism in this century we have come to understand the social and cultural practices that create such silence. As women have begun to gain greater access to educational and economic resources, however, their silence has become interrupted with attempts to speak their own experience; and as they have participated in speaking about their own minds, the so-called intellectual inferiority gradually emerged to be related to systematic social practices, misinterpretations of available data, and other vicissitudes of gender-related emotions.

Until early this century, philosophers and psychologists believed that women were biologically unequipped for superior intelligence, creativity, or moral judgment (Brown & Gilligan, 1992; Labouvie-Vief, 1994). However, the experiences of women often have belied these stereotypes, and throughout the ages women have told of learning to suppress their strong creative urges and their strivings for self-expression, which came to be perceived as a source of disapproval and danger. As Gerda Lerner (1993) notes, historically, claiming the authority to write, and particularly to write about the self, did not fit the cultural mold. A woman asserting authority was a freak and had to deal with that fact in her writing. In medieval women's writings, women often claimed validation by appealing to God as a source of assuming the authority—clearly perceived as deviant—to write. For example, the abbess Hildegard of Bingen (Fox, 1985) claimed that she had received divine inspiration through a series of visions, and only after a long struggle for self-authorization determined to follow her visions. If a woman claimed more human authorization, she had to spend considerable time defending her place and her voice, including (a) asserting she actually was the author of her own work, and (b) that she had a right to her own thought. Often, she dealt with this problem by finding a male sponsor to write a preface to her writing.

Such struggles of women with their own sense of creativity is expressed very poignantly in the lives of many writers of this century, such as Sylvia Plath and Virginia Woolf. Echoing Virginia Wolff's earlier study *A Room of One's Own*, Heilbrun (1988) recently has argued that highly creative women learn to experience their powers as dangerous and as outside the self. Because cultural attitudes belittle and ridicule the striving for power and creative expression in women, they are fearful of having applied to them such labels as "shrill," "angry," and "egotistical." Ashamed of the creative strivings that lead to such labeling, extraordinary women are engaged in a constant struggle to hide the clarity of their minds and the urgency of their creative strivings. Indeed, Heilbrun argues that well into this century, it remained impossible for women to admit in their own autobiographical narratives their claims of achievement, admissions of ambition, or the realization that their own accomplishments may be more than mere luck or the result of others' generosity. She notes that many autobiographies of women of the past indicate that accomplished women tend to describe their exciting lives in a flat and unexciting way, even though there is ample evidence—as can be gleaned, for example, from published correspondence—that this is a one-sided narrative:

> *Their letters and diaries are usually different, reflecting ambitions and struggles in the public sphere; in their published autobiographies, however, they portray themselves as intuitive, nurturing, passive, but never—in spite of the contrary evidence of their accomplishments—managerial. (Heilbrun, 1988, p. 24)*

In her book *Silences,* Olsen (1978) also addresses this conflict. Women, argues Olsen, live under the agony that creation and femininity are incompatible. As an example, Olsen quotes from Anaïs Nin's diaries:

> *The aggressive act of creation; the guilt for creating. I did not want to rival man; to steal man's creation, his thunder. I must protect them, not outshine them. (in Olsen, 1978, p. 49)*

As attention has been drawn to these achievement conflicts in women, research has upheld few objective differences in intellectual status between men and women (see Labouvie-Vief et al., 1995; Maccoby & Jacklin, 1974). Following Leta Hollingsworth's (1926) pioneering early research, what differences do exist often could be explained in terms of differences in educational opportunities and other cultural practices. Yet changes are a matter of degree, and psychological research continues to demonstrate that old patterns persist. Despite evidence that female intellectual endowment does not lag behind that of men, women on average continue to lag in achievement behind men. Moreover, this gender lag increases in the course of development. Indeed, in early childhood, girls *surpass* boys on most measures of school achievement. However, as they grow into adolescence, girls' superiority over boys begins to decline, and they tend to fall back behind boys.

Girls growing up often begin to downgrade and relinquish ambitious career goals and come to deny that they are gifted or special; instead of proud displays of self-exhibition one finds an insistence on normality. Thus girls who early in adolescence were confident and outspoken, become increasingly confused and silent about what they know. Thus as they grow older, girls often are found to retreat from achievement-related challenges; standing out for women becomes a source of conflict and shame, and they attempt to hide their excellence (Brown & Gilligan, 1992; Kerr, 1987).

As girls relinquish a proud sense of self-confidence they also become susceptible to experiences of shame, depression, and powerlessness that are not equally prevalent among boys. As they grow older, boys and girls begin to diverge in their patterns of emotional expression and coping: males increasingly externalize or act out conflict, whereas females increasingly use defenses that internalize conflict, turning aggression and assertiveness inward. As a result, different patterns of vulnerability to disorders of self emerge for men and women. Boys and young men experience more behavioral and acting out disorders, whereas girls and women experience more emotional disorders such as anxiety and depression (Labouvie-Vief et al., 1995).

Of course, insight into the cultural processes that shape different gender-relevant emotional schemata itself is a result of profound cultural changes by which the mind is being de-gendered (see Bem, 1993; Labouvie-Vief, 1994). As contemporary theories are reevaluating old dualisms of abstract–concrete, mind–body, transcendent–immanent, objective–subjective, and reason–emotion, so are they transforming traditional dualisms relating to gender. However, such transformation is far from a uniform process; it may be associated with more mature, advanced forms of development, rather than being an automatic result of cultural changes. Thus, we already noted that Jung believed that early development fosters the formation of dualisms, whereas to transcend those dualisms is specific task of development around and after midlife and beyond. In a similar vein, a number of life span researchers have suggested that the ability to bridge reason–emotion dualisms and to understand their dialectical relationship emerges only in adulthood (see Labouvie-Vief, 1994).

Such movements away from dualistic thinking also appear to characterize thinking about gender. As men and women move into midlife, one often observes a freeing from the cultural constraints of "manhood" or "womanhood." No longer defined as objects to the agency of men, women often move from a world of confinement to one of daring openness, of a release from their earlier interiority. Thus from young adulthood to midlife, women have been found to become less traditionally "feminine" but more dominant, independent, objective, and intellectually oriented. In contrast, men are sometimes found to give up inflated agentic claims. Instead, they elaborate those dimensions of self previously projected onto women as dangerous and uncanny: those related to their intuition and to nonrational dimensions of life, and more generally, to those aspects of experience in which we feel ourselves to be moved and receptive rather than proactive (for review, see Gutmann, 1987; Labouvie-Vief et al., 1995).

V. CONCLUSIONS

I began this chapter by talking about the relationship between two modes of thinking. Most major theories of development in the past proposed a differentiation between a rational and a non-rational mode and

suggested that the latter more strongly reflects the influences of important emotional schemata. This mode was assumed to be replaced in the
course of development by more rational forms of thinking. Using the examples of the domain of gender and thought, I suggested that in contrast,
this hierarchical resolution actually reflects a dissociation of rational and
nonrational forms of thinking. Thus, the latter are not really given up in
development, but rather continue to function in an unregulated form.

An emerging solution to this problem is to view the modes not as oppositional, but rather as interacting with, and mutually informing each
other. Thus as rational structures become more powerful, they can embrace and contain emotions that, at less developed levels, are too disruptive and disorganizing to be integrated. Through this movement,
then, rational structures can inform emotions, rendering them more objective and comprehensible. In turn, another complementary movement
enriches rational structures with emotions: as emotional schemata change
during development, they also can be an occasion to inform rational structures, and form an impetus for further development.

However, such a mutually supportive interaction is not by any means
an automatic outcome of development. The degree to which the two
modes cooperate in a fairly balanced way depends on the degree to which
they are integrated in the surrounding milieu in which individuals develop. This chapter has suggested that the two systems of thought have remained extremely oppositional at the cultural and collective level. This
dualism, in turn, has tended to put a limit on individuals' ability to integrate gender-related emotional experiences and rational views of the
world.

As Bettelheim (1962) argues, strong dualisms may be especially prevalent in past societies in which socialization for violence contributed to extreme gender polarization. In such societies, the capacity to talk about
and conceptualize the underlying emotional realities of conflict between
the genders remains negligible, and destructive emotions are acted out in
the open. However, as world cultures have expanded and begun to form
a worldwide community, more reflection on and conceptualization of the
underlying emotional conflict has occurred. As a result, the natural envy
of one gender for the other can be rationally acknowledged as a condition
of existence, rather than being acted out in ritual and cultural practice.

Interestingly, such a view continues the program begun by Freud
and Piaget, who proposed a dialectic between two systems of thinking,
yet abandoned that dialectic by considering one of those systems less mature. By acknowledging this abandoned system as a dimension that has its
own potentials for growth we can continue to complete the kind of project begun by these theorists. By embracing the full range of human emotions rather than bracketing them as "immature," we not only can ground

rational structures in important organismic systems, but we also can envision new levels of maturity in which, ultimately, the split between reason and emotion is transcended.

REFERENCES

Battersby, C. (1989). *Gender and genius: Towards a feminist aesthetics.* Indianapolis: Indiana University Press.

Bem, S. L. (1993). *The lenses of gender.* New Haven, CT: Yale University Press.

Benjamin, J. (1988). *Bonds of love: Psychoanalysis, feminism, and the problem of domination.* New York: Pantheon Books.

Bernard, J. (1987). *The female world from a global perspective.* Bloomington, IN: Indiana University Press.

Bettelheim, B. (1962). *Symbolic wounds: Puberty rites and the envious male* (rev. ed.). New York: Collier Books.

Brown, L. M., & Gilligan, C. (1992). *Meeting at the crossroads: Women's psychology and girls' development.* Cambridge, MA: Harvard University Press.

Bruner, J. (1986). *Actual minds, possible worlds.* Cambridge, MA: Harvard University Press.

Case, R. (1991). *The role of primitive defenses in the representation and regulation of early attachment relations.* Paper presented at the Society for Research in Child Development, Seattle, WA.

Chodorow, N. (1978). *The reproduction of mothering.* Los Angeles: University of California Press.

Commons, M. L., Richards, F. A., & Armon, C. (1984). *Beyond formal operations: Late adolescent and adult cognitive development.* New York: Praeger.

Damon, W., & Hart, D. (1988). *Self-understanding in childhood & adolescence.* Cambridge, NY: Cambridge University Press.

de Beauvoir, S. (1952). *The second sex.* New York: Alfred A. Knopf.

Duby, G., & Perrot, M. (Eds.) (1992/93). *A history of women in the west.* Vols. 1–4. Cambridge, MA: Harvard University Press.

Epstein, S. (1990). Cognitive-experiential self-theory. In L. A. Pervin (Ed.), *Handbook of personality: Theory and research.* New York: The Guilford Press.

Erikson, E. H. (1951). *Childhood and society.* New York: W. W. Norton.

Fischer, K. W., Shaver, P. R., & Carnochan, P. (1990). How emotions develop and how they organize development. *Cognition and Emotion, 4,* 81–127.

Fox, M. (1985). *Illuminations of Hildegard of Bingen.* Santa Fe, NM: Bear.

Freud, S. (1957). Formulations regarding the two principles in mental functioning. In J. Rickman (Ed.), *A general selection from the works of Sigmund Freud* (pp. 43–44). Garden City, NY: Doubleday. (Original work published in 1911)

Freud, S. (1963). Some psychological consequences of the anatomical differences between the sexes. In P. Rieff (Ed.), *Sexuality and the psychology of love* (pp. 183–193). New York: Macmillan. (Original work published in 1925)

Gergen, K. J. (1992). Psychology in the postmodern era. *Invited address, American Psychological Association.* Washington, DC.

Gergen, K. (1994). *Realities and relationships.* Cambridge, MA: Harvard University Press.

Gilligan, C. (1982). *In a different voice.* Cambridge, MA: Harvard University Press.

Gould, S. J. (1981). *The mismeasure of man.* New York: Norton.

Gutmann, D. (1987). *Reclaimed powers: toward a new psychology of men and women in later life.* New York: Basic Books.

Heilbrun, C. (1988). *Writing a woman's life.* New York: Ballantine Books.

Herdt, G. H. & Stoller, R. J. (1990). *Intimate communications: Erotics and the study of culture.* New York: Columbia University Press.

Hermans, H. J. M., & Kempen, H. J. G. (1983). *The dialogical self: Meaning as movement.* San Diego: Academic Press.

Hollingsworth, L. (1926). *Gifted children: Their nature and nurture.* New York: Macmillan.

Kegan, R. (1982). *The evolving self.* Cambridge, MA: Harvard University Press.

Kerr, B. A. (1987). *Smart girls, gifted women.* Columbus, OH: Ohio Publishing.

Kohlberg, L. (1984). *Essays on moral development: Vol. 2. The psychology of moral development.* San Francisco: Harper & Row.

Labouvie-Vief, G. (1994). *Psyche and eros: Mind and gender in the life course.* New York: Cambridge University Press.

Labouvie-Vief, G., Hakim-Larson, J., Devoe, M., & Schoeberlein, S. (1989). Emotions and self-regulation: A life span view, *Human Development, 32,* 279–299.

Labouvie-Vief, G., Orwoll, L., & Manion, M. (1995). *Narratives of mind, gender, and the life course. Human Development, 38,* 239–257.

Labouvie-Vief, Chiodo, L. M., Goguen, L. A., Diehl, M., & Orwoll, L. (1995). Representations of self across the lifespan. Psychology and the Aging, *10,* 404–415.

Lakoff, G. (1987). *Women, fire & dangerous things.* Chicago, IL: University of Chicago Press.

Lacqueur, T. (1990). *Making sex: Body and gender from the Greeks to Freud.* Cambridge, MA: Harvard University Press.

Lazarus, R. S. (1991). *Emotion and adaptation.* New York: Oxford University Press.

Lerner, G. (1986). *The creation of patriarchy.* New York: Oxford University Press.

Lerner, G. (1993). *The creation of feminist consciousness.* New York: Oxford University Press.

Lloyd, G. (1984). *The man of reason: "Male" and "female" in Western philosophy.* Minneapolis: University of Minnesota Press.

Loevinger, J. (1993). Measurement of personality: True or false. *Psychological Inquiry, 4,* 1–16.

Maccoby, E. E., & Jacklin, C. N. (1974). *The psychology of sex differences.* Stanford, CA: Stanford University Press.

Neumann, E. (1973). *The origins and history of human consciousness.* Princeton, NJ: Princeton University Press.

Noam, G. G. (1988). The self, adult development, and the theory of biography and transformation. In D. K. Lapsley & F. L. Power (Eds.), *Self, ego, and identity: Integrative approaches.* New York: Springer.

Olsen, T. (1978). *Silences.* New York: Delacorte Press/Seymour Lawrence.

Ortner, S. B., & Whitehead, H. (Eds.). (1981). *Sexual meanings: The cultural construction of gender and sexuality.* New York: Cambridge University Press.

Piaget, J. (1955). *The language and thought of the child.* New York: New American Library.

Piaget, J. (1981). *Intelligence and affectivity: Their relationship during child development.* Palo Alto, CA: Annual Reviews.

Rosaldo, M. Z., & Lamphere, L. (1974). *Women in culture and society.* Stanford, CA: Stanford University Press.

Schott, R. M. (1988). *Cognition and eros.* Boston, MA: Beacon Press.

Selman, R. L. (1980). *The growth of interpersonal understanding: Developmental and clinical analyses.* New York: Academic Press.

Simon, B. (1978). *Mind and madness in ancient Greece.* Ithaca, NY: Cornell University Press.

Stern, D. L. (1985). *The interpersonal world of the infant.* New York: Basic Books.

Stoller, R. J. (1985). *Presentations of gender.* New Haven: Yale University Press.

Whitmont, E. C. (1969). *The symbolic quest: basic concepts of analytical psychology.* Princeton, NJ: Princeton University Press.

CHAPTER 7

Emotion and Cognition in Attachment

Victor G. Cicirelli

Department of Psychological Sciences
Purdue University
West Lafayette, Indiana

I. INTRODUCTION

Investigations of attachment phenomena and formulations of attachment theory have increased in recent years in an effort to better understand personality and social development, interpersonal relationships, and psychopathology in both children and adults. The concept of attachment was originally formulated in the attempt to explain the failure of infants to develop normally when separated from their mothers (or principal caregivers) for extended periods of time (Bowlby, 1979, 1988). However, multiple attachments to other family members (such as father or siblings) and nonfamily individuals (such as friends or other caregivers) can develop during childhood and adolescence and coexist with the attachment to the mother.

Also, attachments exist in adulthood and old age either as the emergence in adulthood of new attachments between adults, such as attachment to a spouse or intimate friend (Ainsworth, 1989; Berman & Sperling, 1994) or as a continuation of early attachments (e.g., to the mother or to siblings).

Attachment itself may be defined in various ways (Berman & Sper-

---

ling, 1994) that overlap but emphasize different aspects of the concept. In all cases, however, both emotions and cognitions underlie the content, organization, and processes of attachment. The cognitive content includes memories, knowledge, beliefs, expectancies, and interpretations, whereas the emotion content includes simple, complex, and diffuse emotions (moods), along with feelings (defined here as subjective experiences of emotion).

In the present chapter, the objective is to explore the relationship between emotions and cognitions as they coexist in attachment. Because they are the underlying components of attachment, understanding their relationship will offer insight into the dynamics of the attachment process itself.

II. OVERVIEW OF INFANT–MOTHER ATTACHMENT

At the outset of any exploration of this topic, certain basic concepts of infant–mother attachment must be reviewed briefly to give readers a common background in order to understand multiple and life span attachments. What happens in the individual's initial attachment early in life is regarded as influencing other concurrent and later attachments. For a more detailed discussion, the reader is referred to existing sources (Bretherton, 1985, 1992; Magai & McFadden, 1995; Main, Kaplan, & Cassidy, 1985).

Infant attachment is an inherited propensity, predisposition, or motive to seek or maintain proximity to, and experience emotional security from, a more competent attachment figure (typically the mother) who provides aid and protection when environmental demands are too great for the infant's independent survival or adaptation (Ainsworth, 1989; Bowlby, 1979, 1988). To be attached is to remain physically close or be in the presence of the mother (or able to communicate with her), and to experience concomitant emotional security. Attachment behavior includes any behavior that attempts to bring (or results in bringing) the infant close to or in the presence of the attachment figure; it is the means or vehicle for attaining and maintaining attachment. Attachment style refers to the child's typical overt pattern of attachment behavior: secure attachment, insecure avoidant attachment, insecure anxious/ambivalent attachment, or disoriented/disorganized attachment.

As infant and mother interact, the infant develops an internal working model, in which a subjective representation of self, the mother, and the relationship between them is internalized (Bretherton, 1992; Magai & McFadden, 1995). This internal representation stabilizes the attachment relationship beyond the immediate situation and provides a theoretical basis for the existence of attachment in adulthood.

III. ATTACHMENT IN ADULTHOOD

Some theorists argue that attachment to the mother diminishes or ends with the child's attainment of autonomy in adolescence, because there is no further need for the protection or security afforded by parental caregiving (e.g., Weiss, 1986). Others (Ainsworth, 1989; Berman & Sperling, 1994; Bowlby, 1979; Main et al., 1985; Rothbart & Shaver, 1994) view attachment to others as important throughout life.

Various researchers have obtained evidence regarding life span attachment by proceeding along several different fronts. These research topics include multiple attachments (Ainsworth, 1989; Shaver & Hazan, 1993), adult attachment styles (Main et al., 1985; Shaver & Hazan, 1993), intergenerational transmission of attachment (Main et al., 1985; van IJzendoorn, 1995), attachment and loss (Bowlby, 1980; Rando, 1993), and clinical aspects of disturbed attachment (Bowlby, 1988; Main et al., 1985; Sperling & Berman, 1994). Other research directions include continuation of attachment to the mother (Ainsworth, 1989; Bowlby, 1980; Cicirelli, 1991; Levitt, 1991; Whitbeck, Simons, & Conger, 1991) and care of the aged parent (Antonucci, 1994; Cicirelli, 1991, 1993, 1995). Even in adulthood, individuals appear to have a fundamental need to belong, and to have unique and multiple attachments with others throughout the life span.

A. *Characteristics of Life Span Attachment*

The extension of the concept of attachment between the young child and the mother to include later childhood, adolescence, and the entire life span (Ainsworth, 1989; Bowlby, 1980; Cicirelli, 1991) is a basic proposition of life span attachment theory. A life span attachment has a number of characteristics that will be discussed in turn.

First, attachment to the mother coexists with multiple attachments between the child and others, whether formed early or later in life, and does not preclude other major attachments. Adult children's grief over the death of parents is evidence for such lifelong attachments (Ainsworth, 1989). Also, evidence exists that both the adult child's attachment and the parent's nurturing activities (such as financial or instrumental help, advice, understanding, and emotional support) continue throughout adulthood despite the formation of other attachments (Cicirelli, 1991; Levitt, 1991; Whitbeck et al., 1991).

Second, attachment to the mother coexists with developing autonomy of the child through adolescence and into adulthood. Secure attachment does not prevent the attainment of autonomy.

Third, secure attachment to the mother in adulthood differs from dependency or overattachment (preoccupied attachment); it is neither dysfunctional nor pathological. Levitt's (1991) finding that most adults place their relationship with the mother among their very closest relationships attests to the normative nature of this attachment relationship.

Fourth, attachment is universal at the level of a genetic predisposition to form attachments, although cultural differences exist (van IJzendoorn & Tavecchio, 1987). The lower psychological processes, such as speed of cognitive processing and basic attachment behaviors, are considered to belong to the basic evolutionary equipment of every human being.

Fifth, the attachment to the mother is unique (nonreplaceable), based on shared experiences and feelings in the formative years (Ainsworth, 1989). Shared experiences and feelings between mother and child in the early portion of life have significance that cannot be forgotten, despite new attachments in adulthood.

Sixth, attachment to the mother contributes to the survival and adaptation of the child from an evolutionary and ethological viewpoint, as well as that of the adult child's own children, and the survival of the family gene pool. The mother's continuing nurturance increases the adult child's feelings of security and comfort.

Seventh, the form of attachment behaviors changes as the child grows and matures into adulthood, with a sophisticated system of attachment behaviors developing over time. When direct proximity or contact is not feasible at times of stress, the adult child substitutes symbolic attachment, using the working model to represent closeness to the mother (Bretherton, 1992; Cicirelli, 1991), supplemented by occasional visits and telephone calls. Full-blown separation distress occurs only when the child feels anxious or threatened by certain life situations or when the mother is not available when expected.

Last, the attached child will be motivated to protect the existence of the attachment figure should she become seriously ill or decline in health; it is based on the child's self-interest in preserving a parent whose nurturance helps to maximize the child's adaptation.

B. Adult Attachment and Parent Caregiving

The protective aspect of the adult attachment relationship has been the focus of my recent research. It is theorized that as the adult child's vulnerability to loss of the parent through aging and death increases in late middle age, the adult child is motivated to protect the existence of that parent through caregiving and other forms of helping behavior in order to delay the loss of the parent for as long as possible. That is, a threat to attachment presented by the parent's dependency arouses a motive to protect the attachment figure, which in turn elicits helping or caregiving behavior. Indeed, the majority of adult children provide some form of help to their parents in old age. To conceive of helping or caregiving as a form of protective behavior is to imply not only a commitment by adult children to provide help but to provide sustained help.

An earlier study (Cicirelli, 1983) provided an initial test of the relationship of attachment to protection of the parent by determining the relationship between adult daughters' attachment to elderly mothers, filial obligation, attachment behaviors (visiting and telephoning), and their commitment to provide future help. A path model revealed a direct effect of the adult child's attachment on commitment to provide future help and an indirect effect through its effect on attachment behaviors, whereas obligation showed only an indirect effect that was less than that of attachment. However, the study was limited by use of affection and compatibility as indicators of attachment, in the absence of a suitable measure of adult attachment. Other existing studies support a link between attachment to an elderly parent and caregiving behavior (see Cicirelli, 1993), but also used poor indicators of attachment.

To remedy this deficiency, a measure of the strength of secure attachment to the parent in adulthood based on core aspects of attachment was developed (Cicirelli, 1995); secondary arguments from validity data supported the contention that secure attachment and not preoccupied insecure attachment (Main et al., 1985) was being measured. The instrument was used in a study to clarify the effects of attachment and filial obligation as motives for parent caregiving and their subsequent effects on burden (Cicirelli, 1993). In a path analysis of data from 78 daughters caring for elderly mothers, both attachment and obligation were related to the amount of help provided. However, stronger attachment was related to less subjective burden, whereas stronger obligation was related to greater burden.

IV. EMOTION AND COGNITION IN ADULTHOOD

Bowlby (1979, 1988) conceptualized the internal working model in terms of information processing. Initially, the attachment relationship between the infant and mother can be represented at the enactive level (through motor activity) and then at an image level. However, as further development occurs, information processing occurs in an efficient manner at the verbal level. The infant's memories of self, the mother, and the attachment relationship in different contexts are stored and retrieved. Information about new interactions is interpreted in terms of these memories and ongoing cognitive processes.

Cognitively, the infant develops a hierarchy of knowledge or beliefs about the attachment figure, going from specific details in concrete situations to more abstract or global levels of thought. Further, the content can be organized in a consistent or inconsistent fashion depending on the responsiveness and dependability of the mother. In secure attachment, there should be consistency of thinking as one goes from concrete to abstract levels of thought concerning the attachment figure, and regarding positive and negative traits of the self or the attachment figure. Also, there should be a high level of differentiation and integration of thought about the attachment figure.

The homeostatic control (or attachment behavioral system) operates in a cognitive manner. That is, deviations from a proximity goal in relation to the attachment figure are detected and homeostatic behavior patterns are employed until the norm or proximity goal is attained.

Regardless of whether the attachment is secure or insecure, an infant experiences and expresses a variety of emotions in the course of an attachment relationship, especially during times of separation and reunion with the attachment figure. On the emotional level, the infant experiences feelings of comfort and emotional security when with or close to the mother, feelings of anxiety, anger, or despair when separated from the mother, and feelings of elation or joy upon reunion. Many other feelings are experienced, especially in the various types of insecure attachment. In adulthood too, attachment patterns can be viewed as "strategies for regulating negative affect" in close relationships (Bartholomew, 1993).

However, the role of emotion in relation to cognition has never been sufficiently clarified by attachment theorists. In Bowlby's (1979, 1988) information-processing model, the role of emotions or motivations has not been dealt with adequately despite the fact that the core of attachment is the attainment of emotional security (Bretherton, 1992). Obviously, Bowlby dealt with emotions in attachment theory, but he did not deal with the dynamics of the relationship between emotion and cognition, or how emotions are incorporated into an information-processing approach. Cognition seems to predominate over emotion, but Bowlby does not explain how the information-processing approach deals with emotion. For example, when the infant detects an unacceptably large distance from the mother, does the accompanying emotion motivate attachment behavior to maintain proximity, or is the behavior the result of the cognition? Or, do the two interact somehow?

Before attempting to clarify the roles of cognitions and emotions in attachment, exploration of the relation between cognitions and emotions is needed. In earlier literature, two broad viewpoints are found: (a) cognitions cause or control emotions, and (b) emotions cause or control cognitions. Although later scholars have moved toward a more integrated position, there is still a great deal of disagreement about the relation between cognitions and emotions (see Ekman & Davidson, 1994), and no definitive answer has yet emerged.

V. RELATION BETWEEN COGNITIONS AND EMOTIONS

An emotion can be broadly defined as a preconscious or conscious state of positive or negative feeling, varying in intensity and duration, sometimes manifesting itself in expressive behavior, and functioning to motivate adaptive or maladaptive adjustment to the environment. Such a state of feeling is the result of immediate sensations or perceptions of environmental context, physiological arousal, neurological arousal, and cognitive mediation.

A. Cognition Approach

One traditional approach is that cognition controls or causes emotions. For example, Schachter (1975) theorized that an individual's emotions (or experiences of feelings) come from awareness of body arousal (physiological arousal, which is the same for all emotions) plus the conscious appraisal or evaluation of that arousal. The arousal is cognitively labeled after appraising or evaluating the significance of the stimuli for the self. In short, processing information, evaluating, and using language to label the diffuse sensations to identify and generate (or construct) the emotion are all involved. In this view, although emotions influence thinking, the cognitive appraisal of a situation always precedes and determines the existence of the emotion (Lazarus, 1991).

The extent to which cognition plays a role depends on the complexity of the emotion that is involved. Cognitive appraisal is also important in the regulation of the level and intensity of experienced feelings, the expression or inhibition of emotions depending on appropriateness to the context, and even the extent of physiological arousal.

Mayer and Salovey (1995) posit a continuum of cognitive construction and regulation of emotion. At the lowest level, nonconscious or unconscious construction of emotion occurs either at the neurological level or is automatized and no longer attended to; this may involve biologically programmed physiological experience and at most the most basic cognitions. At intermediate levels of conscious construction, the number and complexity of differentiated emotions increases along with the regulation of emotional expression. At the highest level, there is an extended conscious attempt to understand, define, and enhance emotion, including feelings in the esthetic, moral, and religious domains.

Most scholars (Ekman & Davidson, 1994) agree that cognitive information processing and evaluation of events can provoke emotion. However, a purely cognitive approach cannot easily account for various emotion phenomena occurring prior to any cognitive interpretation, such as (a) differential patterns of brain activity and physiological arousal indicating the presence of different emotions, (b) the existence of more or less universal facial expressions associated with different emotions, (c) the speed of response of certain intense emotions, especially those related to survival, and (d) emotional responses occurring at a young age before language development has taken place.

B. Emotion Approach

The classical position (e.g., Zajonc, 1984) in this general approach is that emotions precede and control cognitions. However, much evidence now exists that this may not be the case. An alternative is the two-system approach as proposed by Berkowitz (1993). In this view, some emotions exist independent of cognition, and others depend on cognition for their form and expression. Such a view is supported by the laboratory animal studies of LeDoux (1986, 1994a), which identified a direct neural pathway for sensory input to the amygdala (the brain structure controlling emotional response), bypassing the cortex. Stimulus sensations via the direct pathway arrive at the amygdala sooner than those via the cortex; thus, a quick emotional response (as to a threat stimulus) is possible, which may then be modified after the cortex has interpreted the stimulus sensation.

Such responding would seem especially applicable to stimuli experienced in infancy when cognitive development is extremely immature. During the first year or so of life, cognitive discrimination ability exists, but little evaluative skill or language development. Later on, such responding might apply to simple or "primitive" emotions (such as anger, fear, joy, and feelings of security or comfort), where differential neurological arousal for different types of emotions leads directly to differential experiences and expressive behavior.

However, there may be problems with such a viewpoint, as some individuals (e.g., Parrott, 1993) claim that infants are well developed to deal with emotions provided one does not equate cognitive maturity with language. According to Lazarus (1994), by 4 months of age an infant whose arm is restrained shows an unmistakable expression of anger. By 7 months, although the infant recognizes that the offending agent is both external and a person, it is unlikely that it recognizes the event to be a threat or regards the offending agent as accountable. Thus, the infant's early expression of anger lacks important appraisal processes.

Izard (1994) regards an associative bond between the image of the mother's face and a feeling of enjoyment as one of the first "affective–cognitive" structures (or schemata) to develop; it depends on the existence of perceptual discrimination, but goes beyond the latter to include some recognition memory, and storage retrieval capacities. Similarly, the infant develops primitive communication ability enabling it to signal the mother when distressed, and sufficient cognitive ability to associate the appearance of the mother with feelings of comfort. Another position (Labouvie-Vief, DeVoe, & Bulka, 1989) is that emotions in infancy are expressed in actions, but that emotions become more linked with cognitive and symbolic processes and more differentiated with increasing maturity.

These examples seem to indicate that neither a cognitive nor an emotion approach alone can account for all phenomena. This situation might indicate another viewpoint, which the author suggests below.

VI. A THREE-LEVEL THEORY OF EMOTIONS AND THE DEVELOPMENT OF ATTACHMENT

From an evolutionary viewpoint, at least some emotions must be universal, as well as emotion-specific neurologically, physiologically, and experientially, if survival of the infant, the species, and the gene pool are to be ensured. In short, some emotions must be immediate, relatively intense, and adaptive. Such emotions would be considered as operating at Level One. They would be elicited by the sensory representation of the environmental stimuli or context, lead to differential neurological and (possibly) physiological arousal, and subsequently to differential subjective experience and expressive behavior for purposes of survival. Such emotional reactions would occur quickly, involuntarily, and immediately, with or without consciousness. Examples of the subjective experience of such emotions would be pain, fear, anxiety, grief, anger, security, and joy. At this level, emotions predominate, and if any cognition exists, it is very weak and immature.

At Level Two, both emotions and cognitions operate, with cognitions being more mature than those found at Level One and exerting at least an equivalent influence. Level Two is found primarily in infancy and early childhood, and involves a "merger" of affective–cognitive structures. The latter would account for the kinds of reactions observed by Lazarus (1994) and Izard (1994). Affective–cognitive structures of this sort, when existing in relation to an attachment figure, can be viewed as the beginnings of the internal working model of attachment.

At Level Three, a higher order of cognitive processes and language abilities is found. Through a history of months of interaction with the mother, a nexus of such affective–cognitive structures develops that constitutes the mental representation of a secure attachment to the mother. (Alternatively, if the mother is inconsistent in responding to the infant's signals of distress or is rejecting or abusive, the infant may come to associate certain negative emotions with the mother, and develop a mental representation of an insecure attachment.) As the child and the mother continue to interact over time, the child uses developing cognitive abilities and stimulus appraisal skills to construct and regulate complex emotions. This new information adds to the earlier internal working model of the attachment relationship.

In summary, the three-level theory proposes that, at Level One, certain universal primitive emotions can be elicited in the infant without cognitive intervention, with rapid reactions for purposes of survival. At Level Two, certain somewhat more complex emotions can be elicited in the infant or young child by stimulus situation, with reactions for purposes of survival and/or optimum adaptation. At this stage, there is a merging or coordination of primitive emotions and cognitive capacities in the form of emotional memories that help the individual appraise the situation. Finally, at Level Three, complex emotions exist by virtue of the child's (or adult's) use of cognitive capacities to construct or generate emotions for purposes of adaptation. All three levels of emotion processing continue to exist within the child but, as development continues over time, Level Three develops greater richness and sophistication as cognitions and emotions become more interwoven (similar to the more mature levels proposed by Labouvie-Vief et al., 1989, and by Mayer & Salovey, 1995). With maturity, there is greater balance and harmony as thoughts become more elaborate and emotions become more complex, leading to more effective adaptation.

However, the infant's initial attachment to the mother is formed at a time when primitive emotions are strongest and dominate cognitions. Consequently, the infant's emotions have a greater influence on the initial infant–mother attachment than immature but developing cognitive abilities. These early emotions influence the cognitions of the infant about the self, the mother (attachment figure), and their relationship, which may be inexact and poorly defined. One can view the internal working model as involving an emotional working memory as well as a cognitive working memory. As such, the initial attachment (whether secure or insecure) is long lasting and may resist modification in adulthood. Most important, since the initial infant attachment is perceived by most researchers as the prototype or template for other concurrent or later multiple attachments, the latter will be indirectly influenced by the domination of the primitive emotions of the initial attachment.

From an ethological-evolutionary perspective (Bowlby, 1988), the infant has a genetic predisposition to form an attachment to a primary attachment figure, as noted earlier. This predisposition, coupled with the strong primitive emotions characteristic of Level One and the affective–cognitive structures represented by Level Two (which become part of the internal working model), helps to account for various attachment phenomena throughout life: the continued existence of the attachment to the mother, use of the original attachment relationship as the template for other attachment relationships in adulthood, grief reactions at loss of the attachment figure, and various clinical manifestations associated with disturbed attachments. In regard to the latter, LeDoux (1994b) found evidence for the existence of two parallel brain systems for memory, one for declarative memory of cognitively mediated materials and one for emotional memory (which is hypothesized to operate at Level Two). (Goleman, 1995, also discusses emotional memory.) Although the former is subject to cognitive construction, the latter is not. Thus, emotional memories can be evoked by stimuli associated with an earlier situation, but do not necessarily match declarative memories.

The existence of a separate system for emotional memories occurring early in life may provide some explanation for the difficulty in altering dysfunctional attachment styles in later childhood or adulthood. However, alteration is possible; Main et al. (1985) found that some adults who were classified as insecurely attached in childhood were able to gain cognitive insights into these early attachment patterns and achieve a coherent (and secure) attachment orientation in adulthood. This suggests the value of cognitive interventions in treating disturbed attachments, especially at Level Three where complex emotions have formed and cognition has a greater role. In secure attachment, the individual develops an effective mature cognitive-emotional system. However, in disturbed attachments, early negative emotions lead to inappropriate and maladaptive cognitive functioning in maturity with poorly regulated emotions. Interventions using cognitive therapy may help the individual to understand and change these maladaptive thinking habits.

From the perspective of both attachment theory and the three-level emotion theory, one can pose many questions for future research studies that will yield greater understanding than research conceptualized from either perspective alone. For example, how are emotions involved in the maintenance and disruption of attachment in comparison to the role of cognitions? How do different attachment styles lead to different psychopathologies and their respective maladaptive cognitive and emotional manifestations? Is there an interaction effect between the content and organization of cognitions in the internal working model, and does this in turn depend upon higher order interactions with different kinds of emotions?

Understanding the mutual influence of cognitive and emotional systems throughout development seems to be essential to fully understand the complexities of attachment relationships over the life span. This task is one that investigators of emotion may find challenging to undertake.

REFERENCES

Ainsworth, M. D. S. (1989). Attachments beyond infancy. *American Psychologist, 44,* 709–716
Antonucci, T. C. (1994). Attachment in adulthood and aging. In M. B. Sperling & W. H. Berman (Eds.), *Attachment in adults: Clinical and developmental perspectives* (pp. 256–272). New York: Guilford Press.
Bartholomew, K. (1993). From childhood to adult relationships: Attachment theory and research. In S. Duck (Ed.), *Learning about relationships* (pp. 30–62). Newbury Park, CA: Sage.
Berkowitz, L. (1993). Towards a general theory of anger and emotional aggression: Implications of the cognitive-neoassociationistic perspective for the analysis of anger and other emotions. In R. S. Wyer, Jr. & T. K. Srull (Eds.), *Advances in social cognition. Vol. VI. Perspectives on anger and emotion* (pp. 1–46). Hillsdale, NJ: Erlbaum.
Berman, W. H., & Sperling, M. B. (1994). The structure and function of adult attachment. In M. B. Sperling & W. H. Berman (Eds.), *Attachment in adults: Clinical and developmental perspectives* (pp. 1–28). New York: Guilford Press.
Bowlby, J. (1979). *The making and breaking of affectional bonds.* London: Tavistock.
Bowlby, J. (1980). *Attachment and loss: Vol. 3. Loss: Sadness and depression.* New York: Basic Books.
Bowlby, J. (1988). *A secure base: Parent-child attachment and healthy human development.* New York: Basic Books.
Bretherton, I. (1985). Attachment theory: Retrospect and prospect. In I. Bretherton & E. Waters (Eds.), *Growing points of attachment theory and research* (pp. 3–38). *Monographs of the Society for Research in Child Development, 50* (1–2, Serial No. 209).
Bretherton, I. (1992). Attachment and bonding. In V. B. Van Hasselt & M. Hersen (Eds.), *Handbook of social development: A lifespan perspective* (pp. 133–155). New York: Plenum Press.
Cicirelli, V. G. (1983). Adult children's attachment and helping behavior to elderly parents: A path model. *Journal of Marriage and the Family, 45,* 815–825.

Cicirelli, V. G. (1991). Attachment theory in old age: Protection of the attached figure. In K. Pillemer & K. McCartney (Eds.), *Parent–child relations across the life span* (pp. 25–42). Hillsdale, NJ: Erlbaum.

Cicirelli, V. G. (1993). Attachment and obligation as daughters' motives for caregiving behavior and subsequent effect on subjective burden. *Psychology and Aging, 8,* 144–155.

Cicirelli, V. G. (1995). A measure of caregiving daughters' attachment to elderly mothers. *Journal of Family Psychology, 9,* 89–94.

Ekman, P., & Davidson, R. J. (1994). Affective science: A research agenda. In P. Ekman & R. J. Davidson (Eds.), *The nature of emotion: Fundamental questions* (pp. 411–430). New York: Oxford University Press.

Goleman, D. (1995). *Emotional intelligence.* New York: Bantam Books.

Izard, C. E. (1994). Intersystem connections. In P. Ekman & R. J. Davidson (Eds.), *The nature of emotion: Fundamental questions* (pp. 356–361). New York: Oxford University Press.

Labouvie-Vief, G., DeVoe, M., & Bulka, D. (1989). Speaking about feelings: Conceptions of emotion across the life span. *Psychology and Aging, 4,* 425–437.

Lazarus, R. S. (1991). Cognition and motivation in emotion. *American Psychologist, 46,* 352–367.

Lazarus, R. S. (1994). Appraisal: The long and the short of it. In P. Ekman & R. J. Davidson (Eds.), *The nature of emotion: Fundamental questions* (pp. 208–215). New York: Oxford University Press.

LeDoux, J. E. (1986). Sensory systems and emotion: A model of affective processing. *Integrative Psychiatry, 4,* 237–248.

LeDoux, J. E. (1994a). Cognitive-emotional interactions in the brain. In P. Ekman & R. J. Davidson (Eds.), *The nature of emotion: Fundamental questions* (pp. 216–223). New York: Oxford University Press.

LeDoux, J. E. (1994b). Memory versus emotional memory in the brain. In P. Ekman & R. J. Davidson (Eds.) *The nature of emotion: Fundamental questions* (pp. 311–312). New York: Oxford University Press.

Levitt, M. J. (1991). Attachment and close relationships: A life-span perspective. In J. L. Gewirtz & W. L. Kurtines (Eds.), *Intersections with attachment* (pp. 183–205). Hillsdale, NJ: Erlbaum.

Magai, C., & McFadden, S. H. (1995). *The role of emotions in social and personality development: History, theory, and research.* New York: Plenum.

Main, M., Kaplan, N., & Cassidy, J. (1985). Security in infancy, childhood, and adulthood: A move to the level of representation. In I. Bretherton & E. Waters (Eds.), *Growing points of attachment theory and research. Monographs of the Society for Research in Child Development* (Vol. 50, pp. 66–104). (1–2, Serial No. 209). Chicago: University of Chicago Press for the Society for Research in Child Development.

Mayer, J. D., & Salovey, P. (1995). Emotional intelligence and the construction and regulation of feelings. *Applied and Preventive Psychology, 4,* 197–208.

Parrott, W. G. (1993). On the scientific study of angry organisms. In R. S. Wyer, Jr., & T. K. Srull (Eds.), *Advances in social cognition. Vol. VI. Perspectives on anger and emotion* (pp. 167–177). Hillsdale, NJ: Erlbaum.

Rando, T. (1993). *Treatment of complicated mourning.* Champaign, IL: Research Press.

Rothbart, J. C., & Shaver, P. C. (1994). Continuity of attachment across the life span. In M. B. Sperling & W. H. Berman (Eds.), *Attachment in adults: Clinical and developmental perspectives* (pp. 31–71). New York: Guilford Press.

Schachter, S. (1975). Cognition and centralist-peripheralist controversies in motivation and emotion. In M. S. Gazzaniga & C. B. Blakemore (Eds.), *Handbook of psychology* (pp. 529–564). New York: Academic Press.

Shaver, P. R., & Hazan, C. (1993). Adult romantic attachment: Theory and evidence. In D. Perlman & W. Jones (Eds.), *Advances in personal relationships* (Vol. 4, pp. 29–70). London: Jessica Kingsley.

Sperling, M. B., & Berman, W. H. (Eds.). (1994). *Attachment in adults: Clinical and developmental perspectives.* New York: Guilford Press.

van IJzendoorn, M. H. (1995). Adult attachment representations, parental responsiveness, and infant attachment: A meta-analysis on the predictive validity of the adult attachment interview. *Psychological Bulletin, 117,* 387–403.

van IJzendoorn, M. H., & Tavecchio, L. W. C. (1987). The development of attachment theory as a Lakatosian research program: Philosophical and methodological aspects. In M. H. van IJzendoorn & L. W. C. Tavecchio (Eds.), *Attachment in social networks: Contributions to the Bowlby-Ainsworth attachment theory* (pp. 3–31). Amsterdam, The Netherlands: Elsevier Science Publishers B.V.

Weiss, R. S. (1986). Continuities and transformations in social relationships from childhood to adulthood. In W. W. Hartup & Z. Rubin (Eds.), *On relationships and development,* (pp. 95–110). Hillsdale, NJ: Erlbaum.

Whitbeck, L. B., Simons, R. L., & Conger, R. D. (1991). The effects of early family relationships on contemporary relationships and assistance patterns between adult children and their parents. *Journal of Gerontology: Social Sciences, 46,* S330–337.

Zajonc, R. B. (1984). On the primacy of effect. *American Psychologist, 39,* 117–123.

CHAPTER 8

Emotion

and

Memory

Kenneth T. Strongman
Department of Psychology
University of Canterbury
Christchurch, New Zealand

I. INTRODUCTION

At first blush it seems obvious that it is appropriate to consider the links between emotion and memory from a developmental perspective. Both emotion and memory change over the life span and various theories of emotion, particularly those of a cognitive persuasion, have a role for memory. Moreover, at the commonsense or folk psychology level it seems self-evident that our memories are affected by our emotions. However, there is a surprising dearth of material of either an empirical or theoretical nature on the topic. Furthermore, on looking into the topic in more depth, there are some murky conceptual issues.

As any researcher in the field of emotion knows, the term *emotion* has proved difficult to define. The reasons for this may go beyond the fact that it indexes a complex area of life; it may be that emotion eludes easy definitional clarity because of its multidimensionality and the differences in nomenclature across the field. In any event, in a number of fields, the terms *emotion* and *affect* are used more or less interchangeably. Here, they will both be used as general terms, with specific emotions and moods (background states of a quieter, more enduring nature) seen as subcategories of affect or emotion.

Even more problematically, what exactly does the idea of links between memory and emotion imply? Is memory affected by the emotional aspects of the event to be remembered? Does one's emotional state at the time of an event affect one's memory for it? Does one's emotional state at the time of recall affect one's memory for an event whether or not the event itself was emotional? And there are more specific questions such as whether the act of trying to recall any events of earlier life is itself emotional.

For present purposes, attention will settle on the various questions that arise from the issue of whether and how emotion affects memory. That memory might affect emotion is more properly considered within a framework of general theories of emotion rather than within the specific context of development. Moreover, because adult memories are sometimes of childhood, and because emotion–memory links have their origins in childhood, this chapter will range from childhood to old age. Treating the early end of the life span may seem odd in a handbook concerned with adult emotion. However, when considering emotion and memory it would be foolish not to make a life span analysis, particularly if part of the aim is to take a theoretical perspective.

II. LIFE SPAN DEVELOPMENT

It is disappointing to report that there is very little research relevant to the links between emotion and memory across the life span. Of course there has been research on early autobiographical memory, mood, and memory in adult subjects, and on reminiscence in old age, but there has been little in the way of research devoted to a life span perspective. In this section I review these bodies of literature; later I will examine what one can extrapolate from these literatures that will inform a developmental perspective.

A. Autobiographical Memories of Early Childhood

An early examination of childhood memory and emotion was conducted by Waldfogel (1948), who showed that the first memories *of* childhood derive from the age of three or four and emotional content of either a positive or negative nature. Many other studies followed. Howes, Siegel, and Brown (1993) provided an interesting discussion of the literature on early memories and suggested that the widespread belief that childhood memories are distorted probably comes from Freud's concern with early traumatic events. This implicit theory has three aspects: the notion that the infantile memory system is weak, that trauma can increase in strength over time, and the fact that memory from very early childhood becomes distorted. They also point to the belief that affect strengthens memory.

Of considerable importance in this context is the "flashbulb" effect described by Brown and Kulik (1977). If someone lives through a strong emotion-provoking event there is long-term recall plus strong memory of various noncentral perceptual aspects of the event. The suggestion is that infantile memories may well be characterized by such effects.

Howes and colleagues (1993) had 300 undergraduates write down whatever they could recall of their earliest memories. Other individuals who had been present at the time of the remembered event were also asked to describe the event. The two accounts were then compared. The researchers also had subjects describe their two earliest memories, make a written record of them, and then answer a questionnaire that asked for very specific information. The results indicated that in general there was not much distortion in the memories, as attested by the concordance between the student's report and the other informant's report. The most common content of the memories was of getting hurt. There was much emotion involved in the recall, but it was just as likely to be positive as negative. It thus seems that *any* powerful affect can strengthen memory. Moreover, the researchers found much remembrance of trivial details, as in the flashbulb effect.

Howes et al. (1993) suggested that early memories are of two sorts, one kind powered by strong emotion, the other by keenly focused attention, though otherwise emotionally neutral. They also felt that they had obtained evidence that affect can be lost from memory; that is, some subjects reported events being neutral, though verifiers recollected the person being highly emotionally aroused at the time. It is possible that although the affect may help to maintain the memory of the event, the affect itself may be forgotten. In the end, Howes et al. concluded that the principal impact of emotion takes place at the time of encoding. Any distortions they found were not large and seemed to be of noncentral aspects of the events.

Given the limitations of space in this chapter and the focus on adulthood and aging, we need not belabor the issue of childhood memories at this time. Suffice to note the conclusions arrived at in the recent working document of the British Psychological Society (1995). This document concludes that (a) normal event memory is largely accurate, though it may contain some distortion and elaboration; (b) virtually nothing can be recalled of events before the first birthday, and little before the second; and (c) though there are many reports of trauma having been forgotten, the mechanisms that underlie the process are not well understood. Further in-depth discussions of the topic can be found in Ceci and Bruck (1993) and Lindsay and Read (1994).

B. Mood and Memory in Adult Subjects

In this section I review studies of the relation between mood and memory; I first deal with laboratory-based studies and then turn to endogenous mood, as in the effects of depression.

1. LABORATORY-BASED STUDIES

Two approaches to the study of mood and memory are found in the literature, one concerning the study of how general emotional arousal (an activated mood) affects memory, and the other addressing the specific properties of particular emotional states or moods. The bulk of work has pursued the latter approach, but before turning to this literature, it is worth noting the general effect of emotional arousal on memory.

Burke, Heuer, and Reisberg (1992) had subjects view slides of an emotionally arousing story or a similar but emotionally neutral story. They were tested on the material either immediately or after some delay. Emotional arousal appeared to influence memory more for details than for central events, and also affected memory for plot-relevant information. Thus, in general, there was a memory advantage for arousing material. The data on retention interval were equivocal, although rehearsal improved performance and more testing led to better memory. Emotional arousal improved memory for the gist of the story, for basic visual information, and for details associated with central events, but undermined memory for background information. However, whether or not the story was arousing interacted with this. Generally, emotion seemed to improve memory for material linked to the action. Burke and colleagues argued that the reason for this is that attention is narrowed during emotional arousal, partly due to the fact that there are resource limitations on the ability to spread attention more widely.

I turn now to the effects of specific emotions and moods on memory. Bower (1987, 1992) was among the first to examine this process within the context of state-dependence and mood-congruence processes in memory. Mood state-dependent memory has it that recall during a given mood is partly determined by what was learned when in that mood. Mood congruence refers to some material being more likely to be stored and/or recalled when in a particular mood because of its emotional value. These effects are couched within a cognitive network theory in which each emotion has a specific node in memory, the nodes linking all memories that are relevant. They are also linked with propositions describing relevant events from life. The nodes can be activated either by physiological or symbolic stimuli. Excitation is transmitted to other nodes that lead to autonomic nervous system (ANS) arousal and emotional behavior. This in turn spreads activation throughout the memory structure, thus influencing later memories.

As Blaney (1986) reported in a review of the literature, there are mixed findings with respect to state-dependent effects in both adults and children. In adults there is a nonrobust effect of mood states being important when meaning cues are vague. With respect to mood congruence, a wide range of effects have been reported.

There are various ways of accounting for mood-congruence effects. They may simply be part of an automatic process; or they may be motivational in nature. For example, depressed people may recall negative material because they are trying to cope with it, or they may be trying to neutralize it. Whatever the explanation, Blaney argued that it is certain that mood-based congruent memory sometimes contributes to the perpetuation of existing mood states, even if it does so only through the screening out of positive material.

There is some evidence that mood-priming effects might be less powerful in children than in adults. Forgas, Burnham, and Trimboli (1988) gave 8 to 10-year-olds either positive or negative audiovisual information about two target children. Beforehand, happy or sad moods were induced. One day later, they were again put into a happy or sad mood and assessments were made of recall, recognition, and impression formation. Memory was better when they were happy in encoding, retrieving, or both, when material was incongruent with the learning mood, when the target characters were in contrasting mood states, and when recall and encoding moods matched. Moreover, a happy mood increased the extremity of positive and negative impressions of the target persons.

According to Forgas and colleagues, these results show that children are different from adults in the influence of transient mood on memory. Generally, happy children learn and remember better than sad children. This is not so in adults, and may be linked to the inability of children to modulate their emotions. It also may be due to the motivational aspects of moods rather than with their cognitive content.

Forgas and colleagues believe that their results with children show some support for Bower's mood state-dependent retrieval hypothesis and suggest that encoding mood is more important than retrieval mood in memory; the children recalled more negative than positive information and more that was incongruent than congruent with the learning mood.

Mood-congruence effects are robust with adults but are not found with children, who, when happy, learn more of both negative and positive material. It is possible that children might not be good at the right kind of processing, or that they might be more sensitive than adults towards contrast between mood and materials. Alternatively, the mood-priming effects may be less powerful because children are less subtle, analytic, interpretative, and inferential in person perception than adults.

Although mood-priming effects might be less powerful in children than in adults, motivational consequences might be more important to them. It is possible that children need more emotional experience before being able to use affect as an aid to memory. Certainly children cannot use mood states as retrieval cues as well as adults, but they do rely on them as aids to motivation and as cues to encoding.

The most recent review of mood state-dependent memory is in the form of a meta-analysis by Ucros (1989). The general finding is that mood state-dependent effects are seen more often with positive than negative moods. Strongest effects are seen in studies that use real-life events, have contrasting moods, have mood states specific to items, last longer, have a smaller sample size, select subjects according to direct mood criteria, pay subjects, and use adults rather than students or children. Of note for this chapter, the older the subjects are the stronger is the mood effect on memory.

In a final comment on the area, Bower concluded (1987) that mood and memory theory has not fared as well as expected; there are a number of successes but also several clear failures—under conditions where it should reasonably have succeeded. Now, it is possible that some of the inconsistencies and failures are due to the fact that we do not adequately understand developmental processes, and have not taken developmental stage adequately into account in these kinds of investigations. In the future, it will be important to undertake developmentally oriented studies. It may well be that mood-congruence effects are not consistent throughout the life span. There is evidently some change that takes place between childhood and adulthood; as well, there could be further changes over the life span. For example, congruence effects might be of greater or less significance in the elderly.

2. ENDOGENOUS MOOD

Links between memory and depression have been studied over many years, although little of the research has been from a developmental perspective. For example, there is a paucity of literature on the relation between memory impairment in the aged and depression. A case in point is a study by O'Hara, Hinrichs, Kahout, Wallace, and Lemke (1986), who examined self-reported memory disturbance in depressed and nondepressed men and women over the age of 65. The subjects were asked to compare themselves with others of their age, and with themselves when they were younger, and to describe the frequency of the trouble they had in remembering names and faces. In general, subjects with high levels of depressive symptoms reported higher levels of memory complaints than did subjects with lower levels of depression, but there were no differences as a function of type of depression diagnosis. There were no differences in free recall between the groups. The authors concluded that it is symptom severity rather than diagnosis of depression that is important to impairment of memory in the depressed elderly.

A meta-analysis of the area of depression and memory impairment is provided by Burt, Zembar, and Niederehe (1995), the results of which show that depression and memory are clearly related, although the causal mechanisms that underlie the relationship are not clear. Interestingly, in the present context, they show that the greatest effects are demonstrated for age and patient status, there being a greater association of impairment with depression in younger than older patients. This might be seen as counter-intuitive to the idea of greater cognitive vulnerability in older versus younger people.

Burt and colleagues suggest four possible explanations for this effect. First, the effects of age might overlap or be confounded with other moderator variables (such as type of depression or medication). Also, the effect may come from age of onset rather than from age of patient. Thus, some of the relatively younger samples might include a greater proportion of patients predisposed to early-onset depression, which in turn might be more related to memory impairment.

Second, late-onset depression is complicated by factors such as co-morbid physical illness. Moreover, depression may account for a greater proportion of cognitive variance in younger patients. Third, there may be floor effects because memory impairment is greater in very old people. And finally, if memory–depression links are partly due to the failure to use memory strategies that require effort, depression may have less impact on such strategies in older people. Whatever the appropriate explanation might be, it is clear that depression leads to more severe memory impairment among younger versus older patients.

A recent analysis of links between emotional disorders of a more general nature and cognition by Mathews and Macleod (1994) is relevant to both mood and depression. In an analysis of the work on mood and memory, they list a number of problems that remain even though mood states might activate memory representations. For example, the mood state-dependent memory effects have not been well replicated; there are instructional effects on bias and mood-incongruent recall; mood-congruent recall is restricted to self-encoded stimuli; and there are different types of cognitive facilitation under different emotions.

Mathews and Macleod also consider autobiographical memory and summarize the literature as showing that with neutral cue words and the instruction to describe the first memory that comes to mind, depressed or anxious subjects report more negative memories than nonanxious or nondepressed subjects. With emotional cues, depressed or anxious people have shorter recall latencies for negative than for positive memories. Are these effects due to differences in past experience or in the retrieval process? Using material to which people have equal access, the effects are weaker and seem dependent on the nature of the encoding task. The evidence for anxious subjects points strongly in both directions, that is, for the enhanced and the impaired recall of negative material. "The weight of empirical evidence suggests strongly that facilitated ability to recall emotionally negative information is a characteristic of elevated depression, but not of elevated anxiety" (Mathews & Macleod, 1994, p. 34).

D. Reminiscence

Individuals of all ages reminisce, though folk theory would have it that the frequency of reminiscence increases with age. However, Webster (1994) demonstrated that age is not a predictor of the frequency of reminiscence, nor of the emotional tone or the type of content of reminiscences. Reminiscence is a life span process; nevertheless, most of the research on reminiscence is undertaken with older people. In general, females tend to reminisce more than males, as do those who are more open to experience. Other personality dimensions also relate to the type of reminiscence.

Wong and Watt (1991) defined reminiscence as "personal memories of a distant past; it consists of long-term memories of events in which the reminiscer is either a participant or an observer" (p. 272). Because many, or even all, of these events are likely to have an emotional component, reminiscence is, in turn, likely to have an emotional aspect. Moreover, reminiscence in general may be pertinent to a person's emotional well-being. The research discussed in this section represents recent directions in this context.

Wong and Watt (1991) identify six types of reminiscence: integrative, instrumental, transmissive, narrative, escapist, and obsessive. They gathered reminiscence data from elderly men and women (65–95 years) either living in the community or in institutions. In general, those who are judged as aging successfully engage in more integrative and instrumental reminiscence, and less of the obsessive type than those who are judged as aging less successfully.

Apart from the categorization of types of reminiscence, the significance of this study lies in the demonstration that some types of reminiscence are beneficial to aging. Successful aging is measured by assessment of mental and physical health and may reasonably be supposed to subsume emotional well-being.

A similar study was conducted by Fry (1991). Again, the research involved a large number of elderly individuals (67–82 years) from the community and from nursing homes. They were given interviews and questionnaires about their reminiscence. Fry found wide variation in the frequency of reminiscence and in the degree of pleasantness associated with it. For many elderly individuals, reminiscence is pleasing and helps to lift self-esteem. Reminiscence is promoted particularly in those who are open to experience. However, Fry found a negative relationship between well-being (the presence of positive and the absence of negative emotion) and frequency of reminiscence. Perhaps depression and anxiety help to bring about reminiscence. Certainly, elderly individuals with a self-perception of well-being have more to do and may therefore simply have less time to reminisce.

This type of finding is extended by Brittlebank, Scott, Williams, and Ferrier (1993). They showed that in clinically depressed individuals (average age 43), overgeneral recall in autobiographical memory, particularly for emotionally positive memories, is correlated with failure to recover from depression. (Overgeneral memory has been associated with defensive processes [Singer & Salovy, 1993]).

Yang and Rehm (1993) compared depressed and nondepressed elderly individuals. The researchers had subjects recall 30 memories and rate them for happiness and sadness and their importance, both at the time of occurrence and at the time of recall. Results of the study are in line with the mood-congruence hypothesis. The nondepressed see greater positive emotional change between then and now. The depressed recall more memories rated as sad now than the nondepressed and also regard both positive and negative memories as becoming more neutral in comparison with the nondepressed. In general, Yang and Rehm argued for reminiscence being self-enhancing, in that recall of happier memories is associated with less depression.

Again, from a more therapeutic perspective, Mills and Coleman (1994) described a case study that demonstrates how reminiscence and counseling skills can be used to stimulate emotional autobiographical memories. They regard this as of possible therapeutic benefit.

This brief overview of some recent studies on reminiscence and autobiographical memory is enough to show further links between emotion and memory. Certainly, the frequency of reminiscence in the elderly and the emotional tone of the reminiscences themselves appear to be related to well-being. In fact, apart from demonstrating various memory–emotion relationships, reminiscence may provide an example of the self-regulation of emotional states, a notion that could have therapeutic implications.

III. GENERAL PERSPECTIVES AND THEORY

In a very useful although very general discussion of emotion and memory in the aging process, Cavanaugh (1989) stressed the importance of individual differences in the feelings induced by autobiographical memories. He pointed out that there was an early literature on this topic (e.g., Meltzer, 1930) but then a decline for many years. He argued that emotion was left out of cognitive research on memory due to a misunderstanding of what Freud said about repression and due to the rise of behaviorism.

Cavanaugh argued that there are three lines of relevant work. First, personality theorists have mentioned a turning inward with age, which may bring greater awareness of affect associated with cognition, in self-evaluation and self-reflection. This is related to reminiscence and the search for the meaning of happy and unhappy experiences. "Accuracy is moot. How you feel about memory is what matters" (Cavanaugh, 1989, p. 601). Second, Cavanaugh suggested that what is important in reminiscence is attempts to deal with the separation-individuation process; how one sees oneself and how one sees oneself in relation to others might become increasingly important with age. Third, there is one's self-perception of one's own ability as a rememberer. Defenses may develop if and when older people believe that their memory is fading, a matter which is probably more emotionally laden for older than for younger adults.

Interestingly, Cavanaugh is one of the few researchers to make use of the idea of nostalgia, a notion that is of considerable everyday import and which is clearly relevant to emotion–memory links. As he put it, remembering the past is reminiscence, whereas adding in bittersweet emotions to this is nostalgia. Nostalgia helps to maintain identity and relationships with part of the self from former times, as well as providing a measure of personal change. This is an area in need of study.

By far the most penetrating general perspective on developmental aspects of emotion and memory has been given by Leichtman, Ceci, and Ornstein (1992). They sorted out five perspectives on emotion–memory links, each representing a distinct view of the memory system, and took a life span developmental viewpoint.

The first and most obvious account of emotion–memory links is through network theory, in which information is thought to be stored in a network of related representations, nodes, pathways, and so on, with affective state being given nodal status. An affective node can act as a retrieval cue so there might be chains of nodes from points concerned with either positive or negative emotion. Leichtman et al. quoted particularly from the work of Isen (1987) in this context. They described the acquisition of emotional nodes as something that apparently begins at an early age. If children in the first grade have a positive mood induced, they are more likely to work things out on an affective dimension first when given a choice. Also, with 3–4-year-olds, positive emotion promotes the ability to see new connections between stimuli.

The problem for network theory is that negative affect does not show symmetrically opposite effects to that found with positive affect. Negative affect either fails to facilitate the recall of negative material or provides a less effective retrieval cue than positive affect. A possible reason for this is that the structures that represent positive affect are more loosely represented in memory than those that represent negative affect, so when they are activated they spread more widely. The main function of positive affect seems to be to broaden the context for the interpretation of stimuli. However, a further problem for network theory is that when emotional arousal is extreme, either positive or negative, there are amnesic results.

The second way of accounting for emotion–memory effects according to Leichtman et al. is through level of arousal. In brief, the argument is that because attention is always limited, there is less available at encoding time in conditions where high arousal is making heavy demands. The result is more forgetting. High arousal might have greater memorial effects on children than adults, perhaps because highly emotional events sap more of a young child's relatively limited-capacity resources than those of adults.

A third possible way of viewing emotion–memory effects related to arousal is energy, following the finding that high levels of emotion at the time of encoding somehow empower the memory system. There are two possible examples of this: flashbulb memories, already referred to earlier, for personal circumstances that obtained at the time of receiving shocking information going into a "permastore" from which the system is energized; or, the possibility that the low energies of depressed persons undermine recall. Data relevant to this view come from studies on eye-witness memory in children (e.g., Peters, 1991). The general finding is that the flashbulb effect plus stress from harrowing experiences under-mines recall.

A fourth view is that emotion–memory links are enhanced by or work through motivational and attentional channels. People who are in a positive, relaxed frame of mind are more willing to take chances and put in the sort of effort that might benefit all performance, including mem-ory. In fact, it is possible to reinterpret a number of studies along the lines that affective states might have an effect on children's recall through motivation and attention by altering their view of the world.

Finally, Leichtman et al. drew attention to integrated trace accounts of emotion–memory links. This suggests that the emotion–memory rela-tionship is inherent in human information processing; one analyzes stim-uli while making a pattern recognition analysis that includes emotional responses to stimuli. Any memory trace is made up of both cognitive and affective features so emotionally based remembering may work through this integrated memory trace.

Leichtman et al. concluded that there is no clear picture of how emo-tion influences the developing memory system, other than to say that emotion is important both during encoding and retrieval. Many factors are likely to be involved in any effects, from level of arousal to the con-text in which the event is occurring.

IV. NOW AND THE FUTURE

As with any area that has not been well excavated by researchers, ei-ther empirically or theoretically, conclusions are hard to form. Crucially missing is any life span developmental study of the links between emo-tion and memory. In most existing studies, investigators have concen-trated on the early and the late years with almost nothing in between other than what might be gleaned fortuitously from the ever-present un-dergraduate student. Moreover, some researchers have taken the real-life-based autobiographical memory approach, and others have used artificially generated materials in laboratory experiments. Rapproche-ment between the two is not easy.

It is possible to say that there are some links between emotion and memory and between mood and memory, and that they occur both at the time of encoding and at recall, although the evidence is more persuasive at encoding. The only emotions that have been studied have been happiness and sadness (mostly manipulated), depression and anxiety (mostly occurring naturally). Whatever the specific effects, such as "flashbulb" memories for personal aspects of more shocking events, there is strong evidence for the social construction of early memories (Bretherton, 1993; Nelson, 1993)—which accounts for the distinct gender differences that have been observed in children (Fivush, 1993). There are also differences between emotion–memory links in the young and the old.

These are not the most powerful conclusions with which to end a chapter such as this. What remains, of course, is the future. Both theory and research need to take a life span developmental perspective with respect to emotion–memory links. Comparisons need to be made of the effects of specific emotions, such as, say shame or guilt or love on memory at different ages or stages of development. Comparisons need to be made of the effects of depressive illnesses and of the more ordinary everyday depressions that most people experience. Bridges have to be built between autobiographical and experimental approaches, and nostalgia, which is so important in everyday life, might also be considered.

Any such work would perhaps be best achieved through an analysis of narrative and discourse in autobiographical memory over the life span. This would bring about a rapprochement between folk psychology and "scientific" psychology, which would give an area such as this increasing credibility. There has been sketchy experimentation and sketchy theorizing. The field is ripe for more intense investigation.

REFERENCES

Blaney, P. H. (1986). Affect and memory: A review. *Psychological Bulletin, 99,* 229–246.

Bower, G. H. (1987). Commentary on mood and memory. *Behavior Research and Therapy, 25,* 443–455.

Bower, G. H. (1992). How might emotions affect learning? In S. A. Christianson (Ed.), *Handbook of emotion and memory* (pp. 3–32). Hillsdale, NJ: Erlbaum.

Bretherton, I. (1993). From dialogue to internal working models: The co-construction of self in relationships. In C. A. Nelson (Ed.), *The Minnesota Symposia on Child Development* (Vol. 26, pp. 237–262). Hillsdale, NJ: Erlbaum.

British Psychological Society (1995). *Recorded memories. Report of the Working Party.* Exeter: B.P.S. Publications.

Brittlebank, A. D., Scott, J., Williams, J. M. G., & Ferrier, I. N. (1993). Autobiographical memory in depression: State or trait marker? *British Journal of Psychiatry, 162,* 118–121.

Brown, R., & Kulik, J. (1977). Flashbulb memories. *Cognition, 5,* 73–99.

Burke, A., Heuer, F., & Reisberg, D. (1992). Remembering emotional events. *Memory and Cognition, 20,* 277–290.

Burt, D. B., Zembar, M. J., & Niederehe, G. (1995). Depression and memory impairment: A meta-analysis of the association, its pattern, and specificity. *Psychological Bulletin, 117,* 286–305.

Cavanaugh, J. C. (1989). I have this feeling about everyday memory and aging. *Educational Gerontology, 15,* 597–605.

Ceci, S. J., & Bruck, M. (1986). Suggestibility of the child witness: A historical review and synthesis. *Psychological Bulletin, 113,* 403–439.

Fivush, R. (1993). Emotional content of parent–child conversations about the past. In C. A. Nelson (Ed.), *The Minnesota Symposia on Child Psychology* (Vol. 26, pp. 25–77). Hillsdale, NJ: Erlbaum.

Forgas, J. P., Burnham, D. K., & Trimboli, C. (1988). Mood, memory, and social judgments in children. *Journal of Personality and Social Psychology, 54,* 697–703.

Fry, P. S. (1991). Individual differences in reminiscence among older adults: Predictors of frequency and pleasantness ratings of reminiscence activity. *International Journal of Aging and Human Development, 33,* 311–326.

Howes, M., Siegel, M., & Brown, F. (1993). Early childhood memories: Accuracy and affect. *Cognition, 47,* 95–119.

Isen, A. M. (1987). Positive affect, cognitive processes, and social behavior. *Advances in Experimental Social Psychology, 20,* 203–253.

Leichtman, M. D., Ceci, S. J., & Ornstein, P. J. (1992). The influence of affect on memory: Mechanism and development. In S. A. Christianson (Ed.), *The handbook of emotion and memory research and theory.* Hillsdale, NJ: Erlbaum.

Lindsay, D. S., & Read, J. D. (1994). Psychotherapy and memories of childhood sexual abuse: A cognitive perspective. *Applied cognitive psychology, 8,* 281–338.

Manning, S. K., & Julian, L. (1975). Recall of emotional words. *Journal of General Psychology, 92,* 237–244.

Mathews, A., & MacLeod, C. (1994). Cognitive approaches to emotion and emotional disorders. *Annual Review of Psychology, 45,* 25–50.

Meltzer, H. (1930). The present status of experimental studies on the relationship of feeling to memory. *Psychological Review, 37,* 124–139.

Mills, M. A., & Coleman, P. G. (1994). Nostalgic memories in dementia: A case study. *International Journal of Aging and Human Development, 38,* 203–219.

Nelson, L. (1993). Events, narratives, memory: What develops? In C. A. Nelson (Ed.), *The Minnesota Symposia on Child Psychology (Vol. 26,* pp. 1–24). Hillsdale, NJ: Erlbaum.

O'Hara, M. W., Hinrichs, J. V., Kohout, F. J., Wallace, R. B., & Lemke, J. H. (1986). Memory complaint and memory performance in the depressed elderly. *Psychology and Aging, 1,* 208–214.

Peters, D. (1991). The influence of stress and arousal on the child witness. In J. Doris (Ed.), *The suggestibility of children's recollections* (pp. 60–70). Washington, DC: American Psychological Association.

Singer, J. A., & Salovey, P. (1993). *The remembered self: Emotion and memory in personality.* New York: The Free Press.

Terwogt, M. M., Schene, J., & Harris, P. (1986). Self-control of emotional reactions by young children. *Journal of Child Psychology and Psychiatry, 27,* 357–366.

Ucros, C. G. (1989). Mood state-dependent memory: A meta-analysis. *Cognition and emotion, 3,* 139–167.

Wong, P. T. P., & Watt, L. M. (1991). What types of reminiscence are associated with successful aging? *Psychology and Aging, 6,* 272–279.

Waldfogel, S. (1948). The frequency and affective character of childhood memories. *Psychological Monographs, 62,* Whole No. 291.

Webster, J. D. (1994). Predictors of reminiscence: A lifespan perspective. *Canadian Journal on Aging, 13,* 66–78.

Yang, J. A., & Rehm, L. P. (1993). A study of autobiographical memories in depressed and nondepressed elderly individuals. *International Journal of Aging and Human Development, 36,* 39–55.

CHAPTER 9

Emotion and Everyday Problem Solving in Adult Development

Fredda Blanchard-Fields
Department of Psychology
Georgia Institute of Technology
Atlanta, Georgia

I. INTRODUCTION

Although there is a rich and diverse literature on cognitive changes with aging, the understanding of the structure and functional impact of emotion–cognition relationships in adulthood and aging is only beginning to develop. The majority of studies on emotion–cognition relationships in the gerontological literature have focused on the extent to which empirically observed age differences in cognitive tasks reflect confounded age differences in arousal or affect, as opposed to being a function of age changes in basic cognitive processes (e.g., Kausler, 1990). For example, research has examined whether or not anxiety inhibits the use of more flexible decision criteria (Geen, 1985). In addition, the classic studies by Eisdorfer and colleagues (see Eisdorfer, 1968) argued that age differences in verbal learning could be an artifact of overarousal of older adults in test situations. Thus, the past literature reflects the fact that primary questions about the role of emotion in cognitive functioning and aging came primarily from those interested in cognitive processes. From this point of view, emotional constructs were really little more than nuisance factors representing possible confounding influences on studies designed to measure age changes in cognition.

Instead of viewing emotion as a separate domain of research or a "nuisance" variable in cognitive research, many researchers now have openly questioned whether emotion can be separated from cognition, either theoretically or empirically (e.g., Bower, 1981). Emotions represent an important influence on cognition in the laboratory and in everyday life (e.g., Bower, 1981; Labouvie-Vief, 1992; Sinnott, 1989). Of particular interest to this chapter is the role of emotion in the everyday reasoning of adults across the latter half of the life span.

There has been widespread interest in examining alternative conceptualizations of intelligence (i.e., practical intelligence), which take into account specific competencies associated with everyday problem solving that are not represented in traditional tests of intellectual ability (e.g., Cornelius & Caspi, 1987; Sternberg & Wagner, 1986). Many questions of central interest do not necessarily focus on normative changes in cognitive processing mechanisms per se, but on how individuals access and use information under particular kinds of situational demands. For example, one's beliefs about whether marriage should come before a career will influence a person's interpretation of everyday marital problems (e.g., attributions as to who or what caused the problem) and the subsequent strategies used to solve those problems.

Research on practical intelligence underscores the importance of explicitly emphasizing the study of cognition in actual everyday and social situations and a concern with psychosocial and affective components of reasoning. Social cognitive research that examines emotions in aging persons attempts to determine the extent to which the dynamic interaction between emotion and cognition either provides alternative models for understanding psychological reality or represents new belief systems that could influence adults' perceptions and behaviors.

II. CONCEPTUALIZATIONS OF EVERYDAY PROBLEM SOLVING IN A SOCIAL CONTEXT

The research on traditional problem solving and aging has been criticized in that the abstract tasks used lack ecological validity and ignore problems embedded in a social context. Problem situations in a social context are primarily ill structured and involve strategies that are highly dependent upon the particular context and individuals' life goals (Baltes, Dittmann-Kohli, & Dixon, 1984; Berg & Klaczynski, 1996). As a function of the social content inherent in these situations, ill-structured problems are unpredictable and are continually in transformation. The dynamic interplay of factors inherent in such problems produces ambiguity with respect to differing individual perspectives. Thus, individuals must generate their own interpretation of a problem situation rather than rely on the structure imposed by others. Not only are there multiple definitions of a problem space, but there are multiple alternative solutions to ill-structured problems. Each solution is potentially efficacious depending upon the compromises one is willing to make.

Current research utilizing this approach calls attention to the importance of emotions and other psychosocial factors involved in solving problems (Blanchard-Fields, Jahnke, & Camp, 1995; Meacham & Emont, 1989; Sinnott, 1989). For example, studies demonstrate that as adults grow older, their problem-solving goals become more concerned with other people, intimacy, and generativity (Sansone & Berg, 1993). In sum, the ill-structured and social nature of task structures tend to be more representative of problems encountered in everyday life. Before discussing the literature on age differences in this type of everyday problem solving, the problem-solving process itself needs to be specified.

A. The Problem-Solving Process

In order to select the appropriate strategies to solve everyday problem situations, the problem solver must first specify the set of conditions she or he perceives as needing a resolution. The problem solver must define the nature of the problem, which is reflected in specific goals set to achieve a desired outcome. Specific elements of this process can include (a) determining what caused the problem, (b) establishing the degree to which the individual has control over the cause and means to solve the problem, and (c) defining the important facets of the problem situation (e.g., pleasing others, eliminating obstacles, proving oneself). How the individual defines a problem has an impact on the strategies perceived to be effective, the desirability of these strategies, as well as the strategies actually selected to solve the problem (Berg & Calderone, 1994; Sinnott, 1989).

The majority of research examining developmental trajectories of problem-solving ability in adulthood have focused on strategy selection and problem-solving efficacy. However, there is a recent increase in studies examining developmental differences in problem interpretations and goals and how they relate to the selection of problem-solving strategies. These will be explored later. In general, the findings from studies examining developmental trajectories of the efficacy of everyday problem-solving strategies are less than consistent. These inconsistent findings may be explained within a contextual perspective on everyday problem solving and the variations in criteria used to judge problem-solving efficacy.

B. A Contextual Perspective on Everyday Problem Solving

A contextual perspective stresses the importance of considering how changing contextual demands influence how individuals appraise, interpret, and are motivated to employ specific strategies to solve a problem. Researchers suggest that successful problem solving can be conceived in a context of adaptive cognition where cognitive and affective functioning as well as physical characteristics of the environment interact or are embedded in cultural values, attitudes, and sociocultural institutions (Baltes et al., 1984; Labouvie-Vief, 1992). As a result, criteria unique to everyday problem solving in adulthood as a function of contextual demands need to be specified. For example, well-structured, single-criterion problems may be encountered frequently for youth in academic contexts. Thus, more traditional modes of problem solving are adaptive in this context. However, situations reflecting multiple criteria for potential solutions are more prominent in the problems of everyday living faced by older adults. There are several researchers who have attempted to specify these criteria from various theoretical perspectives.

For example, adaptive problem solving in an everyday context has been purported to entail (a) an awareness that the veracity of the solution to a particular problem is relative to differing perspectives and goals of the individual (Labouvie-Vief, 1992; Sinnott, 1989); (b) an awareness of the role of self in interpreting problems (Berg, Klaczynski, Calderone, & Strough, 1994; Labouvie-Vief, 1992); and (c) a recognition that logical reasoning is embedded in a sociocultural matrix (Labouvie-Vief, 1992; Meacham & Emont, 1989; Sebby & Papini, 1989). In other words, in order for an individual to exercise good judgment in problems reflecting uncertainty and ambiguity, she or he needs to take into consideration a contextual perspective. From this framework, effective problem solving in an everyday context involves an "openness" to perspectives and solutions in order to meet the adaptive demands of one's environment in addition to an organizational structure to maintain continuity. It also suggests an "openness" on the part of assessment criteria to take into consideration whether or not a problem-solving strategy is effective as a function of the demands of the environment and the goals of the problem solver in that particular context (e.g., Adams, 1991; Blanchard-Fields & Camp, 1990).

C. Criteria for Judging Problem-Solving Efficacy

The measures used most often in the problem-solving literature have been primarily quantitative in nature, such as the number of solutions generated, the number of steps to arrive at a solution, or the lack of redundancy in responding. In this case, both responses and criteria for efficacy of the solution have been generated by experimenters. It has been suggested by some that these types of measures may obscure qualitative differences inherent in the solutions themselves (Adams, 1991; Blanchard-Fields & Camp, 1990).

Another criteria for judging problem-solving efficacy captures the individual's own perspective on problem-solving competence. Individuals rate the efficacy of their own solutions. In this way, the criteria for problem-solving efficacy is determined by what the individual perceives to be effective given that she or he is living in the particular context in question. Along the same lines, researchers have used a criterion group of judges to determine problem-solving efficacy (e.g., individuals' solutions are compared to the ratings provided by adult judges). In essence, this approach provides a prototype (by means of the judges' efficacy ratings) of what is adaptive in a particular context. Solutions generated by participants in the study can be compared to this prototype. However, both self- or judge-perceived scales may be too global to delineate the qualitatively different form and content of an individual's solutions.

Until recently, relatively little effort has focused on the sensitivity of the dependent measures used to capture possible developmental differences in how the individual structures reality and approaches everyday problems. In this case, it is necessary to use problem-solving tasks requiring the individual to generate her or his own interpretation of the problem situation. This approach considers qualitative differences in the form and content of solutions. For example, scoring systems may assess the type of problem-solving strategy used in particular situations (e.g., problem-focused strategies, cognitive reevaluations, emotional regulation). By contrast, other scoring systems examine the development of relativistic thinking in problem solving, (i.e., the ability to consider and coordinate multiple perspectives in a problem situation). Embedded in these approaches is the assumption that one level of problem solving is invariably better than another. This not only requires further empirical support, it needs to be reconciled with the contextualist notion that superiority of a problem-solving strategy is relative to how adaptive it is given the particular demands of the context.

III. ADULT DEVELOPMENTAL DIFFERENCES IN PROBLEM SOLVING

In accordance with the varying criteria used to judge the efficacy of everyday problem-solving solutions, there are diverse findings as to the developmental trajectory of everyday problem solving in adulthood and aging (see Berg & Klaczynski, 1996 for a review). When quantitative criteria are used to assess age differences in adults' everyday problem solving, findings indicate that middle-aged adults outperform younger and older adults (who do not differ from each other) (Denney, 1989; Denney & Pearce, 1989). In this case, adults were asked to generate solutions for hypothetical practical problems (e.g., When you open the refrigerator up, you notice that it is not cold inside; but rather it is warm. What would you do?). Criteria for effective problem solving included number of "safe and effective" solutions as well as number of "self-initiated" solutions. Other studies have corroborated this finding in the areas of decision making with respect to automobile purchase (Hartley, 1989) and in problems using the criterion of experimenters' ratings of solution efficacy (Camp et al., 1989).

Other studies find no age differences in problem-solving efficacy or demonstrate older adults' adeptness in solving everyday problems (Berg et al., 1994; Sinnott, 1989). For example, when comparing criteria used for determining problem-solving efficacy, younger and older adults differed on type of strategy used to solve everyday problems, yet age groups did not differ in perceived effectiveness of their strategies (Berg et al., 1994; Camp et al., 1989).

Studies that have found progression in problem-solving efficacy with age have used criteria such as comparison to the performance of a group of adult judges. For example, Cornelius and Caspi (1987) assessed practical problem solving in everyday situations including home management, interpersonal conflicts, conflicts with co-workers, home management, and so on. Effective performance on their problem-solving inventory increased with age, whereas performance on more traditional problem-solving tasks declined after middle age. Other studies demonstrating progression in problem-solving effectiveness assessed qualitative differences in problem-solving strategy as indexed by level of cognitive maturity (e.g., flexibility in responding, complexity of problem interpretation, mature vs. defensive strategies) (Blanchard-Fields & Irion, 1988a; Diehl, Coyle, & Labouvie-Vief, 1994). For example, youths engaged in self-blame when responding to a stressor, and, thus dealt with this blame by avoiding the situation or by hostilely reacting toward the situation (Blanchard-Fields & Irion, 1988b). On the other hand, older adults perceived the source of stress as located within the self resulting in conscious, reflective appraisal. Similarly, other researchers found that young adults blame a stressful outcome on others or circumstances in the environment and do not take personal responsibility for the role they played in a stressful conflict. With maturity, older adults consciously reflect and appraise each stressful situation and make a decision or evaluation on the basis of autonomous standards and values (Labouvie-Vief, Hakim-Larson, & Hobart, 1987).

Finally, Blanchard-Fields and Camp (1990) examined age differences in the use of qualitatively different strategies as a function of the type of problem-solving domain (e.g., family, relationship, consumer problems). They found different styles of problem solving in adolescence through older adulthood. There were no age differences in problem-solving style for consumer and home-management domains. In addition, all age groups tended to use more direct problem-focused strategies (i.e., confronting and fixing the problem at hand). Older adults produced more strategies such as passively accepting the situation at hand or avoiding direct confrontation more often than younger age groups. However, they reported these strategies more so in domains involving interpersonal conflict with family or friends. By contrast, younger adults adopted more of a problem-focused or cognitive analytic approach to all problems. It appears that older adults evinced an awareness of when to avoid or passively accept a situation within interpersonal domains as compared to more instrumental problem domains (e.g., consumer matters) (Blanchard-Fields & Camp, 1990). Perhaps older adults engage in a more differentiated approach to problem situations in that they use diverse strategies in dealing with problems depending upon the type of situation.

In sum, it appears that problem-solving efficacy in older adults is influenced by (a) the criteria employed (i.e., qualitative vs. quantitative, self-perceived vs. experimenter-perceived efficacy), (b) the problem-solving domain (e.g., instrumental vs. interpersonal), and (c) mediating factors such as personal relevance and emotional salience. I now address these mediating factors, and in particular, explore older adults' problem-solving effectiveness in more emotionally salient and interpersonal contexts.

IV. THE ROLE OF EMOTION IN EVERYDAY PROBLEM SOLVING

One of the defining characteristics of everyday problem solving is its interpersonal nature. In this domain, age differences in strategy preference are most evident. Studies suggest that older adults interpret everyday problems differently than younger adults in that they focus on interpersonal concerns of the problem (e.g., Sinnott, 1989). Given the inherent ambiguity in interpersonal problem situations, some propose that mature thinking involves the redefinition of the problem space by accepting inherent uncertainties and resolving them (e.g., Arlin, 1984). Similarly, other researchers suggest that this interpretive process in adulthood is characterized by increased awareness of self as interpreter or the ability to consider multiple perspectives in reasoning tasks of an interpersonal nature and high emotional salience (Berg et al., 1994; Blanchard-Fields, 1986, 1994; Labouvie-Vief, 1984).

A focus on interpersonal and/or social problem solving suggests a number of ways in which problem solving and emotion are related. For example, Showers and Cantor (1985) discussed how mood states direct decision-making strategies and the importance of the role emotion plays in how the individual construes a problem space. This, in turn, affects problem-solving strategy preference. They stressed the need to examine both the emotional and cognitive aspects of the individual in constructing multiple interpretations of the problem definition.

The role of emotion in everyday problem solving can be explored at many different levels. These are exemplified in research suggesting that (a) as adults grow older, they are better able to integrate both emotional and cognitive aspects of reality (Labouvie-Vief, 1992); (b) goals related to the importance of emotion regulation change from childhood to adulthood (Carstensen, 1992; Lawton, Kleban, Rajagopal, & Dean, 1992); (c) emotional well-being is an important outcome of everyday problem solving (Spivack, Platt, & Shure, 1976); or (d) that emotional salience influences problem-solving strategy selection (Blanchard-Fields et al., 1995; Prohaska, Leventhal, Leventhal, & Keller, 1985).

From a developmental perspective, changes in adult reasoning can reflect an integration and consistency in reasoning across cognitive and affective domains. For example, Blanchard-Fields (1986) found that adolescents resolved interpretive discrepancies in interpersonal dilemmas low in emotional salience as well as younger and middle-aged adults. However, for emotionally salient problems, adolescents were less effective at deriving good resolutions or unbiased interpretations than their adult counterparts. It appears that with increasing cognitive maturity, affective content may pose less of a disruption on cognitive performance. Other studies suggest that the coordination of cognition and affect represents a critical element in further progression in adult development. For example, Kramer (1990) demonstrated that older adults with high affective intensity demonstrate more dialectical thinking. Higher levels of ego maturity involving emotional regulation and openness to affective experience are found to relate to more mature coping mechanisms and social cognitive reasoning (Blanchard-Fields, 1986; Labouvie-Vief et al., 1987). Older adults are found to be more effective in regulating their emotions (Labouvie-Vief et al., 1987; Lawton et al., 1992). Finally, Folkman and Lazarus (1988) demonstrated that emotional salience plays an important role in age differences in coping with stress. These studies suggest that there are qualitative changes in the ways individuals perceive and structure everyday problems, and increased efficacy in regulating affective responses with increasing age.

A. Problem Interpretation and Goals

As noted earlier, the goals of older adults in problem situations focus more on interpersonal and emotional concerns. Carstensen (1992) found that older adults place a greater value on quality of relationships and, thus, intensify intimacy with a limited few. Similarly, Sansone and Berg (1993) found that adults have more interpersonal goals than children and focus on the importance of regulating affect. As noted above, older adults tend to have goals related to the regulation of affect (Lawton et al., 1992).

It seems, then, that there are multiple potential influences of emotion on construction of the problem space in everyday problem solving (e.g., awareness of emotions in self, cognitive representations of emotions, cognitive appraisal, affect intensity changes). In addition, the relationship between emotion and problem representation may change both quantitatively and qualitatively across the life span. Consistent with this reasoning I have conducted a program of research examining age differences in causal attributions from adolescence through older adulthood. The area of causal attributions provides a task domain where ill-structured or ambiguous tasks are the norm, thus, taking into account how an individual structures an everyday problem-solving situation. The social psychology literature is replete with examples of attributional biases made by college-age students in these situations (Kelley & Michela, 1980; Nisbett & Ross, 1980). These biases occur as a function of the outcome valence of the situation (e.g., high versus low emotionality); the degree of ambiguity of social information given about causal factors; controllability of the situation, and more.

It is of primary interest to delineate and validate the idea of adaptive cognition in adulthood as characterized by a change in causal attributions. Adaptive cognition is, for the purposes of this research, reflected in the ability to engage in a relativistic approach (i.e., coordinating multiple factors of causation) when making causal attributions. Of particular interest here is how relativistic causal attributions are influenced by the emotional salience of situations. For example, do individuals confronted with an emotionally laden context, such as a relationship dilemma, display more or less relativistic causal attributions, and is this related to age differences?

In several studies, my colleagues and I found that when situations were ambiguous with respect to the causal factors of an event outcome

and reflected negative, interpersonal content, older adults made more interactive attributions (i.e., viewing the cause of an event as a combination
of external and internal causes) than younger adults (Blanchard-Fields,
1994; Blanchard-Fields & Norris, 1994). However, older adults also attributed blame to the primary protagonist more than younger age groups,
again, primarily in negative relationship situations. The increase in interactive attributions reflects a relativistic orientation (i.e., the ability to
perceive and coordinate multiple perspectives), which in the adult development literature is considered a more mature form of thinking (Kramer,
Kahlbaugh, & Goldston, 1992; Labouvie-Vief, 1992). However, the greater
use of dispositional attributions by older adults suggests that, in some
cases, they also overemphasized dispositional information. To further
examine this issue, Blanchard-Fields and Norris (1994) examined dialectical attributional processing in adolescence through older adulthood using a qualitative analysis. They found that middle-age adults
scored higher on dialectical attributional reasoning (considering dispositional and situational factors in relation to each other, mutually determined and codefined) than adolescents, youth, and younger and older
adults. However, older adults and adolescents scored lowest on dialectical reasoning.

In order to explain why older adults were (a) more predisposed to
making the dispositional attributions and (b) engaged in less dialectical
reasoning in negative relationship situations, the socioemotional content
of the experimental stimuli (negative relationship vignettes) was examined further. It was hypothesized that the pattern of responding on the
part of older adults was driven by social schemas evoked by the particular vignettes' content. Research suggests that schemas representing past
situational experiences and social knowledge structures influence the
causal inferences made about situations or events (Bargh, 1989; Fiske, &
Pavelchak, 1986). Over the life span, life experiences and social knowledge are accumulated and provide well-instantiated processes whereby problem interpretations are invoked. It may be the case that social
schemas were evoked in the above studies as a function of the value-
laden content of several of the vignettes. Such social schemas may have
been particularly salient for older adults given their experience, life
stage, and cohort.

This hypothesis was corroborated when we reexamined the qualitative essays written on emotionally salient vignettes. The events involving a
husband who "works too much" and a love triangle, in particular, evoked
emotionally laden attitudes amongst individuals ranging in age from 15
to 68 years of age. For example, older adults, and older women in particular, strongly endorsed the schema, "a marriage comes first before one's
career," compared to the other age groups. For the vignette involving a

youthful marriage, the schemas "parents should have talked not pro-voked the young couple" and "they were too young and got lucky" dis-played a curvilinear relationship with age. It is also interesting to note that the "relationship rule" as to when one is too young to marry was conceptually linked to the attribution "they got lucky." This illustrates the premise that schemas are conceptually linked and evoke particular types of attributions. It appears that affectively laden values were evoked from these vignettes, and in turn, could have influenced attributional assessment. Thus, greater dispositional attributions and less dialectical thinking may be, in part, a result of the activation of relationship and role-related schemas associated with particular vignettes. Dialectical rea-soning (e.g., considering multiple perspectives) could have been sup-pressed given the strong influence of an individual's causal schemas as-sociated with a particular event. More research is needed to validate this assumption.

This research suggests an important relationship between cognitive appraisal and emotion. Along this line, research finds that emotions are associated with distinctive patterns of cognitive appraisal (Manstead & Tetlock, 1989; Smith & Ellsworth, 1985). Recent research has examined this relationship from a developmental perspective. For example, Weiner and Graham (1989) found elicited affect mediated the relationship be-tween perceptions of causal control over a problem situation and an in-tended helping behavior. They concluded that linkages between emo-tion, thinking, and behavior remain stable in healthy older adults.

Blanchard-Fields and Norris (1994) examined causal attributions as a function of the emotional salience of problem situations. In order to examine the issue of emotional salience, they had respondents ranging in age from adolescents to older adulthood rate each vignette in terms of how emotionally salient the situation was for them (in addition to the at-tribution ratings described earlier). Vignettes were separated into three levels of emotional salience: high, medium, and low. They then exam-ined age group differences on the relativistic rating measures as a func-tion of level of emotional salience. Although adolescents were lower on relativistic ratings overall, these differences were primarily a function of the level of emotional salience (i.e., adolescents scored lower on interac-tive attributions only for medium and high levels of emotional salience).

B. The Influence of Emotion on Problem-Solving Strategy Selection and Efficacy

It is important to consider the role of emotion in how an individual construes a problem, and, in turn, adopts a problem-solving strategy. For example, Weiner and Graham (1989) found that emotions rather than thoughts are the main direct determinant of action. Similarly, Folkman and Lazarus (1988) found a relationship between elicited emotion and intended action (i.e., coping). Different styles of coping were associated with changes in types of emotions. Age differences revealed that younger adults' use of positive reappraisal was related to a decrease in feelings of disgust and anger and an increase in pleasure and confidence. Older adults' use of positive reappraisal was associated with an increase in worry and fear. Young adults' use of confrontive coping was associated with lower levels of anger and disgust, but it was not related to either positive or negative emotions in older adults. They argued that older adults could be more temperate when dealing with negative emotional affect.

In a recent study, we directly examined the emotional salience of problems (ranging from high to medium to low) as a determinant of the degree to which adolescents through older adults produced particular problem-solving strategies (Blanchard-Fields et al., 1995). In low and high emotionally salient situations, there were no age differences in the use of instrumental and proactive problem-solving strategies (i.e., directly confronting a problem situation and implementing a particular strategy). However, in high emotionally salient situations, older adults endorsed more passive-dependent and avoidant strategies than either young or middle-aged adults. These findings tend to support the premise that older adults' responses are related to the emotional impact of the problem situation encountered. Older adults, like young and middle-aged adults, used more problem-focused strategies in less emotionally salient and more instrumental task situations (e.g., returning defective merchandise). When the situations were higher in emotional salience (e.g., moving to a new town, taking care of an older parent) older adults used more emotion-regulating strategies (e.g., suppressing emotions, not trying to alter an uncontrollable situation). Again, this relates back to the research demonstrating that older adults are better able to regulate negative affect in life situations (Carstensen, 1992; Lawton et al., 1992). Similarly, older adults have been shown to use more emotion-focused strategies when problem situations are appraised as uncontrollable (Blanchard-Fields & Irion, 1988b; Labouvie-Vief et al., 1987).

V. CONCLUSIONS, IMPLICATIONS, AND FUTURE DIRECTIONS

The research reviewed in this chapter suggests that affect plays an important role in everyday problem solving. In fact, adult developmental differences were amplified in emotionally laden problem contexts. It was shown that affect directs and is directed by interpretation and representation of the problem situation. In turn, the nature of this process affects problem-solving strategy selection. This underscores the need to examine the emotional and cognitive interface when individuals construct interpretations of social situations, or a problem space. It was also shown that older adults may have greater flexibility in responding to situations high in emotional salience. Similarly, the social cognition literature suggests that social intelligence involves the ability to construct multiple alternatives of a situation and use affective appraisal and emotional regulation as coping mechanisms, thus, allowing flexibility in adapting old strategies and learning new strategies (Cantor & Kihlstrom, 1989).

Despite the mounting research on emotion and everyday problem solving, there are still many areas that need further elaboration and examination. The existing evidence for changes in adulthood in affect intensity, the use of affective appraisal, the social knowledge base, and emotional regulation stress the importance for future research to examine everyday problem solving within an emotional context. Future research on developmental changes in emotional intensity as well as emotional understanding are needed given that these changes result in differences in problem-solving interpretation and strategy preferences. In addition to manipulating the emotional salience of a situation, it would be useful to focus on the individual's phenomenological experience of emotion (i.e., an analysis of the current level of functioning of emotional self-experience from early to later adulthood).

The study of causal attributions and problem appraisal is an important avenue in assessing the relationship between emotion and everyday problem solving. Much of the activity involved in everyday problem solving involves understanding causes of outcomes and/or evaluating the controllability of managing outcomes. Whether it be life tasks or social schemas, there is a need to link social or everyday problem solving solutions to individual differences in emotional and motivational appraisal.

Finally, when examining domains high in emotional saliency, ambiguity, and ecological validity, progressive changes in the developing adult are more likely to be documented, and these changes seem to be related to qualitative differences in the way the individual perceives and structures everyday problems. In contrast, studies examining problem solving in relatively abstract, low emotionally salient tasks demonstrate decreasing problem-solving ability with increasing age. It is important to consider both research perspectives to gain a more complete picture of developmental variation in problem-solving ability. Developmental differences with respect to gains and losses can exist concurrently, and in a complementary fashion (Baltes, 1987).

ACKNOWLEDGMENTS

Some of the research reported in this chapter was supported by National Institute on Aging research grant AG-7607 awarded to Fredda Blanchard-Fields.

REFERENCES

Adams, C. (1991). Qualitative age differences in memory for text: A life-span developmental perspective. *Psychology and Aging, 6,* 323–336.

Arlin, P. (1984). Adolescent and adult thought: A structural interpretation. In M. L. Commons, F. Richards, & C. Armon (Eds.), *Beyond formal operations* (pp. 258–271). New York: Praeger.

Baltes, P. B. (1987). Theoretical propositions of life-span developmental psychology: On the dynamics between growth and decline. *Developmental Psychology, 23,* 611–626.

Baltes, P. B., Dittmann-Kohli, F., & Dixon, R. A. (1984). New perspectives on the development of intelligence in adulthood: Toward a dual-process conception and a model of selective optimization with compensation. In P. B. Baltes & O. G. Brim (Eds.), *Life-span development and behavior* (vol. 6, pp. 33–76). New York: Academic Press.

Bargh, J. A. (1989). Conditional automaticity: Varieties of automatic influence in social perception and cognition. In J. S. Uleman & J. A. Bargh (Eds.), *Unintended thought: Causes and consequences for judgment, emotion, and behavior* (pp. 3–51). New York: Guilford.

Berg, C. A., & Calderone, K. (1994). The role of problem interpretations in understanding the development of everyday problem solving. In R. J. Sternberg & R. K. Wagner (Eds.), *Mind in context: Interactionist perspectives on human intelligence* (pp. 105–132). New York: Cambridge University Press.

Berg, C. A., & Klaczynski, P. (1996). Practical intelligence and problem solving: Searching for perspectives. In F. Blanchard-Fields & T. Hess (Eds.), *Perspectives on cognitive change in adulthood and aging* (pp. 323–357). New York: McGraw-Hill.

Berg, C., Klaczynski, P., Calderone, K., & Strough, J. (1994). Adult age differences in cognitive strategies: Adaptive or deficient? In J. Sinnott (Ed.), *Handbook of adult lifespan learning* (pp. 371–388). Westport, CT: Greenwood.

Blanchard-Fields, F. (1986). Reasoning on social dilemmas varying in emotional saliency: An adult developmental perspective. *Psychology and Aging, 1,* 325–333.

Blanchard-Fields, F. (1994). Age differences in causal attributions from an adult developmental perspective. *Journal of Gerontology: Psychological Sciences, 49,* P43–P51.

Blanchard-Fields, F., & Camp, C. J. (1990). Affect, individual differences, and real world problem solving across the adult life span. In T. Hess (Ed.), *Aging and cognition: Knowledge organization and utilization* (pp. 461–497). Amsterdam: North Holland.

Blanchard-Fields, F., & Irion, J. (1988a). Coping strategies from the perspective of two developmental markers: Age and social reasoning. *Journal of Genetic Psychology, 149,* 141–152.

Blanchard-Fields, F., & Irion, J. (1988b). The relation between locus of control and coping in two contexts: Age as a moderator variable. *Psychology and Aging, 3,* 197–203.

Blanchard-Fields, F., Jahnke, H., & Camp, C. (1995). Age differences in problem solving style: The role of emotional salience. *Psychology and Aging, 10,* 173–180.

Blanchard-Fields, F., & Norris, L. (1994). Causal attributions from adolescence through adulthood: Age differences, ego level, and generalized response style. *Aging and Cognition, 1,* 67–86.

Bower, G. H. (1981). Mood and memory. *American Psychologist, 36,* 129–148.

Camp, C. J., Doherty, K, Moody-Thomas, S., & Denney, N. W. (1989). Practical problem solving in adults: A comparison of problem types and scoring methods. In J. D. Sinnott (Ed.), *Everyday problem solving: Theory and applications* (pp. 211–228). New York: Praeger.

Cantor, N., & Kihlstrom, J. F. (1989). Social intelligence and cognitive assessments of personality. In R. Wyer & T. Srull (Eds.), *Advances in social cognition* (vol. 2, pp. 1–60). Hillsdale, NJ: Erlbaum.

Carstensen, L. L. (1992). Selectivity theory: Social activity in life-span context *Annual Review of Gerontology and Geriatrics, 11,* 195–217.

Cornelius, S. W., & Caspi, A. (1987). Everyday problem solving in adulthood and old age. *Psychology and Aging, 2,* 144–153.

Denney, N. W. (1989). Everyday problem-solving: Methodological issues, research findings and a model. In L. W. Poon, D. C. Rubin, & B. A. Wilson (Eds.), *Everyday cognition in adulthood and later life* (pp. 330–351). New York: Cambridge Press.

Denney, N. W., & Pearce, K. A. (1989). A developmental study of practical problem solving in adults. *Psychology and Aging, 4,* 432–442.

Diehl, M., Coyle, N., & Labouvie-Vief, G. (1994). *Age and gender differences in strategies of coping and defense across the life span.* Unpublished manuscript.

Eisdorfer, C. (1968). Arousal and performance: Experiments in verbal learning and a tentative theory. In G. Talland (Ed.), *Human behavior and aging: Recent advances in research and theory* (pp. 189–216). New York: Academic Press.

Fiske, S. T., & Pavelchak, M. A. (1986). Category-based versus piecemeal-based affective responses: Developments in schema-triggered affect. In R. M. Sorrentino & E. T. Higgins (Eds.), *Handbook of motivation and cognition: Foundations of social behavior* (pp. 167–203). New York: Guilford Press.

Folkman, S., & Lazarus, R. (1988). Coping as a mediator of emotion. *Journal of Personality and Social Psychology, 54,* 466–475.

Geen, R. G. (1985). Test anxiety and visual vigilance. *Journal of Personality and Social Psychology, 49,* 963–970.

Hartley, A. A. (1989). The cognitive ecology of problem solving. In L. W. Poon, D. C. Rubin, & B. A. Wilson (Eds.), *Everyday cognition in adulthood and late life* (pp. 300–329). New York: Cambridge University Press.

Kausler, D. (1990). Motivation, human aging, and cognitive performance. In J. E. Birren & K. W. Schaie (Eds.), *Handbook of the psychology of aging* (3rd ed.) (pp. 171–182). New York: Academic Press.

Kelley, H. H., & Michela, J. L. (1980). Attribution theory and research. *Annual Review of Psychology, 31,* 457–501.

Kramer, D. A. (1990). Conceptualizing wisdom: The primacy of affect-cognition relations. In R. Sternberg (Ed.), *Wisdom: Its nature, origins, and development* (pp. 279–316). Cambridge, UK: Cambridge University Press.

Kramer, D. A., Kahlbaugh, P. E., & Goldston, R. B. (1992). A measure of paradigm beliefs about the social world. *Journal of Gerontology, 47,* 180–189.

Labouvie-Vief, G. (1984). Logic and self-regulation from youth to maturity. In M. Commons, F. Richards, & C. Armon (Eds.), *Beyond formal operations* (pp. 158–179). New York: Praeger.

Labouvie-Vief, G. (1992). A neo-Piagetian perspective on adult cognitive development. In R. J. Sternberg & C. A. Berg (Eds.), *Intellectual development* (pp. 52–86). New York: Cambridge University Press.

Labouvie-Vief, G., Hakim-Larson, J., & Hobart, C. J. (1987). Age, ego level, and the life-span development of coping and defense processes. *Psychology and Aging, 2,* 286–293.

Lawton, M. P., Kleban, M. H., Rajagopal, D., & Dean, J. (1992). Dimensions of affective experience in three age groups. *Psychology and Aging, 7,* 171–184.

Manstead, A. S. R., & Tetlock, P. E. (1989). Cognitive appraisals and emotional experience: Further evidence. *Cognition and Emotion, 3,* 225–240.

Meacham, J., & Emont, N. (1989). The interpersonal basis of everyday problem solving. In J. D. Sinnott (Ed.), *Everyday problem solving: Theory and applications* (pp. 7–23). New York: Praeger.

Nisbett, R., & Ross, L. (1980). *Human inference: Strategies and shortcomings of social judgment.* Englewood Cliffs, NJ: Prentice-Hall, Inc.

Prohaska, T. R., Leventhal, E. A., Leventhal, H., & Keller, M. L. (1985). Health practices and illness cognition in young, middle-aged, and elderly adults. *Journal of Gerontology, 40,* 569–578.

Sansone, C., & Berg, C. A. (1993). Adapting to the environment across the life span: Different process or different inputs? *International Journal of Behavioral Development, 16,* 215–241.

Sebby, R., & Papini, D. (1989). Problems in everyday problem solving research: A framework for conceptualizing solutions to everyday problems. In J. D. Sinnott (Ed.), *Everyday problem solving: Theory and applications* (pp. 55–71). New York: Praeger.

Showers, C., & Cantor, N. (1985). Social cognition: A look at motivated strategies. In M. Rosenzweig & L. W. Porter (Eds.), *Annual review of psychology* (vol. 36, pp. 275–305). Palo Alto, CA: Annual Reviews.

Sinnott, J. (1989). *Everyday problem solving: Theory and applications.* New York: Praeger.

Smith, C. A., & Ellsworth, P. C. (1985). Patterns of cognitive appraisal in emotion. *Journal of Personality and Social Psychology, 48,* 813–838.

Spivack, G., Platt, J., & Shure, M. (1976). *The problem-solving approach to adjustment.* San Francisco: Jossey-Bass.

Sternberg, R. J., & Wagner, R. K. (Eds.). (1986). *Practical intelligence.* New York: Cambridge University Press.

Wiener, B., & Graham, S. (1989). Understanding the motivational role of affect: Life-span research from an attributional perspective. *Cognition and Emotion, 3,* 401–419.

CHAPTER 10

Emotion in the Construction of Autobiography

Jan-Erik Ruth *and* Anni Vilkko
Department of Social Policy
University of Helsinki
Helsinki, Finland

I. INTRODUCTION

In this chapter we will discuss the life lived, and also life as experienced and narrated, and how these interact in the construction of a life story. We also discuss the origin of emotions (i.e., the expressive, reflective, and reevaluative nature of emotions in personal accounts). A theoretical postulate in the discussion is the intersubjective nature of emotions: that it is possible for the reader of narratives to detect and to understand emotional expressions based on cultural communality of reaction. The presentation focuses on how the collective subjectivity is reflected in gender- and class-specific narratives as well as in accounts from different periods of life. How emotions can be regulated by the use of symbolic expressions or expressions from the cultural repertory is also discussed.

II. THE "SELF" AND "EMOTION" AS NARRATIVE CONSTRUCTS

We tend to understand our lives as if they were stories, and in the events and episodes of a life as well as in life stories the narrating self can be seen (Bruner, 1990). Hence, a life story is not only a reflection of the life course, but also of the personality features of the narrator. This leads us to presume that narrators differ substantially in the emotionality their narrating selves convey. Lives differ as to the episodes they contain and persons differ in the significance they ascribe to their life events. Self-reflective judgments are especially sensitive to emotions where narrators' self-esteem and their beliefs about their abilities are concerned (Singer & Salovey, 1993).

Narration is a verbal construction, however, and there is considerable freedom for the narrator to choose what to present and what to conceal in accounts of life. The picture we get of the development of the narrating self through the life is thus quite selective: some episodes can be omitted or their relevance denied, some others may be given a considerable significance and they may appear repeatedly in the life story. Furthermore, several stories can be created and re-created about a life, all out of the needs of the self at the moment of narration (Kenyon, 1996).

The concept of emotion in narrative research is conceived in quite a broad way, in contrast to the usual psychologically narrow descriptions of emotions as temporary states. Mader (1996) has eloquently depicted emotion in narrative research as "similar to language, a process disposition with its own intentionality directed towards values and a valued future. It is experienced as a psycho-physical subjectivity (such as pleasure vs. displeasure, tension vs. release, calm vs. excitation) and it includes a cultural structure" (Mader, 1996, p. 47). Mader further described emotionality as a sense of balance or a social sonar for positioning persons in the power field of cultural expectations, norms, and values. Emotion seems to be tightly bound with memory. "The experience of emotion changes the way individuals organize information about and evaluate the self" (Singer & Salovey, 1993, p. 131). The narrative approach to understanding emotions has been advocated because "emotion is not just part of the story, it is the story" (Wood, 1986, p. 206, see also Sarbin, 1986).

The emotional episodes in people's accounts of life are often quite extended in time, one example being the feelings of abandonment, anger, and inadequacy after a divorce or of grief after the loss of a loved one. These emotional episodes can go on for several years (Averill, 1988, Magai & McFadden, 1995). Emotions are used by the self for self-regulating as well as self-supporting processes, and through a continuous appraisal of relevance and context the meaning ascribed to life events may change through time (Carstensen, 1991; Mader, 1995). The feelings of inadequacy instigated by a divorce proceeding may later be replaced by self-assurance and satisfaction over the self's power to make seminal decisions that can turn the troubled life around. Looking back, it is impossible to say which of these two emotional states tied to the same life situation should be considered "the right" or "the true one."

Autobiographical remembering is a cognitive process where the possibility of aroused emotional states is always present. As in therapy, the act of putting the disparate experiences into words and creating a coherent plot out of them adds to the personal understanding of the emotional content of life episodes (Polkinghorne, 1991, 1996). The remembered life events act as inner triggers for emotions, emotions that are relived and reexperienced. Personally important, unique, and emotional life events constitute events that will be significantly better remembered (Cohen, 1993). But emotions can also acquire a new emotional content if the events are reevaluated out of later biographical insights (Crawford, Kippax, Onyx, Gault, & Benton, 1992). Recollections and judgments are likely to be thematically congruent with the narrator's mood states while reflecting on their lives (Singer & Salovey, 1993).

The act of telling or writing about one's life also elicits emotional states that are partly dependent on outer triggers, such as the presumed listener or reader. The situation or the social context in which the remembered event is expressed is a third factor that will affect emotional content. It has been shown that the type of discourse in reminiscence groups is essential for the way the self will be constructed and presented as well as for the interpretation of the emotional meaning of life events (Buchanan & Middleton, 1993; Saarenheimo, 1994).

Reminiscing and narrating episodes of one's life or telling one's whole life story is affected by language as well as the social conventions guiding discourse. This context also affects the variability of the emotions that can be described (Wood, 1986). The reciprocal act of telling and listening also have an impact on how the emotions will be transposed or transfered (Cohler & Cole, 1996).

When we use biographical methods, we are interested in precisely these subjective interpretations and reinterpretations, the individual meaning-giving process of life episodes, the experience of growing and aging, the social construction of the self, and the discourse by which emotional states are produced as well as the reciprocal act of telling and listening (Ruth & Kenyon, 1996).

III. THE COLLECTIVE SUBJECTIVITY OF GENDER AND CLASS

The collective subjectivity in many stories can form patterns that differentiate groups according to gender, class, cohort, geographical area, or the historical time period under which the narrators construct their stories. Comparisons can be made based on the diverging ways of constructing and telling life themes (Ruth & Birren, 1995). In this chapter, the emotional tone in life stories is tied to gender and class issues; in addition, overarching life themes will be addressed by examples from recent research. The narrative data presented in what follows is based on the Finnish study, "The Way of Life, Aging and Well-Being" by Jan-Erik Ruth and Peter Öberg (1992, 1996) and two works on women's autobiographies by Anni Vilkko (1994a,b).

We can ask whether there are gender-specific patterns revealed in emotional content of telling about one's life. The question seems to get an affirmative answer in narratives. The female narrator shows a "relational self" with constant reference to significant others. Women often use "we" instead of "I" when describing how their lives evolved and often also describe themselves as objects rather than subjects in their lives. The women of the cohort of "the wars and the Depression" (Roos, 1985) were socialized into a caretaking and emotional leader role, and their narrational selves are more personal and intimate than those of the men (see also Miller, 1991).

In many of the life stories of men, a more proactive self can be seen, a self that is socialized to the provider and careerist role and which in some instances look much more like curricula vitae:

"I would say that the chief architect (of my life) is myself."
"Even from our republic's point of view I must have made a difference."

The above might constitute a general rule, but there are many exceptions. Male narrators who coped well and whose lives developed as they wished also very readily put themselves in charge of how their lives developed and they often refrained from mentioning life projects that did not succeed as well. Men who had lost a grip on life, or those who never had the feeling of inner control, took a less active and assertive but sometimes even more emotionally charged position:

"This [life] has not turned out as I wished. Like that bitch, damn it, that was a big mistake! . . . because our daughter was on her way."
"Nobody is the master of one's own fate."

The class dimension of the narration is clearly visible, even overriding the above-mentioned gender differences. When the "collective subjectivity" of class is expressed, it is often very vividly accounted for as well as highly emotionally charged. The emotional tone and the linguistic and expressive style are central characteristics when coding for class themes in narratives. This is true for women as well as men. This can be seen in the accounts of two women from the working class:

"We who moved into cities from the country, the victims of rural depopulation and change, we were put down. We were exploited. . . . We were crushed. "'Housewife'? Nay, they never called us bitches that then."

Two upper-class men express themselves in quite a different way. The accounts may be as filled with emotion as in the above-mentioned examples from the working class but the expressional style is quite different:

"What do I remember from my childhood? Sunny days, like all kids do."
"My life has been so colorful and rewarding . . . so filled with important things to do. My wife was so wonderful, so blessed, so gifted, gave me six super-gifted children." (Ruth & Öberg, 1992, 1996).

IV. CONTINUITY AND DISCONTINUITY OF EMOTION IN LIFE STORIES

When looking for overarching life themes in narratives, the emotional tone and its continuity versus discontinuity in the life stories might constitute a fruitful dimension for analysis. The Finnish study (Ruth & Öberg, 1992, 1996) produced six different lifestyles of the aged: four showed continuity concerning the emotional tone of the narration, whereas two patterns of life were characterized by discontinuity. Four of the patterns of life were characterized by more or less positive accounts, whereas two resulted in problematic and dysfunctional old age.

In **the bitter life,** hardships, emotional problems, and illness were described from childhood, to middle age, to old age. The future was described as continuously problematic:

"It was just a struggle for survival, there was no choice."
"My life has just been mistakes, it has been so petty that it has been nothing."
"I suppose it [the future] is a stroke. . . . The neighbors won't notice until weeks after and they'll find me with black flies in the window."

The same continuity could be found in the opposite pattern: **the sweet life.** The "sunny days" from childhood persisted and life turned out to be a sweet dream. If there were problems, they were not stressed, but what was stressed was how they were overcome. Old age was rewarding and the future seemed bright:

"In my heart I feel that every day is a joy."
"When I look at others of my age I think, oh dear, you haven't taken your vitamin C. . . . You won't keep in good shape, as I do."
"I am not bitter, like so many others. I still laugh very easily."

Emotional continuity was also expressed in ways of **life as a job career,** typical of well-educated males, and **the devoted, silenced life,** typical of some working- and middle-class women.

In **life as a trapping pit** and **life as a hurdle race** the emotional tone in the narratives from childhood and youth changed rather dramatically when the respondents approached maturity and old age. For the former, accumulated negative turning points in life formed "trapping pits" where coping was not successful, control of life was gradually lost, and emotional problems accumulated. Old age turned into the most miserable period of life:

> *"I see an old woman who could have taken better care of herself. Now the mirror only makes me feel bad that I'm so old."*

For the type of **life as a hurdle race,** problems created by loss of father or husband because of the wars or economic hardships in youth caused by the Depression were gradually overcome. By never giving up, these fighters became the heroes of their own lives. They regained control over life, and with more fulfilling human relationships (e.g., after the death of a violent spouse) old age finally constituted the prime time of life:

> *"When he [the husband] died I felt like a big dictator had died. I felt like a bird turned free from the cage."*
> *"This is the best time of life, if I can stay healthy."*
> *"The 1990s look good, I have nothing to complain about."*

V. THE STRUCTURE OF EXPRESSED FEELINGS

The discrepancy between the actual life event and the moment when it is recalled explains the constructive nature of narration in an autobiography. The dynamics between these time levels re-create the narrated memory every time it is told. In the autobiography this can be observed by examining the emotional depth of the memory and the relationship between the recalled and the factual events. The concept of "structure of feeling" (Williams, 1977) reproduces the role of emotions and the original emotional experience. Carolyn Steedman (1986) introduced it in relation to autobiography (see also Bristow, 1991).

The basic idea here is that although the narrator who assesses the memory is fully aware that some essential parts may be missing, the recalled memory is constructed on the basis of previously experienced "original" feelings (e.g., pity, fear, hatred, happiness). In this process, the emotional content of the memory either repeats that which was previously experienced or is reassessed. The emotional force of the narrated memory, according to Steedman's way of thinking, is the factor that makes the narrator and the reader feel and think, and makes them generalize from an individual event to general knowledge based on historical and cultural experience. A strongly felt loneliness and recurrent emotional state in later life can be seen in the autobiography of a Finnish woman:

> *"I can't remember it word for word but I will never forget how those words made my heart run cold. . . . I don't know how my mother felt when she said that, all I know is how I felt. Those words opened the door to loneliness once and for all. Those words that my mother maybe didn't even notice became my lifelong companion."*

It is not always easy to convey emotional experiences through language. The narrator can use conventional methods of biographical narration and can also describe and name emotions. The experienced emotions can be transmitted to the reader of the biography through the interpretation of the structure of the text. For example, the consecutiveness and interrelationships of sentences and themes can convey a strong affective experience without the narrator naming the emotions. An emotionally charged event can represent a turning point in life (e.g., leaving in anger or staying out of pity), and thus, gain an emphasized, symbolic status in the structure of the narration. A single affective memory in a life history can symbolize a whole period of life:

> *"My granny and I used to walk in the forest and collect wood for the fire, little sticks that would clatter against each other when Granny tied them together with a rope. I can still remember that when I see broken twigs in the woods. Sometimes I pick one up and take it home. It's like my childhood, Granny and the spirit of the forest were right there."*

In order to emphasize the emotional content, a memory can also turn toward nostalgia or idealization (e.g., longing for a place and time that are no more). A nostalgic charge can be created when independent elements are connected in a generalizing way:

> *"I can see the scenery, hear the birds, feel that sensitive atmosphere, that unique Karelian enchantment, even now when I'm turning grey."*

The cultural conventions of biographical narration provide an opportunity to express emotional experiences. Parallel to this is the use of conventions and conventional expressions to protect, ignore, or overcome emotional experiences that are not considered a part of autobiographical narration or which the narrator does not want to or cannot reproduce. One conventional way to avoid telling about difficult memories in autobiographies is to build on the culturally based understanding between the storyteller and the reader by reciting an appropriate poem, proverb, or aphorism (Vilkko, 1994a).

VI. EMOTIONS, METAPHORS, AND CULTURAL CONVENTIONS

A biographical convention for expressing emotions in narratives is the use of root metaphors for producing condensed tales. A metaphoric language sensitively touches upon the experience world of the reader or listener. The metaphoric expressions appeal to the fantasy of the receiver helping to identify and decipher the emotional content of the message (Cohen, 1979). Offering a possibility for identification, the metaphor reveals not only the individual and unique experience but also provides a frame of reference within which historical, local, and cultural experiences can be understood (Kenyon, Birren, & Schroots 1991; Lakoff & Johnson, 1980).

In the autobiographies of Finnish women, metaphors for individual lives can be found that reflect typical cultural and national configurations (Vilkko 1994a,b). The journey metaphors (a path, a road, a stream), arch metaphors (the seasons, the rainbow), and fabric metaphors (a cloth, a quilt) are general ones and recognizable cross-culturally. But among these groups of metaphors some Finnish, national ones can also be found, like those reflecting poverty and the hardships of living (duckboards or rag rugs).

The most expressive metaphors, the ones that most appeal to the emotions of the reader, are those root metaphors that are used throughout the account, reflecting the central logic of a life course. The narration of a life story can be seen as an act in which the narrator creates a new metaphor of her or himself, a fresh perspective to her or his life. While consciously making use of conventional metaphors so common in storytelling, the author creates new metaphors on her or his life events as well. Clearly individual metaphors or ones borrowed from the cultural repertory bring out the flavor of the life lived. Simultaneously, these images reflect the highly emotional process of reminiscence—the process that is only partly visible in the narrated life story. The logic of a reconstructed life in a written life story can be expressed by using such metaphors as a river, a painting, a blackboard, a jigsaw puzzle, or a Pandora's box (Vilkko, 1994b).

VII. EMOTIONAL THEMES AND STORY TYPES OF THE LIFE COURSE

When discussing biographical research and life span issues, one central question concerns the different age periods of life. Are certain themes and emotional expressions typical of the childhood years and others of adulthood, middle age, and old age? It stands to reason that this would be the case, and some narrative data confirm this thought.

In childhood the life story themes and plots gradually develop out of the myths from fairy tales, classical mythology, and drama, but also from modern myths encountered in films, TV, and literature (McAdams, 1993). One of the early childhood themes seems to be the wish to be helped by the parents. During the first school years the themes concern avoiding conflict and negative emotions with parents and same-sex peers (Thorne & Klohnen, 1993). Value systems, gender roles, and intimacy constitute some of the themes of youth (Erikson, 1963). In young adulthood the main themes in accounts of life are centered around power relations and love relations (McAdams, 1993). In middle age both individuation and commitment themes arise as well as generativity and balance–harmony themes (Erikson, 1963; McAdams, 1993). The main themes of the old concern compensations, reconciliation, and transcendence (Erikson, Erikson, & Kivnick, 1986; McAdams, 1996; Tornstam, 1994).

The narratives of life also differ as far as their form is concerned. In stories depicting emotional issues of childhood, two different types of narratives have been found: coherent stories with a visible plot and impressionistic depictions of "moments-in-time" (Hudson, Gebelt, Haviland, & Bentivegna, 1992). Especially in the latter, the function of the narration seems to be to express the whole emotional richness of the experienced moment, not to give a coherent account of some past life episodes.

In the accounts of adult life these two types of narratives occur concomitantly, even if the typical story of adulthood seems to be a rather lengthy and detailed one. But even in the more situationally oriented depictions, an evaluative component is added, representing the more critical stance of adulthood (Labov, 1977; Labov & Waletzky, 1967).

> *"I can still sense that sunny day, when Pa came from his meadow, with wonderful red wild strawberries in his cap. Those were the peak experiences of my childhood, and they did not consist of more than ordinary fatherly love."*

The aging narrator often actively strives to regulate the emotional content of the story and to emphasize memories with a positive emotional tone. The aim of the aging narrating self, especially when approaching death, seems to be to refrain from telling about negative memories. Often much to the narrator's own astonishment, however, a considerable amount of negatively charged memories still float to the surface. In an accompanying letter to her autobiography, an elderly woman reflects upon this:

> *"As I started my writing, I had in mind all the nice things that happened on the paths and roads of childhood. But it all turned out in quite another way."*

Autobiography is, after all, a genre where there are many means of controlling the emotions. Parts can easily be erased or reconstructed in written accounts. But the act of reminiscing and producing an autobiography sometimes brings up emotionally charged memories, as if the narrating self is reliving the original moments. The psycho-dynamical discourse between the respondent and the interviewer in tape-recorded life stories adds to this effect, producing vivid memories that can be expressed in the present tense or based on interjections. The interviewer may be ascribed the role of "a representative other" to whom the respondent has strong feelings attached:

> *"I don't know what ethnic group you are or what part of the country you come from, but I do not love or approve of the easteners. They are so full of themselves . . ." [the respondent describes the easteners in the military, and shouts out]: "Attention! You damned bulls! He took the club and hit me." [because the eastener thought the respondent would hit him]. "I said, Mr. Captain," [the respondent shouts, gets up off his chair and clenches his fists at the interviewer], "I have played so much baseball, that I could strike right on target in that case."*

There is, in most cases, a visible contrast between the emotional tone that the aging self produces in accounts of childhood and in accounts of late old age. The childhood memories tend to get a rather positive or nostalgic emotional tone, whereas the memories of old age sometimes are depicted in a more commonplace or emotionally flat way. The life stories told by middle-aged persons, however, contain both critical commentary and vivid, dramatic memories, and the negative emotions are not avoided in the same way as they are for the aged. The reason for this state of affairs is not clear, however. One hypothesis is that the developmental task of old age is reconciliation, as Erikson (1963) stated. Another hypothesis is that this is just a reflection of the way the elderly of today have been socialized. Concerning this issue, the age-cohort question is still unsolved. The third hypothesis pertains to the ways of asking for memories across the life span. The distribution of elicited memories seems to be extremely sensitive to the method of prompting. Thus it has been shown that a "reminiscence peak" from late childhood to adolescence will occur if the informant is instructed to tell his or her life story starting with childhood, whereas memories from old age will prevail if the importance of starting with the present (old age) is stressed (Cohen, 1993; Rubin, Wetzler, & Nebes, 1986).

VIII. NARRATIVES OF THE AGING BODY AND THE AGELESS SELF

A modern social gerontological paradox is the absent body in narrative studies of the aging self (Öberg, in press). Kaufman began describing the "ageless self" she found in the life stories of elderly persons around San Francisco as early as 1986. In these stories the body remained subordinate or invisible. The split between body and mind adds to the feeling of continuity in the self (Mader, 1991, 1995). The body may age and vivid descriptions of the changing body may be found in narratives of old age, but the narrating self may, at the same time, dissociate itself from the aging corporality and remain young or middle-aged. In the Finnish study (Ruth & Öberg, 1992, 1996, Öberg, in press) this ambivalence can be seen in a woman's description of her reflection:

> *"That isn't my reflection. I know myself pretty well. . . . Spiritually I don't feel*
> *old, you know. Sure I'm old and all that. But I can see it in the way I look."*

When the body image is portrayed in the life stories, it is in the context of the emotional tone of the life as a whole that binds the episodes of life together (Polkinghorne, 1991). Persons with a problem-filled life and a hopeless old age are struck by the bodily betrayals of old age (Öberg, in press):

> *"The feelings of nausea came from angina pectoris. . . . The calcium deficiency*
> *causes depression, sleeplessness, and lack of appetite. . . . It is like a vicious circle."*

In life stories of a successful life and a happy aging, the body is more integrated into the story and the positive aspects of a mature face is described by a man as follows:

> *"I see an aging man (in the mirror). But I am happy and proud that I still don't*
> *look like an old person. . . . I should say that I see an elderly gentleman. . . .*
> *That a person retains his culture."*

Also in autobiographical accounts of the frail elderly in institutions, the problems of institutional life are not always incorporated into the stories told by the narrating self. Evidently, hope is maintained in late old age by occasional repression of the awareness of the present, relying instead on the memory of a younger, more active and well-functioning self (Ruth & Coleman, 1996).

IX. SUMMARY AND CONCLUSIONS

Even if autobiography can be conceived as a reminiscence process of a cognitive nature, the possibility of evoked emotions is there. The use of emotional expressions in autobiographical accounts seems to fulfill many different purposes. They add to the understanding of unique experiences for individual narrators; they convey the collective subjectivity of groups of individuals; they reveal cultural canons, and they touch upon issues that characterize humans in general.

The emotional content in autobiographies may be openly stated or only hinted at by the concealment of emotions under seemingly neutral expressions. In the latter case, the emotions may be transmitted by the expressive style or the narrative structure of the account. The narrating self has an abundance of possibilities for regulating emotion: for example, active repression or reconstruction of the account. Symbolic or conventional expressions are also quite useful when the narrating self wants to protect itself, to bypass or overcome emotionality in the account.

Emotions in narratives often attain an enlarged meaning that extends the short psychophysiological state that is the starting point for the definition of affect in psychology at large. Seemingly limited emotional moments may well be found in accounts. But many of these emotional moments at the same time seem to convey a symbolic or poetic meaning that characterize extended episodes, life projects, or even whole stages of life.

The emotional tone or language used in the individual account can also represent something larger, such as the collective subjectivity of gender, class, a way of life, or even the experiences of a cohort. The continuity the narrating self ascribes to disparate experiences and episodes of life helps to create the overarching themes in the plot line of a life story. This has basically a self-supporting function, but it also, clearly, has a reference group function.

There seem to be age-typical themes in the accounts of life a well as age-typical styles of narration. It is still unclear, however, as to what extent these age-related differences are developmental and to what extent they are cohort and culture bound. A third uncertainty pertains to the methods used in prompting for memories across the life span. Memories will prevail from the period from which the narrator is asked to start his account.

The metaphoric or symbolic use of emotional expressions are even more evidently tied to social conventions by which life experiences can be told in certain cultures or at certain sociohistorical points in time. But the use of root metaphors for the human condition or the life course also makes some of the emotional expressions global and understandable cross-culturally.

REFERENCES

Averill, J. R. (1988). A Ptolemaic theory of emotion. *Cognition and Emotion, 2,* 81–87.

Bristow, J. (1991). Life stories. Carolyn Steedman's history writing. *New Formation, 13,* 113–131.

Bruner, J. (1990). *Acts of meaning.* London: Harvard University Press.

Buchanan, K., & Middleton, D. (1993). Discoursively formulating the significance of reminiscence in later life. In N. Coupland & J. F. Nussbaum (Eds.), *Discourse and life-span identity.* Newbury Park: Sage.

Carstensen, L. L. (1991). Selectivity theory. Social activity in a life-span context. In K. W. Schaie & M. P. Lawton (Eds.), *Annual review of gerontology and geriatrics* (Vol II, pp. 195–217). New York: Springer.

Cohen, G. (1993). *Memory in the real world.* Hillsdale, NJ: Lawrence Erlbaum Associates.

Cohen, T. (1979). Metaphor and the cultivation of intimacy. In S. Sacks (Ed.), *On metaphor* (pp. 1–10). Chicago: The University of Chicago Press.

Cohler, B. J., & Cole, T. R. (1996). Studying older lives: Reciprocal acts of telling and listening. In J. E. Birren, G. Kenyon, J. E. Ruth, J. J. F. Schroots, & T. Svensson (Eds.), *Aging and biography: Explorations in adult development* (pp. 61–76). New York: Springer.

Crawford, J., Kippax, S., Onyx, J., Gault, U., & Benton, P. (1992). *Emotion and gender. Constructing meaning from memory.* London: Sage.

Erikson, E. H. (1963). *Childhood and society.* New York: Norton.

Erikson, E. H., Erikson, J., & Kivnick, H. (1986). *Vital involvement in old age.* New York: Norton.

Hudson, J. A., Gebelt, J., Haviland, J., & Bentivegna, C. (1992). Emotion and narrative structure in young children's personal accounts. *Journal of Narrative and Life History, 2* (2), 129–150.

Kaufman, S. (1986). *The ageless self: Sources of meaning in late life.* Madison: The University of Wisconsin Press.

Kenyon, G. (1996). The meaning-value of personal storytelling. In J. E. Birren, G. Kenyon, J. E. Ruth, J. J. F. Schroots, & T. Svensson (Eds.), *Aging and biography: Explorations in adult development* (pp. 21–38). New York: Springer.

Kenyon, G., Birren, J. E., & Schroots, J. J. F. (1991). *Metaphors of aging in science and the humanities.* New York: Springer.

Labov, W. (1977). *Language in the inner city. Studies in black English vernacular.* Oxford: Blackwell.

Labov, W., & Waletzky, J. (1967). Narrative analysis: Oral versions of personal experience. In J. Helm (Ed.), *Essays on the verbal and visual arts* (pp. 12–44). Seattle: University of Washington Press.

Lakoff, G. & Johnson, M. (1980). *Metaphors we live by.* Chicago: The University of Chicago Press.

Mader, W. (1991). Aging and the metaphor of narcissism. In G. Kenyon, J. E. Birren, & J. J. F. Schroots (Eds.), *Metaphors of aging in science and the humanities.* New York: Springer.

Mader, W. (1996). Emotionality and continuity in biographical contexts. in J. E. Birren, G. Kenyon, J. E. Ruth, J. J. F. Schroots, & T. Svensson (Eds.), *Aging and biography: Explorations in adult development* (pp. 39–60). New York: Springer.

Magai, C., & McFadden, S. H. (1995). *The role of emotions in social and personality development. History, theory, and research.* New York: Plenum Press.

McAdams, D. P. (1993). *The stories we live by: Personal myths and the making of the self.* New York: Morrow.

McAdams, D. P. (1996). Narrating the self in adulthood. In J. E. Birren, G. Kenyon, J. E. Ruth, J. J. F. Schroots, & T. Svensson (Eds.), *Aging and biography: Explorations in adult development* (pp. 131–148). New York: Springer.

Miller, N. (1991). *Getting personal. Feminist occasions and other autobiographical acts.* New York: Routledge.

Öberg, P. (in press). The absent body—A social gerontological paradox. *Ageing and Society, 6.*

Polkinghorne, D. E. (1991). Narrative and self-concept. *Journal of Narrative and Life History, 1,* (2&3), 135–153.

Polkinghorne, D. E. (1996). Narrative knowing and the study of lives. In J. E. Birren, G. Kenyon, J. E. Ruth, J. J. F. Schroots, & T. Svensson (Eds.), *Aging and biography: Explorations in adult development* (pp. 77–99). New York: Springer.

Roos, J. P. (1985). Life stories of social change: Four generations in Finland. *International Journal of Oral History, 3,* 179–190.

Rubin, D. C., Wetzler, S. E., & Nebes, R. D. (1986). Autobiographical memory across the life span. In D. C. Rubin (Ed.), *Autobiographical memory.* Cambridge, UK: Cambridge University Press.

Ruth, J. E., & Birren, J. E. (1995). Personality and aging: Modes of coping and the meaning of stress. In A. Kruse & R. Schmitz-Scherzer (Eds.), *Psychologie des Lebenslaufs. Festschrift für Hans Thomae.* Darmstadt: Steinkopf.

Ruth, J. E., & Coleman, P. (1996). Personality and aging: Coping and management of the self in later life. In J. E. Birren & K. W. Schaie (Eds.), *Handbook of the psychology of aging* (pp. 308–322). San Diego: Academic Press.

Ruth, J. E., & Kenyon, G. (1996). Biography in adult development and aging. In J. E. Birren, G. Kenyon, J. E. Ruth, J. J. F. Schroots, & T. Svensson (Eds.), *Aging and biography: Explorations in adult development* (pp. 1–20). New York: Springer.

Ruth, J. E., & Öberg, P. (1992). Expressions of aggression in the life stories of elderly women. In K. Björkqvist & P. Niemelä (Eds.), *Of mice and women: Aspects of female aggression* (pp. 133–146). San Diego: Academic Press.

Ruth, J. E., & Öberg, P. (1996). Ways of life—old age in a life history perspective. In J. E. Birren, G. Kenyon, J. E. Ruth, J. J. F. Schroots, & T. Svensson (Eds.), *Aging and biography: Explorations in adult development* (pp. 167–186). New York: Springer.

Saarenheimo, M. (1994). Theories of reminiscence—do we need them? In P. Öberg, P. Pohjolainen, & I. Ruoppila (Eds.), *Experiencing aging. Festschrift to J-E Ruth* (pp. 57–73). Helsinki: SSKH Skrifter, 4.

Sarbin, T. R. (1986). Emotion and act: Roles and rhetoric. In R. Harre (Ed.), *The social construction of emotions* (pp. 83–97). Oxford: Blackwell.

Singer, J. A., & Salovey, P. (1993). *The remembered self. Emotion and memory in personality.* New York: The Free Press.

Steedman, C. (1986). *Landscape for a good woman. A story of two lives.* London: Virago Press.

Thorne, A., & Klohnen, E. (1993). Interpersonal memories as maps for personality constancy. In D. C. Funder, G. Ross, R. D. Parke, C. Tomlinson-Keasey & K. Widaman (Eds.), *Studying lives through time. Personality and development* (pp. 223–253). Washington, DC: American Psychological Association.

Tornstam, L. (1994). Gero-transcendence—A theoretical and empirical exploration. In L. E. Thomas & S. A. Eisenhandler (Eds.), *Aging and the religious dimension* (pp. 203–225). Westport, CT: Greenwood.

Vilkko, A. (1994a). Homespun life. Metaphors on the course of life in women's autobiographies. *Cultural Studies, 8* (2), 269–278.

Vilkko, A. (1994b, July). *Metaphors on life in women's autobiographies.* Paper presented in the XIII World Congress of Sociology, Bielefeld, Germany.

Williams, R. (1977). *Marxism and literature.* Oxford: Oxford University Press.

Wood, L. A. (1986). Loneliness. In R. Harre (Ed.), *The social construction of emotions* (pp. 184–208). Oxford: Blackwell.

PART III

Emotion and Relationships

CHAPTER 11

Connections between Parents and Their Adult Children

Lillian E. Troll   *and*
Medical Anthropology Department
University of California, San Francisco
San Francisco, California

Karen L. Fingerman
Department of Human Development
and Family Studies
Pennsylvania State University
University Park, Pennsylvania

I. INTRODUCTION

Three principal questions emerge from the current literature on adult parent–child relationships. First, are adult relationships continuations of those formed when the child was an infant, changing in behavior perhaps but not in kind or affect? Second, what accounts for differences in "attachment bonds?" Is it gender, proximity, context, stage of life, or underlying psychological characteristics? Third, is there a generational difference; are parents more "attached" to their children than their children are to them? If so, why? Subsuming these questions are those dealing with the nature of attachment bonds themselves.

The concept of attachment originated from examinations of relationships between parents and infants and has only recently been applied to relationships between adults (e.g., Antonucci, 1976; Cicirelli, 1983; Troll & Smith, 1976). The focus of the present chapter is on the emotional aspects of parent–child relationships over the life span. Both John Bowlby (1969, 1980) and Mary Ainsworth (1991), the pioneers in attachment theory and research, have argued for persistence of attachments, citing phenomena like emotional closeness in adult parent–child pairs and grief accompanying death. The work of Mary Main (1991) and her followers tends to suggest, in fact, that these persisting bonds retain their early character, at least so far as remaining secure, anxious, or ambivalent. There has even been preliminary work on transmission of attachment patterns across generations (Benoit & Parker, 1994).

Parent–child attachment in adulthood goes against one of the most deeply held values of Western culture, that of independence (see F. A. Johnson, 1993). This view assumes that adults who are too strongly tied to their parents—or to anyone other than a spouse or small children—are "dependent" and thus inadequate human beings. Others, though, have argued that mutuality and interdependence should be developmental goals rather than independence (e.g., Hartup & Lempers, 1973). Given the preliminary state of the field, we prefer to remain tentative about the use of the term "attachment" in referring to adult relationships, particularly because the underlying mechanisms and ties have not been articulated clearly.

II. ISSUES OF DEFINITION

The first question in this chapter pertains to persistence of parent–child bonds. So far, efforts to find continuities between infant–mother and adult parent–child relationships, while heuristic, have opened up some basic definitional issues. These include the nature of the bond, the relation of parent–child bonds to other close ties, and the quality of bonding.

A. Unit of Bond: Individual or Dyad

Adult parent–child connections can be viewed as personality attributes of the individuals involved, of the system formed by the parent and child together, or of larger family systems. From one theoretical point of view, the middle perspective would be the most meaningful. By conceptualizing each of the four parent–child dyads (mother–daughter, mother–son, father–daughter, and father–son) as an independent unit, different from the individuals who compose it as well as from other family dyads or the encompassing family system, dyadic relationships could be considered exclusive and unique. Moreover, the features of the attachment, including emotion, could be viewed not as personal properties of the individuals involved but as epiphenomena of the relationships themselves (Troll, 1994).

So far, however, it is difficult to conceptualize dyads as having feelings. Ainsworth (1991) made the distinction between relationships, which are dyadic, and affectional bonds (including attachments), which are characteristics of individuals. Thus, she sees attachments as properties of individuals, not of dyads. Bowlby's (1969, 1980) conception of attachment considers the interactions between parent and child in infancy as a bank account from which the child draws emotional experiences throughout life. He sees early attachment patterns as products of the relationship, but later patterns as the property of the child. These later patterns include both personality characteristics and the emotions that go with them, and which become increasingly resistant to change. Although there is an extensive literature on mother–daughter bonds in later life (e.g., Thompson & Walker, 1984; Troll, 1987), there is little differentiation of emotional features by kind of dyad.

B. Dyads in Context

A focus on the parent–child dyad seems appropriate for a life span perspective. The initial bond between mother and infant has an emotional quality that appears to be dyadically bounded. As children grow into middle childhood and adolescence, however, this dyadic boundary may loosen and parent–child emotions become influenced by interactions with peers, teachers, and others in a wider social context. Adult offspring possess an array of social contacts independent of their connection to their parents. Efforts to understand adult parent–child "attachment," therefore, might well focus on the context of the relationship, the emotions experienced by both dyad members, and changes not only in the structure of the relationship, but in its emotional quality and its members' emotional experiences.

III. BEHAVIOR AND EMOTIONS

A. Early Attachment Behavior and Emotion

Infant–mother attachments are usually described both in terms of behavior (proximity-seeking) and affect (feelings of security) (Ainsworth, 1991). Adult connections are similarly described in terms of behavior (amount of contact or help) and feelings (affectional closeness) (e.g.,

Rossi & Rossi, 1990). The behavioral manifestations of secure early attachments are complex, involving both approach and avoidance (Ainsworth, 1983). The behaviors involved in adult "attachment" to parents have not been discussed per se. Rather, the quality and strength of the relationship has been assessed by activities like provision of support, residential proximity, and frequency of contact (e.g., Rossi & Rossi, 1990). Thus, most research in the literature on both early childhood and later-life parent–child bonds has been based on behavior rather than affect.

When Ainsworth (1964) invented the "strange situation" to assess infants' attachments to their caretakers, she classified their responses as either secure, avoidant, or anxious/ambivalent based on the infants' behaviors. Main (Main, Kaplan, & Cassidy, 1985) adapted this classification to assess adults' attachments to their mothers, and her classification scheme—and its interpretation—is now used by many psychologists (e.g. Levitt, 1991; Rothbard & Shaver, 1994). Main's system is based both on the content of the retrospective accounts and on their style, a behavioral indicator.

Allen and Walker (1992) argued that the behaviors of caregiving daughters fill the same functions in the lives of their aging mothers that their mothers' behaviors earlier served for them: preserving life, fostering growth, and ensuring acceptability in society. Just as children elicit care because they are vulnerable, frail elders may elicit care because they are vulnerable. Such research suggests a motivation for adults' concerns for their parents, but it does not explore the emotional quality of these concerns. Cicirelli (1991) has gone beyond behavioral indicators in mentioning psychological kinds of attachment behavior on the part of adult children: yearning to be with the parent, feelings of anxiety or concern about being away, and provision of advice and other help.

B. Complex Emotions

Across the life span, parents and offspring experience increasingly complex emotions in their relationships. Yet most sociological findings (e.g., Bengtson, 1987; Rossi & Rossi, 1990), anchored to survey questions about emotional closeness and sharing of values, show overwhelmingly positive feelings. In fact, a majority of writers have restricted their definitions of attachment to relationships involving positive feelings, implying that negative feelings indicate lack of attachment (e.g., Cicerelli, 1991).

From another line of thought, it is possible, however, to view negative feelings not as absence of connection but as demonstrations of connection as much as positive feelings are. Troll and Smith (1976) early suggested that we disregard valence and look at strength of affect. Their hypothesis was that dyad members who entertain strong feelings of any kind for their partners are strongly "attached." Those whose feelings, either positive or negative, are weak or nonexistent are minimally attached. In fact, they suggest, strong love goes together with strong hate. Consistently positive attitudes might even suggest minimal love. Diener, Sandvik, and Larsen (1985) lend support to this hypothesis.

Others have stated that the essence of parent–child relations is the complexity of emotions involved. If so, understanding attachment between adult offspring and their parents would require consideration of an array of emotions. For example, Hess and Waring (1978) suggested that the aging of parents might reawaken strong negative and conflictual feelings. When Weishaus (1978) examined the Berkeley longitudinal data, she found that women experienced negative emotions toward their mothers even in middle age. Cairns (1977) described parent–child relationships as emotionally intense, both in adulthood and in childhood. On the one hand, there can be love, admiration, and respect, and on the other guilt, shame, anger, irritation, hurt, and even repulsion if unwelcome parts of oneself are seen in the other. Fingerman (1995) found that healthy older mothers and their adult daughters generally described their relationships as strong and important, yet both mothers and daughters were able to think of a recent visit in which they felt irritated, hurt, or annoyed. Talbott (1990) provided qualitative accounts of widows' complaints about their children and grandchildren. The widows complained even while they valued these relationships.

C. Persistence of Bonds

How can one understand the persistence of ties that are characterized by such emotional complexity? Could it be that parents and children, throughout life, are held together by a sense of belonging that overrides discomfort and anger? Negative emotions that would have ended their relationship if it were like friendship (Blieszner & Adams, 1995) rarely do so. Hagestad (1981) noted in her Chicago three-generation study that adult parents and children operated as if their interactions were in a demilitarized zone (DMZ). Conflict-prone topics were avoided in the service of continued relations. Fingerman (1995) found that it was difficult for middle-aged mothers even to recognize conflict or negative feelings toward their young-adult daughters—although their daughters' did not have as much difficulty doing so. In other words, the emotions parents and children experience in their relationship over life appear to be distinct from those experienced in other types of relationships. This topic will be touched on later.

IV. DEVELOPMENTAL CHANGE IN EMOTION OVER LIFE

A. *Continuity of Attachment from Infancy to Adulthood*

What aspects of the infant–mother relationship carry over into adulthood and what aspects change as children leave home and establish their own social networks? Attachment in infancy has been examined as a predictor of later behavior, personality, and interaction styles. Much of this interest, though, has been focused on problems associated with poor attachment (Spitz, 1945). The clinical background—largely psychoanalysis—from which much of the study of family relationships emerged has led to a biased interest in pathological outcomes. Infants who do not exhibit stranger anxiety, for instance, are considered not to be securely attached and are expected to exhibit inadequate personality traits later in life and in their own parenting. At the same time, adults who are too securely attached are seen as dependent and thus inadequate human beings. Cicirelli (1995) addressed this dilemma by saying that attachment differs from dependency or over-attachment in that it is not dysfunctional, thus distinguishing different degrees or kinds of attachment but still maintaining that there can be too much of a good thing. The fundamental issue should be not what parents can do to "mess up" their children from infancy but how parents and children experience the closeness most of them undoubtedly feel.

In accord with the child-centered researchers like Ainsworth (1991) and Bowlby (1969, 1980), a number of investigators of adult behavior now conclude that parent–child relationships in later years are continuations of early relationships (e.g. Cicirelli, 1991; Levitt, 1991; Rossi & Rossi, 1990). Levitt attributed such persistence to the establishment and maintenance of relationship expectations, to familiarity with partners and mutually contingent feedback, to cultural norms, and to past relationship experience. She does expect changes over time because of changes in cognitive abilities, the development of the ability to modulate conflict, and age-related social norms that dictate appropriate behaviors. Nonetheless, she sees continuity as an important element in understanding attachment.

Cicirelli (1991 and chap. 7, this volume) is another researcher who noted continuity in adult attachment. He believes it is more symbolic than overt, however. Mental representations of the attachment figure, something like identifications, are used to achieve feelings of psychological closeness and security even when there is no longer direct contact. He hypothesized that children—or adults—make their parents a part of their own personality, and in this way achieve feelings of closeness and contact. When Magai, Distel, and Liker (1995) examined associations between attachment style and adult emotional traits of college students, they found continuity of emotional quality, from attachment experiences apparently deriving from childhood to present emotional traits. For example, avoidant attachment was associated with suppressed hostility.

B. Transmission of Attachment

There is also a budding literature examining transmission of attachment styles across generations. In a study of the beginnings of parental attachments (Bretherton, Biringen, & Ridgeway, 1991), some of the new mothers wanted to re-create the kind of relationship they had experienced with their own mothers, whereas others who had not worked out a comfortable relation with their mothers wanted to achieve a better one with their child. Earlier interaction patterns may, nevertheless, prove difficult to alter, as the work of Benoit and Parker (1994) suggests.

C. Genetic Influences

Although evidence of generational transmission points to continuity in relationships over time, it also suggests the possibility of temperament or genetic influences. Some writers have hinted that there may be a "hard-wired drive" for humans to bond (see Goldsmith & Alansky 1987). Others have scorned this proposal and argued for behaviorist or sociological dynamics. Gewirtz (1976), for example, argued that attachment can be explained by mechanisms like reinforcement of crying by caretakers rather than any "mystical" bonding.

D. Fluctuations in Feelings

Although there may be continuity in attachment quality or style, feelings probably fluctuate over life, both in intensity and in the balance between positive and negative. In general, though, negative affect is less likely to be reported—or perhaps even felt—in later life. Rossi and Rossi (1990), who surveyed the attitudes of two cohorts of parent–child dyads in Boston, reported that common developmental trends as well as the influences of historical events can be observed. For example, the decline in adolescents' feelings of closeness to their parents was greater in those who grew up in the 1960s and 1970s than in those who grew up a decade or two earlier. But both earlier and counter-culture cohorts show some dip in positive feelings. The Rossis further found that the later attitudes of both cohorts toward their parents seemed unaffected by their negative attitudes during adolescence. Older offspring, according to the Rossis, reported consistently close feelings. Reports of intimacy, in fact, increased with age.

Coding of interview data from the Berkeley longitudinal study (Carstensen, 1992) showed that interaction frequency, emotional closeness, and satisfaction with the relationship with their parents all increased from 17 to 50, although this trend was not found for less significant relationships. Nydegger (1991), in her study of fathering, claims that there are two dimensions of parental maturity, distancing and comprehending. Children, she concluded, must establish their own identities and achieve emotional emancipation from parents while still remaining engaged as sons or daughters. Fathers must also distance themselves. The end result is increased positive and decreased negative feelings between fathers and their children. Fingerman (in press) found that when middle-aged daughters were able to take a more distanced stance toward their problems with their mothers, they felt better about the relationship. When they took their mothers' behavior or remarks personally, they rated the relationship more negatively. As children mature, their adolescent feelings of repulsion, rejection, or disgust usually become less ambivalent and less intense. Meanwhile parents, while still seeing their children as a legacy, become less involved with them although still finding them a source of emotional gratification.

E. Changes in Parent–Child Emotion in Old Age

Changes in emotion between parents and offspring in later life may reflect general changes in emotions with aging. The work of Levenson (Levenson, Carstensen, Friesen, & Ekman, 1991) showed a decrease in intensity of affect in later life, or at least a decrease in physiological arousal. Similarly, Labouvie-Vief and her colleagues (Labouvie-Vief, Hakim-Larson, De Voe, & Schoeberlein, 1989) and Lawton and his colleagues (M. P. Lawton, Kleban, Rajagopal, & Dean, 1992) found enhanced self-regulation of emotion with age, with less lability and more moderation of responsiveness. Labouvie-Vief and De Voe (1991) reported that older people develop complex cognitive categories that integrate affective and cognitive modes of thought. At the same time, Carstensen (1993) found evidence among old respondents for increasing affective involvement with significant others, such as their children. She concluded that as we get older, we optimize positive emotional experience and minimize negative. We interact increasingly with close relatives who generally make us feel good, and less frequently with more peripheral people. Less familiar people, on the other hand, are often more appealing to younger people who get nonaffective kinds of gratification (like information) from them.

F. Bereavement

Bowlby's (1969, 1980) observations of adults' grief on the death of their parents significantly affected his ideas about persistence of early attachments. (See Bretherton, 1991, for history of attachment theory.) Recent findings on the effect of the death of old parents (e.g., Klapper, Rubinstein, Moss, & Moss, 1990; Scharlach, 1990) are consistent with this view, as are data on adults' spontaneous mentions of family members (Troll, 1994). Not only does the death of parents who are very old have strong effects on their children and grandchildren, but the people most frequently mentioned by adults of three generations—and presumably therefore the people most "on their minds"—are their parents, even when the respondents themselves are in their 80s.

Changes in the emotional quality of the relationship can take place even before the parent dies. As children anticipate their parents' poor health or death, they may experience increasing anxiety (Cicirelli, 1988). Several writers have reported that the need to cope with parental frailty at the end of life can lead to psychological distancing (Johnson & Catalano, 1981) and decline in positive feelings (Baruch & Barnett, 1983; E. S. Johnson & Bursk, 1972).

Although adults expect to lose their parents at some point, elderly parents in the modern world sometimes outlive their children. In a sample of the "oldest-old"—people over the age of 85—one-third had lost a child (C. L. Johnson & Troll, 1992). Although attachment in infancy is defined as children's grieving upon separation from their parents (Ainsworth, 1964), Weiss (1991) speaks of the opposite, grief of parents on loss of children.

Much has been said recently about the increase of the "beanpole family" with fewer members per generation and more generations surviving. Rossi and Rossi (1990) addressed this issue of increasing prevalence of multigenerational families in their Boston study of family relationships and found that only 4% over the age of 50 had a father living and only 17% a mother. Three generations was the modal lineage depth and 1% percent of respondents had five generations.

V. STRUCTURE AND CONTEXT
OF PARENT–CHILD CONTACT

The second question in this chapter addresses variation in parent–child bonds. Accounts of attachment in early childhood presume that parents and infants reside together and that their relationship is insular and close. At the other end of the life span, it is difficult to separate the quality of the parent–child bond from the context in which it is embedded. It seems that strength of bonds and valence (positive or negative) of bonds are contingent upon both social and psychological circumstances.

A. *Family Structure*

From birth, parent–child dyads are inevitably embedded within larger family structures that involve an array of other people who affect the relationship within the dyad. There is another parent or stepparent, grandparents, siblings, aunts and uncles, and fictive kin who all may have an impact on the emotional quality of the dyadic relationship. Cooney (1994) concluded, from her study of parent–child relations after divorce, that members of intact families form an interconnected network. She even argued that discussion of the quality of dyadic relationships is irrelevant to "normal" family relationship patterns. Dyadic relationships as such, she argued, occur only in disturbed or separated families. Although few researchers have gone to this extreme, most of their efforts to examine parent–child bonds in adulthood have focused on contextual factors, almost to the exclusion of trying to understand the dyad itself.

1. FAMILY STRUCTURE AND EARLY CHILDHOOD PARENT–CHILD BONDS

The study of infant–mother bonding has considered the psychological context more than the social—for example, maternal and child sensitivity—but the study of parent–child bonding among adults has paid more attention to the social context: residential contiguity, frequency of contact, and exchange of help. Bengtson and Black (1973) introduced the overarching construct of "solidarity" that combines association (contact), consensus (value similarity), and affect (positive). This construct has dominated the study of adult parent–child relationships, notably in Bengtson's own work in the University of Southern California longitudinal studies of intergenerational relationships (e.g., Roberts & Bengtson, 1990), but also in that of Atkinson, Kivett, and Campbell (1986) and Rossi and Rossi (1990). For example, Rossi and Rossi used as measures of parent–child solidarity frequency of visiting, of phoning, and of helping.

Not surprisingly, they found that geographic distance proved to be negatively related to all these measures of association and particularly to amount of help.

2. CONTEXT OF ADULT PARENT–CHILD BONDS

These structural indicators may be useful, but they do not appear to explain underlying emotional qualities of parent–child ties. For example, geographic distance is not related either to affective closeness or value consensus. These have been consistent findings since the 1960s (Troll, 1971; Troll & Bengtson, 1979; Troll, Miller, & Atchley, 1979).

Studies of the influence of family structure on parent–child relations have been interested in size of family, marital status, educational level, health, geographic proximity, communication, and gender. For example, "beanpole family" structures resulting from greater life expectancy have been said to make for more intense parent–child relations because of longer duration of the dyad and fewer competing dyads (see Riley, 1983; Rossi & Rossi, 1990). Having more children has been associated with greater likelihood of family caregiving in old age (Aldous & Klein, 1991). Certainly, relationships with children's spouses are important (Fischer, 1981). In an American Association of Retired Persons (AARP) survey of 1500 adults (L. Lawton, Silverstein, & Bengtson, 1994), Blacks reported closer relations with their mother than did Whites, but there were no race differences for relations with fathers. People with less income and greater education said they had more contact with fathers.

3. PARENTAL MARITAL QUALITY

A number of recent studies have looked at parental marital quality and parental divorce (e.g., Amato & Keith, 1991; Booth & Amato, 1994; Rossi & Rossi, 1990). Essentially, divorce seems to have more effect on younger children than on older (L. Lawton et al., 1994). In fact, parental marital quality is almost as influential on parent–child relations as divorce itself (Booth & Amato, 1994), although the negative effect varies markedly by gender, both of parent and child (Booth & Amato, 1994; L. Lawton et al., 1994; Rossi & Rossi, 1990). These gender differences will be reviewed in the section on gender below. Economic resources affect the relationship in many ways. Thus the research of social gerontologists, often large-scale and longitudinal, have contributed a great deal to understanding the behavioral aspects of relationships, but they have not told us much about the complex emotions that accompany them. In fact, as mentioned previously, their definition of family cohesion or solidarity as positive affect ignores guilt, shame, and other emotions that are also associated with seeking proximity.

B. Gender

There has been general consensus that the mother–daughter bond is stronger than the other three (Fischer, 1981; Troll, 1989). This phenomenon has been attributed both to differential socialization and inborn genetic differences. Rossi and Rossi (1990), for example, stated that women have a greater developmental stake to maintain close relationships with their parents and children than do men because the probabilities are much higher that women will need help and emotional support from them. Daughters feel closer to parents than sons (Cicirelli, 1983), and daughters are their parents' favorite children (Aldous, Klaus, & Klein, 1985). Daughters have a higher rate of visiting parents than do sons (Marini, 1985) and more involved relationships with them (Greene and Boxer, 1986). Mothers help their adult children more on a daily basis than do fathers (Huyck, 1991).

Across adulthood, the mother–daughter bond has been found to have a profound meaning for both individuals. From adolescence on, according to Rossi and Rossi (1990), there seems to be a growing gap between women's and men's ratings of intimacy with their adult children; with the women—mothers and daughters—reporting higher intimacy levels than the men—fathers and sons. A study of Radcliffe 1964 graduates (Welsh & Stewart, 1995) reported that the quality of 43-year-old women's relationships with their mothers was related to their self-esteem five years later. Sholomskas and Axelrod (1986) reported that mothers' career values influenced their daughters' career choices. Stewart and Healy (1989) had found that women who felt similar to their mothers were higher on emotional adaptation after the birth of their first child than those who did not feel similar. However, this pattern was reversed 28 months later.

Relations with fathers appear to be less intense, and perhaps more complicated. Noncareer daughters' relationships with their fathers appear warm but lack communication (Nydegger & Mitteness, 1991). Given the definition of bonds as involving strong affect, both positive and negative, these noncareer daughters seemed to have fairly distant relationships with their fathers. Career daughters' relationships with their fathers were like those of sons, characterized by shared interests rather than strong emotions. Sons' relationships with their fathers involve contact and mutuality but lack the complex intimacy of mother–daughter ties. Their temporary withdrawal from their fathers during the early years of their marriage and career could become estrangement, although the fact that they share the male world of work counteracts this.

Aside from differences in mothers' and fathers' and daughters' and sons' relationships with one another, there appear to be gender differences in the experience of life transitions. It could be that men have a more precarious bond to their families in general, as has been observed from early years on (Troll, 1986). For example, the happiness of the parents' marriage affects fathers' closeness to daughters, though it appears to have no effect on relationships between mothers and sons (L. Lawton et al., 1994; Rossi & Rossi, 1990). The Rossis note that when there is marital tension, fathers move to the periphery of family affection, regardless of later divorce. Finally, at least one study (Umberson, 1990) found that death of a mother had more impact on both psychological distress and self-reported adaptation than did death of a father, although Scharlach (1990) did not find such a difference.

VI. GENERATIONAL DIFFERENCES IN ATTACHMENT

The third introductory question to this chapter asks whether parents might not be more "attached" to their child than their child to them. The early attachment research, focused on infant development, essentially ignored the mother's behavior and feelings except for her responsiveness to infants' cues. This oversight is being remedied. Mothers appear to have emotional connections to their children even before they are born. A paper by Glogger-Tippelt (1989) reported that maternal bonds were evident during pregnancy, concurring with Zeenah, Keener, Stewart, and Anders (1985). When Bretherton and her associates (Bretherton, Biringen, & Ridgeway, 1991) interviewed 37 mothers of 18-month old infants about their feelings at the child's birth, 30 used strong emotional words like "ecstatic" and "elated."

A. Parents' Greater Investment

Much of the adult literature reports stronger and less ambivalent feelings on the part of parents than of their children. Bengtson and Kuypers (1971) talked about the "generational stake"—parents' greater investment in their children than vice versa—which would make them see less difference between their children and themselves than actually existed. They concluded that parents strive for continuity, but their children for distinctiveness. Hagestad (1987) found that parents report more positive relationships than their children, that younger generations were more ready to report strain and conflict, and parents were less likely to report changes in their relationship. Similarly, Fingerman (1995) found that older mothers underestimated their middle-aged daughters' use of destructive behaviors and in general had a rosier view of their daughters' behaviors and feelings than the daughters did.

B. Childrens' Success and Parental Well-Being

Not only do parents appear to maintain a strong sense of connection and compatibility with offspring, their own emotional state and mood seems to be affected by their perceptions of their children's achievements and well-being. According to Ryff and her colleagues (Ryff, Lee, Essex, & Schmutte, 1994), middle-aged parents perceive their adult children as part of their own well-being. Parents come to terms with their children being separate from themselves, but their perceptions of how their grown children turned out influences them strongly. Parental status and the mere existence of children is not automatically associated with positive feelings (Glenn & McLanahan, 1981), however. Nor does mere contact with children appear to be associated with positive emotions for parents of grown children (or probably with children of any age).

In older as in younger attachment, behavioral indicators may be manifest in times of stress. Thus, older parents may have greater contact with their children when there is trouble in the family (Troll, 1983). Moreover, associations with children in trouble may have a negative influence on parents' well-being. When Pillemer and Suitor (1991) interviewed 100 Massachusetts parents over 65, they found that those whose children had problems reported more distress and had higher levels of depression than those whose children did not. They viewed their children's difficulties as signs of their own failure. Aging parents' relationship to their children may involve strong ties, but the effect of these ties may be either positive or negative.

C. Children's Feelings for Parents

Adult children seem to be less emotionally invested in their parents than their parents are in them. Nevertheless, they experience complex emotions in these relationships. Negative emotions may dissipate in adulthood, freeing them to "invest" in their parents. Hagestad's term "DMZ" to describe the efforts of adult children to avoid potentially disruptive feelings with their parents, shows that they still care for their approval (Brody, 1990; Troll, 1987). On the other hand, they have to come to terms with their parents as distinct individuals (Blenkner, 1965; Nydegger, 1991) in the process of what Blenkner called "filial maturity." Moreover, offspring who provide care for frail or cognitively impaired parents demonstrate their commitment to their parents through their actions. At the same time, data on caregiving by children speak loudly about burden. Troll, Miller, and Atchley (1979) speculated that part of the help given by some adult children to their aging parents might be attributable to feelings of obligation and shame rather than fondness and concern.

VII. MEASUREMENT

Saying that significant relationships between parents and children persist from infancy and childhood throughout the years of life does not provide clear operational constructs that could be used across cultures and human conditions. "Solidarity," the construct offered by Bengtson and his colleagues, is a first big step in this direction. These authors provide an heuristic framework that has been adopted by many investigators, particularly sociologists. One of its problems, however, is the assumption of positive affect as a sine qua non of close relationship. The affective component of family solidarity has been examined primarily as a unidimensional construct, ignoring the diversity and complexity of emotions in adulthood, particularly between parents and children. Another problem is deciding whether such variables as association, consensus, and affect is the same as perceived closeness or intimacy, and whether it indexes the attachment bond described by Ainsworth and Bowlby, or beyond that, whether contact frequency or value consensus or the combination called solidarity is the same as striving for contact. Much of what is known about parent–child ties in later life is based on behavior rather than affect.

Adult attachment scales like those of Main, Cicirelli, and Cooney are all self-report instruments that rely on retrospective accounts. But ingenious new approaches like those used to study emotions (e.g., those of Magai (Magai et al., 1995), Carstensen (Carstensen & Turk-Charles, 1994), and Labouvie-Vief (Labouvie-Vief et al., 1989) promise more exciting avenues, and it is hoped that their techniques will be applied specifically to parent–child issues. The observational approach of Fingerman (1995) also forges the way to more meaningful data.

VIII. CONCLUSION

In summary, the parent–child relationship involves complex emotions that serve to bond parents to children and children to parents throughout life. A combination of positive and negative emotions exists. So far, most efforts to examine bonds between parents and offspring have focused on behavioral indicators, whether at the psychological level in terms of behavior in infancy or at the sociological level in terms of structure in adulthood. The nature of parents' and children' behaviors throughout life may reflect a sense of connection based on belonging. Perhaps we may have to move back from a focus on behavior of either individuals or dyads to emotions.

REFERENCES

Ainsworth, M. D. S. (1964). Patterns of attachment behavior shown by the infant in interaction with his mother. *Merrill-Palmer Quarterly, 10,* 51–58.

Ainsworth, M. D. S. (1983). Patterns of infant–mother attachment as related to maternal care: Their early history and their contribution. In D. Magnusson & V. L. Allen (Eds.), *Human development: An interactional perspective* (pp. 35–57). New York: Academic Press.

Ainsworth, M. D. S. (1991). Attachments and other affectional bonds across the life cycle. In C. M. Parkes, J. Stevenson-Hinde, & P. Marris (Eds.), *Attachment across the life cycle* (pp. 33–51). London: Routledge.

Aldous, J., & Klein, D. (1991). Models of intergenerational relations in mid-life. *Journal of Marriage and the Family, 53* (3), 595–608.

Aldous, J., Klaus, E., & Klein, D. (1985). The understanding heart: Aging parents and their favorite children. *Child Development, 56,* 303–316.

Allen, K. R., & Walker, A. J. (1992). Attentive love: A feminist perspective on the caregiving of adult daughters, *Family Relations, 41,* 284–289.

Amato, P. R., & Keith, B. (1991). Consequences of parental divorce for children's well-being. A meta-analysis. *Psychological Bulletin, 110,* 26–46.

Antonucci, T. (1976). Attachment: A life-span concept. In T. Antonucci (Ed.), *Attachment: A life-span concept,* Symposium of the American Psychological Association, New Orleans, 1974. *Human development, 19*(3), 135–142.

Atkinson, M. P., Kivett, V. R. S., & Campbell, R. T. (1986). Intergenerational solidarity: An examination of a theoretical model. *Journal of Gerontology, 41,* 408–416.

Baruch, G., & Barnett, R. C. (1983). Adult daughters' relationships with their mothers. *Journal of Marriage and the Family, 45,* (3), 601–606.

Bengtson, V. L. (1987). Parenting, grandparenting, and intergenerational continuity. In J. B. Lancaster, J. Altmann, A. S. Rossi, & L. R. Sherrod (Eds.), *Parenting across the slife span: Biosocial dimensions* (pp. 435–456). Hawthorne, NY: Aldine De Gruyter.

Bengtson, V. L., & Black, K. D. (1973) *Solidarity between parents and children: Four perspectives on theory development.* Paper presented at the Preconference Workshop on Theory and Methodology, National Council on Family Relations, Toronto.

Bengtson, V. L., & Kuypers, J. A. (1971). Generational difference and the developmental stake. *Aging and Human Development, 2,* 249–260.

Benoit, D., & Parker, K. C. H. (1994). Stability and transmission of attachment across three generations. *Child Development, 65,* 1444–1456.

Blenkner, M. (1965). Social work and family relationships in later life with some thoughts on filial maturity. In E. Shanas & G. Streib (Eds.), *Social structure and the family: Generational relations* (pp. 46–59). Englewood Cliffs, NJ: Prentice-Hall.

Blieszner, R., & Adams, R. G. (1995, November). *The causes and consequences of problems with friends in old age.* Paper presented at the annual meeting of the Gerontological Society of America, Los Angeles.

Booth, A., & Amato, P. R. (1994). Parental marital quality, parental divorce, and relations with parents, *Journal of Marriage and the Family, 56,* 21–34.

Bowlby, J. (1969). *Attachment and loss,* Vol. I. London: Hogarth.

Bowlby, J. (1980). *Attachment and loss,* Vol. 3. London: Hogarth.

Bowlby, J. (1988). Developmental psychiatry comes of age. *American Journal of Psychiatry, 145,* 1–10.

Bretherton, I. (1991). The roots and growing points of attachment theory. In C. M. Parkes, J. Stevenson-Hinde, & P. Marris (Eds.), *Attachment across the life cycle* (pp. 9–32). London: Routledge.

Bretherton, I., Biringen, Z., & Ridgeway, D. (1991). The parental side of attachment. In K. Pillemer & K. McCartney (Eds.), *Parent–child relations throughout life* (pp. 1–24). Hillsdale, N.J.: Erlbaum.

Brody, E. (1990). Role reversal: An inaccurate and destructive concept. *Journal of Gerontological Social Work, 15,* 15–23.

Cairns, R. B. (1977). Beyond social attachment. The dynamics of interactional development. In T. Alloway, P. Pliner, & L. Krames (Eds.), *Attachment behavior* (pp. 1–24). New York: Plenum.

Carstensen, L. L. (1992). Social and emotional patterns in adulthood: Support for socioemotional selectivity theory, *Psychology and aging, 7*(3), 331–338.

Carstensen, L. L. (1993). Motivation for social contact across the life span: A theory of socioemotional selectivity. In J. E. Jacobs (Ed.), *Nebraska symposium on motivation, 1993* (pp. 209–254). Lincoln: University of Nebraska Press.

Carstensen, L. L., & Turk-Charles, S. (1994). The salience of emotion across the adult life span, *Psychology and aging, 9* (2), 259–264.

Cicirelli, V. G. (1983). Adult children's attachment and helping behavior to elderly parents: A path model. *Journal of Marriage and the Family, 45,* 815–825.

Cicirelli, V. G. (1988). A measure of filial anxiety regarding anticipated care of elderly parents. *The Gerontologist, 28,* 478–482.

Cicirelli, V. G. (1991). Attachment theory in old age: Protection of the attached figure. In K. Pillemer & K. McCartney (Eds.), *Parent–child relations throughout life* (pp. 25–42). Hillsdale, NJ: Erlbaum.

Cicirelli, V. G. (1995). A measure of caregiving daughters' attachment to elderly mothers. *Journal of Family Psychology, 9,* 89–94.

Cooney, T. M. (1994). Young adults' relations with parents: The influence of recent parental divorce, *Journal of Marriage and the Family, 56* 45–56.

Diener, E., Sandvik, E., & Larsen, R. J. (1985). Age and sex effects for emotional intensity. *Developmental Psychology, 21* (3), 542–546.

Fingerman, K. L. (1995). Aging mothers and their adult daughters' perceptions of conflict behaviors. *Psychology and Aging, 10* (4), 639–649.

Fingerman, K. L. (in press). Sources of tension in the aging mother and adult daughter relationship. *Psychology and Aging.*

Fischer, L. R. (1981). Transitions in the mother–daughter relationship. *Journal of Marriage and the Family, 43* (3), 613–622.

Gewirtz, J. L. (1976). The attachment acquisition process as evidenced in the maternal conditioning of cued infant responding (particularly crying). In T. Antonucci (Ed.), *Attachment: A life-span concept,* Symposium of the American Psychological Association, New Orleans, 1974. *Human Development, 19* (3), 143–155.

Glenn, N. D., & McLanahan, S. (1982). Children and marital happiness: A further specification of the relationship. *Journal of Marriage and the Family, 44,* 63–72.

Glogger-Tippelt, G. (1989, July). *Mothers' conceptions of their child during the transition to parenthood.* Paper presented at the 10th biennial meetings of the International Society for the Study of Behavioral Development, Jyvaskyla, Finland.

Goldsmith, H. H., & Alansky, J. A. (1987). Maternal and infant temperamantal predictors of attachment: A meta-analytic review. *Journal of Consulting and Clinical Psychology, 55,* 805–816.

Greene, A. L., & Boxer, A. M. (1986). Daughters and sons as young adults: Restructuring the ties that bind. In N. Datan, A. L. Greene, & H. W. Reese (Eds.), *Life-span developmental psychology* (pp. 125–150). Hillsdale, NJ: Lawrence Erlbaum.

Hagestad, G. O. (1981). Problems and promises in the social psychology of intergenerational relations. In R. W. Fogel & J. G. March (Eds.), *Stability and change in the family* (pp. 11–46). New York: Academic Press.

Hagestad, G. O. (1987). Parent–child relations in later life: Trends and gaps in past research. In J. B. Lancaster, J. Altmann, A. S. Rossi, & L. R. Sherrod (Eds.), *Parenting across the life span: Biosocial dimensions* (pp. 405–434). New York: Aldine de Gruyter.

Hartup, W. W., & Lempers, J. (1973). A problem in life-span development. The interactional analysis of family attachments. In P. Baltes & W. Schaie (Eds.), *Life-span developmental psychology. Personality and socialization* (pp. 235–252). New York: Academic Press.

Hess, B., & Waring, J. M. (1978). Parent and child in later life: Rethinking the relationship. In R. Lerner & G. Spanier (Eds.), *Child influences on marital and family interaction* (pp. 241–273). New York: Academic Press.

Huyck, M. H. (1991). Gender-linked self-attributions and mental health among middle-aged parents. *Journal of Aging Studies, 5* (1), 111–123.

Johnson, C. L., & Catalano, D. (1981). Childless elderly and their family supports. *The Gerontologist, 21* (6), 610–618.

Johnson, C. L., & Troll, L. E. (1992). Family functioning in late late life. *Journal of Gerontology Social Sciences, 47* (2), 566–572.

Johnson, E. S., & Bursk, B. (1977). Relationships between the elderly and their adult children. *The Gerontologist, 17* (1), 90–96.

Johnson, F. A. (1993). *Dependency and Japanese socialization: Psychoanalytic and anthropological investigations into Amae.* New York: New York University Press.

Klapper, J., Rubinstein, R. L., Moss, S., & Moss, S. M. (1990, November). *Patterns of grief among adult daughters who have lost a parent.* Paper presented at the annual meeting of the Gerontological Society of America, Boston.

Labouvie-Vief, G., & De Voe, M. (1991). Emotional regulation in adulthood and later life. In W. Schaie, (Ed.), *Annual review of gerontology and geriatrics* (Vol. II, pp. 172–194). New York: Springer.

Labouvie-Vief, G., Hakim-Larson, J., De Voe, M., & Schoeberlein, S. (1989). Emotions and self-regulation: A life span view. *Human Development, 32,* 279–299.

Lawton, L., Silverstein, M., & Bengtson, V. (1994). Affection, social contact, and geographic distance between adult children and their parents. *Journal of Marriage and the Family, 56,* 57–68.

Lawton, M. P., Kleban, M. H., Rajagopal, D., & Dean, J. (1992). Dimensions of affective experience in three age groups. *Psychology and Aging, 7,* 171–184.

Levenson, R. W., Carstensen, L. L., Friesen, W. V., & Ekman, P. (1991). Emotion, physiology, and expression in old age, *Psychology and Aging, 5* (No. 1), 28–35.

Levitt, M. J. (1991). Attachment and close relationships: A life-span perspective. In J. L. Gewirtz & W. F. Kurtines (Eds.), *Interceptions with attachment* (pp. 183–205). Hillsdale, NJ: Erlbaum.

Magai, C., Distel, N., & Liker, R. (1995). Emotion socialization, attachment, and patterns of adult emotional traits. *Cognition and Emotion, 9,* 461–481.

Main, M. (1991). Metacognitive knowledge, metacognitive monitoring, and singular (coherent) vs. multiple (incoherent) model of attachment: Findings and directions for future research. In C. M. Parkes & J. Stevenson-Hinde (Eds.), *Attachment across the life cycle* (pp. 127–159). London: Routledge.

Main, M., Kaplan, N., & Cassidy, J. (1985). Security in infancy, childhood, and adulthood: A move to the level of representation. In I. Bretherton & E. Waters (Eds.), Growing points of attachment theory and research. *Monographs for the Society for Research in Child Development 50 (1–2), Serial No. 209*

Marini, M. M. (1985). Determinants of the timing of adult role entry. *Social Science Research, 14,* 309–350.

Nydegger, C. N. (1991). The development of paternal and filial maturity. In K. Pillemer & K. McCartney (Eds.), *Parent-child relations throughout life* (pp. 93–110). Hillsdale, NJ: Erlbaum.

Nydegger, C. N., & Mitteness, L. (1991). Fathers and their adult sons and daughters. In S. Pfeifer & M. Sussman (Eds.), Families: Intergenerational and generational connections. (Special issue). *Marriage and Family Review, 16,* 249–263.

Pillemer, K., & Suitor, J. J. (1991). Relationships with children and distress in the elderly. In K. Pillemer & K. McCartney (Eds.), *Parent–child relations throughout life* (pp. 163–178). Hillsdale, NJ: Erlbaum.

Riley, M. (1983). The family in an aging society: A matrix of latent relationships. *Journal of family issues, 4,* 439–454.

Roberts, R. E. L., & Bengtson, V. L. (1990). Is family solidarity a unidimensional construct? A second test of a formal model. *Journal of Gerontology, 45,* S12–S20.

Rossi, A. S., & Rossi, P. H. (1990). *Of human bonding: Parent–child relations across the life course.* New York: Aldine de Gruyter.

Rothbard, J. C., & Shaver, P. R. (1994) Continuity of attachment across the life span. In M. B. Sperling & W. H. Berman (Eds.), *Attachment in adults: Clinical and developmental perspectives* (pp. 31–71). New York: Guilford.

Ryff, C. D., Lee, Y. H., Essex, M. J., & Schmutte, P. S. (1995). My children and me: Midlife evaluations of grown children and of self. *Psychology and Aging, 9* (2), 195–205.

Scharlach, A. (1990, November). *Predictors of filial grief following the death of a parent.* Paper presented at annual meeting of Gerontological Society of America, Boston.

Sholomskas, D., & Axelrod, R. (1986). The influence of mother–daughter relationships on women's sense of self and current role choices. *Psychology of Women Quarterly, 10,* 171–182.

Spitz, R. (1945). Hospitalism: An inquiry into the genesis of psychiatric conditions in early childhood. In O. Fenichel (Ed.), *The psychoanalytic study of the child* (Vol. 1, pp. 53–74). New York: International Universities Press.

Stewart, A. J., & Healy, J. (1989). Linking individual development and social change. *American Psychologist, 44,* 30–42.

Talbott, M. M. (1990). The negative side of the relationship between older widows and their adult children: The mothers' perspective. *The Gerontologist, 30,* 595–603.

Thompson, L., & Walker, A. J. (1984). Mothers and daughters: Aid patterns and attachment. *Journal of Marriage and the Family, 46,* 313–322.

Troll, L. (1971). Family of later life: A decade review. In C. Broderick (Ed.), *A decade of family research and action. National Council of Family Relations* (pp. 187–214). National Council on Family Relations.

Troll, L. E. (1983). Grandparents: The family watchdogs. In T. Brubaker (Ed.), *Family relationships in later life* (pp. 63–74). Beverly Hills, CA: Sage.

Troll, L. E. (Ed.) (1986). *Family issues in current gerontology.* New York: Springer.

Troll, L. E. (1987). Mother-daughter relationships through the life span. In S. Oskamp (Ed.), *Family processes and problems: Social psychological aspects* (pp. 284–306). Newbury Park, CA: Sage.

Troll, L. E. (1989). Myths of midlife intergenerational relationships. In S. Hunter & M. Sundel (Eds.), *Midlife myths: Issues, findings, and practice implications* (pp. 210–232). Beverly Hills, CA: Sage.

Troll, L. E. (1994). Family connectedness of old women: Attachments in later life. In B. F. Turner & L. E. Troll (Eds.), *Women growing older: Psychological perspectives* (pp. 169–201). Thousand Oaks, CA: Sage.

Troll, L. E., & Bengtson, V. L. (1979). Generations in the family. In W. Burr, R. Hill, F. Nye, & I. Reiss (Eds.), *Contemporary theories about the family* (pp. 127–161). New York: Free Press.

Troll, L. E., Miller, S. J., & Atchley, R. C. (1979). *Families in later life.* Belmont, CA: Wadsworth.

Troll, L. E., & Smith, J. (1976). Attachment through the life span: Some questions about dyadic bonds among adults. In T. Antonucci (Ed.), *Attachment: A life-span concept,* Symposium of the American Psychological Association, New Orleans, 1974. *Human Development, 19,* 156–170.

Umberson, D. (1990, November). *The impact of death of a parent on adult children's psychological well-being: A prospective study.* Paper presented at the annual meeting of the Gerontological Society of America, Boston.

Weishaus, S. S. (1978). *Determinants of affect of middle-aged women towards their aging mothers.* Unpublished doctoral dissertation, University of Southern California, Los Angeles.

Weiss, R. W. (1991). The attachment bond in childhood and adulthood. In C. M. Parkes, J. Stevenson-Hinde, & P. Marris (Eds.), *Attachment across the life cycle* (pp. 66–76). London: Routledge.

Welsh, W. M., & Stewart, A. J. (1995). Relationships between women and their parents: Implications for midlife well-being. *Psychology and Aging, 10* (2), 181–190.

Zeenah, C. H., Keener, M. A., Stewart, L., & Anders, T. F. (1985). Prenatal perception of infant personality: A preliminary investigation. *Journal of the American Academy of Child Psychiatry, 24,* 204–210.

CHAPTER 12

Affect and Sibling Relationships in Adulthood

Victoria Hilkevitch Bedford *and* Paula Smith Avioli
Bahvioral Sciences Department   *Kean College of New Jersey*
University of Indianapolis   *Union, New Jersey*
Indianapolis, Indiana

I'VE NEVER BEEN AFRAID OR ALONE IN MY LIFE.
—*Bessie Delany, coauthor of* Having Our Say: The First 100 Years, *with reference to having lived for the past 104 years with her sister.*
New York Times, *1993*

WE DIDN'T DRIVE BACK IN SILENCE BUT IN RAGE. RAGE IS QUIETER.
—*Alice Friman, "Sisters," 1995*

I. INTRODUCTION

Sibling relationships may be the quintessential emotional relationship; they are highly emotional and largely irrational (Bank & Kahn, 1982). All too often, laypeople and social scientists alike equate "sibling relationships" with "sibling rivalry" on the one hand, and to teary-eyed sentimentality associated with the terms "sisterhood" and "brotherhood" on the other hand. The challenge of the present chapter is to integrate trends in affect development, particularly in adulthood and old age, with what is known about the quality of sibling relationships. We achieve this integration by locating sibling research with respect to affect concepts related to adult development. Next, we review empirical studies about sibling affect, guided by concepts developed by adult affect researchers. Finally, we consider whether sibling study has anything to contribute to affect study in general.

A. Defining "Siblings"

As family forms become increasingly complex, and a multicultural perspective further broadens conceptions of family, the definition of siblings becomes more varied. Most research cited in this chapter, however, does not specify how the siblings in their studies are related. No doubt, in these studies siblings refers to those related biologically or adopted. Rarely are step-, half-, foster or socially designated (fictive) siblings included in sibling research. Furthermore, the prevalence of such siblings is unknown even though half of all marriages in the United States today are remarriages, and nearly two-thirds of them involve step- and half-siblings (White & Riedman, 1992a). Current knowledge about the quality of sibling alliance, therefore, is far from inclusive of the many variations of sibling relationships.

B. Importance of Sibling Affect Study

Separation from the family of origin is a norm of dominant Western societies that suggests siblings are mostly irrelevant to the activities, thoughts, and feelings of adults. The societal emphasis on vertical family ties (intergenerational) over horizontal ones (intragenerational) also helps to explain both a professional and personal neglect of sibling relationships. Yet, there now exists ample evidence of sibling importance, particularly to the emotional lives of adults. The reasons for their importance are still being explored, but an obvious one is their ubiquitousness. About 90% of children have at least one sibling, and figures for adults range from 93 to 79% depending on the study (Cicirelli, 1982). As expected, sibling loss increases substantially with age, resulting in fewer living siblings (see Cicirelli, 1995). In Johnson and Troll's (1996) San Francisco sample, 34% of those in their 70s had no living siblings, whereas 55% of those aged 85 to 90 had none; the number increases to 65% without siblings after age 90. For women, however, having a sibling is still much more likely than having a spouse in later years. For instance, in their longitudinal study of San Franciscans who are 85 years and older, Johnson and Barer (1996) found that half of the men, but only 11% of women had a spouse, whereas among the childless oldest-old, 35% of Whites and 47% of Blacks had at least one sibling. Although having children is more likely than both spouse and sibling in later years, a remarkable number of people have survived their children or never had any. Again, in the oldest-old sample, only 68% of Whites and 55% of Blacks had at least one child (Johnson & Barer, 1996). Unique to siblings compared to other kin is the meaning of siblings in late life: siblings are typically the last vestige of one's family of origin, and the relationship represents much of one's early and shared past (Avioli, 1989).

But it is not just having a sibling but rather the quality of the sibling relationship that is important. Mancini and Blieszner (1989) have argued that relationship quality is an end in itself and its importance need not be demonstrated further. Well-being measures, however, have been related to the quality of sibling relationships, particularly with sisters. These studies will be reviewed in the final section of this chapter.

In conclusion, the high prevalence of siblings combined with the affect-laden nature of the relationship indicate that feelings about siblings have an important place in the affective life of adults, which might continue throughout the life course and warrant investigation.

C. Sibling Affect and Affect Concepts in Adult Development

Affect is thought to be manifested in three domains, experiential (felt emotions), physiological (internal arousal), and motoric (expressions of affect) (Schultz, 1985). Adult sibling research is almost exclusively limited to felt emotions. In contrast, studies of children are increasingly using observational data to infer feelings from verbal and nonverbal interactions (e.g., Denham, 1986). Physiological and motoric responses as well as thematic coding of verbal interactions have recently been launched, based upon John Gottman's experience with marital couples (Shortt, 1995).

Affect can be a state that motivates behavior or it can be a simple response (Schultz, 1985). In sibling research, affect is assumed to be linked to memories of events in the relationship, whether the events occurred recently, in the distant past, or at all. Sibling affect, then, originates as a response, whether averaged, compounded, or selected from a lifetime of events with or related to the sibling, but it functions as a state that might inform future interactions with the sibling as well as other behaviors and states.

Affect researchers have disputed whether affects are discrete, independent states (monopolar) or whether they are interrelated, varying only with respect to two bipolar dimensions: pleasure/displeasure and intensity (Schultz, 1985). Sibling relationships are often described in terms of discrete independent states in clinical studies and anecdotal accounts, but most systematic studies of siblings focus on interrelated positive affects and a few include a cluster of negative affects as well (see Bedford, 1989c, 1995; Lowenthal, Thurnher, & Chiriboga, 1975; Moss & Moss, 1989; Ross & Milgram, 1982; Vandell, Minnett, & Santrock, 1987). Specific findings will be discussed in section II.

Schultz (1985) proposed six dynamics of affect that might change with age and, therefore, might be relevant to a description of the development of affect in adulthood. Specifically, the dynamics proposed with respect to emotional experiences are intensity, duration, variability, frequency, quality, and elicitors or instigators.

The study of elicitors of sibling affect, positive or negative, has particular relevance for planning interventions to facilitate sibling social support and caregiving. In other words, understanding how to instigate positive affect and to avoid eliciting negative affect might encourage sibling inclusion in social networks and sibling participation in shared parent care as well as participation in sibling care.

A related issue concerns the constraints and facilitators of sibling affect. According to Blieszner (1988), "a person's level of development influences the nature of relationships" (p. 143). Thus, normative patterns of continuity and change in affective capacities across the adult years might set limits and open new possibilities for the affective nature of the sibling relationship over the years. Both Tomkins (1963) and Labouvie-Vief, Hakim-Larson, DeVoe, and Schoeberlein (1989) have theorized about such patterns. From the perspective of affect expression, Schultz, O'Brien, and Tomkins (1994) reasoned that with age, negative affect would increase and affective states would become blunted and constricted. Focusing on affect regulation, Labouvie-Vief et al. (1989) suggested that with age, people become more aware of their affective experiences (compared to adolescents), more accepting of their own and others' emotional experiences, and better able to use reflection to gain control over these feelings. Thus, it seems that although the expression of affect might appear blunted, due to greater control, in actuality the inner experience of affect might become richer, as demonstrated in the language used to describe emotional experiences. In support of these findings of greater control with age, Lawton, Kleban, Rajagopal, and Dean (1992) described age differences in affective expression. Cross-sectional analyses revealed that older subjects had greater emotional control and mood stability due to more moderate positive affect, low surges of positive feeling, lower psychophysiological responsiveness, and less sensation seeking, as compared to younger subjects.

II. EMPIRICAL FINDINGS ON AFFECTIVE STATES TOWARD SIBLINGS

A. Dimensions of Sibling Affect

Positive affects dominated early studies of siblings. In the very first empirical investigation of sibling affect in adulthood, the sibling bond was described as important and close, second only to the parent–child relationship among middle–aged and late–life adults (spouses were excluded from the ratings) (Cumming & Schneider, 1961). Similarly, in other studies, the sibling relationship itself has often been described in positive affect-laden terms, such as close, friend-like (Connidis, 1989), best friendship (e.g., Allan, 1977; White & Riedmann, 1992b), showing solidarity (Johnson, 1982), emotionally supportive (Moss & Moss, 1989), and intimate (Gold, 1989a). Predominately positive typologies of sibling relationships have also been identified. For example, the Mosses (1989) delineated the intimate and the loyal, whereas Gold (1989a) described the intimate and the congenial based on her finding that closeness, psychological involvement, and acceptance or approval form a single factor.

There are several reasons why negative affects in adult sibling relationships are more difficult to assess than positive affects (Bedford, 1989b), particularly in later life (Bedford, 1993a). Much of the early work on sibling relationships is suspected of being biased due to desirability effects (Scott, 1983). In addition, negative affects may not have been recorded, as pointed out by Bedford (1989a), because adults may not be aware of such feelings towards their siblings. Thus, she urged the use of "sensitive assessment," those procedures that take pains to create a supportive environment in assessing sibling affect (Bedford, 1989a, 1989b). In fact, most studies that report negative affect in sibling relationships used such methods, including supportive discussion groups (Ross & Milgram, 1982), lengthy unstructured personal interviews (Rubenstein, Alexander, Goodman, & Luborsky, 1991), and/or projective tests (Bedford, 1989a, 1989b, 1990a, 1990b). Comparing self-report ratings of positive and negative affect toward sibling with affect theme frequencies derived from projective tests. Bedford (1989b) found that women at the empty-nest phase were consistent, men at this phase were inconsistent on both negative and positive affect, men at the child-rearing phase were inconsistent on positive affect, whereas women during this phase were inconsistent on negative affect. These results suggest that there are distinct life phases during which men and women are more aware of or are more willing to acknowledge positive and negative feelings toward siblings. Notably, the gender differences in these patterns coincide with Gutmann's

(1987) formulation of personality characteristics elicited and suppressed by the parental imperative and its aftermath.

Negative emotions describing the sibling relationship include hostility, jealousy (Gold, 1989a), and rivalry (Moss & Moss, 1989; Ross & Milgram, 1982). Gold (1989a) described the hostile and apathetic typologies of sibling relationships as unambivalently negative. These sibling relations exhibited high levels of rejection, intense resentment, rare contact, no psychological involvement, and no support of sibling (Gold, 1989a). However, they were relatively rare, each describing 10% of the sample. Allan (1977) found that typically congenial siblings expected conflict to erupt between them should they have to live together again. Close reinvolvement between siblings in service of parent care bore out this expectation in Suitor and Pillemer's (1993) study of married daughters caring for parents with dementia in which "siblings were overwhelmingly the most important source of interpersonal stress" (p. S1).

Until recently, positive and negative affect were considered opposite ends of the same continuum, but greater attention to eliminating desirability effects has resulted in separating these affects into two independent dimensions (Bedford, 1989a; Lowenthal et al., 1975). This separation allows for more emotionally ambivalent sibling relationships to emerge. Lowenthal et al. (1975) found high levels of both positive and negative feelings simultaneously in the relations between sisters, and more than between brothers. Gold's loyal type (the most prevalent, 35% of her aged sample) experienced simultaneously low levels of positive and negative feelings toward their siblings. Specifically, loyals manifested low levels of closeness, modest resentment and envy, and infrequent contact (Gold, 1989a).

Some studies of sibling relationships have delineated additional affect dimensions. For instance, indifference has been studied as a discrete dimension of affect (Cicirelli, 1985; Gold, 1989a). Bedford (1989a) attempted to capture a theoretically defined feeling of separateness, which combined indifference, estrangement, and longing, corresponding to the category "moving away from siblings," based on Horney's (1945) model. "Moving against" siblings included only those negative feelings that involved engagement with the sibling, at least symbolically, namely, conflict (rivalry, envy, jealousy, disappointment, annoyance, etc.). Clinical studies tend to focus on specific affects toward siblings, as though they were independent dimensions. Of particular concern to clinicians are sexual feelings, fear, aggression, and jealousy related to siblings, given that they are sometimes implicated in various psychopathologies.

In the first published study of sibling affect using observational and physiological data, some affects were sampled that are not readily available from self-report data. Warmth included interest, validation, humor, and affection. Conflict included anger, sadness, contempt, and tension. Power included dominance, belligerence, and defensiveness (Shortt, 1995). Shortt did not determine whether the young adults in this study were aware of these feelings.

B. *Dynamics of Sibling Affect*

1. FREQUENCY

The frequency of experiencing a particular affect gives misleading impressions of the quality of sibling relationships, because most adult siblings have little contact with each other, averaging about once a month. Furthermore, contact frequency has proven to be a poor proxy for the socioemotional quality of sibling relationships (McGhee, 1985). In fact, contact sometimes interferes with the psychosocial adjustment of late-life siblings if it is perceived as threatening to personal autonomy or the equitable and voluntary nature of the relationship (Sussman, 1985). Sibling relationships are thought to be largely symbolic, in that they do not cease in the absence of contact (Bedford, 1989a; Wellman & Wortley, 1989). If frequency of particular feelings for siblings are to be studied, diary studies or experience sampling methods are needed to access frequency of affect with respect to the symbolic sibling relationships, as in relation to thoughts and conversations with others about the sibling (Auhagen, 1990).

2. INTENSITY

Intensity is a useful dynamic of sibling affect that has been captured at its nadir in the loyal and apathetic types and at its zenith positively and negatively in the intimate and hostile types, respectively (Gold, 1989a). Bedford (1989b) found women used extreme intensity ratings more often than men. More research is needed to ascertain whether this sex difference indicates differences in response style or in the actual emotional experience of women. Lowenthal et al. (1975) suggested that this greater intensity of feeling between sisters relates to higher levels of conflict, a point to be expanded upon later.

"High access" siblings who are age-near and shared much in childhood are likely to experience more intense levels of affect toward one another (Bank & Kahn, 1982). This association reflects not only high levels of involvement when young, but also a greater perceived resiliency in the sibling relationship compared to other primary relationships. Whereas rude or selfish conduct weakens friendships, it does not alter the quality of ascribed relationships, such as that of sibling relationships (Schneider, 1980).

3. ELICITORS

Elicitors of sibling affect are divided into contemporary and past events. Past events reside in memory and may or may not be accessible to conscious awareness. Related to elicitors are various predictors of sibling affect that might provide clues to unidentified elicitors.

Bedford (1989c) investigated contemporary sources of satisfaction and conflict in sibling relationships across adulthood and the frequency at which such events occurred. Only the variable *shared interests* was significantly related to felt satisfaction with the sibling, and this was true for all ages (20 to 79). Significant sources of sibling conflict were *giving help, being outdone,* and *sibling's bossiness;* levels of conflict elicited by these events were greater for older than for younger subjects. On the other hand, these conflict-eliciting events occurred much less frequently in the lives of older than younger subjects, perhaps due to their active efforts to avoid this unpleasant experience.

Early experiences in the history of the sibling relationship have been viewed as elicitors of sibling affect, often based on psychoanalytic formulations about early sibling rivalry. Findings indicate that feelings of closeness between siblings in adulthood are not likely to surface if the siblings were not close when children (Scott, 1983). Connidis (1989) suggested that the sibling bond may be shaped by or interpreted in relation to the intergenerational tie between parent and child. Research on child sibling relations has demonstrated that parents are an important early determinant (Boer, Goedhart, & Treffers, 1992; Dunn, 1988; Hetherington, 1988).

Notably, it is not the absolute level of parental behavior, but, rather, the degree of discrepancy in their behaviors toward offspring that is an important source of parental influence on sibling relations (Dunn, 1988; Hetherington, 1988). These discrepancies typically result in poorer sibling relationships (e.g., more negative, aggressive, and rivalrous interactions), characterized by fewer prosocial behaviors. Moreover, the sibling emotions elicited by differential parental treatment in childhood apparently continue into adulthood (Brody, Stoneman, & McCoy, 1994; Stocker, Dunn, & Plomin, 1989). In fact, adults predominantly attribute their feelings of sibling rivalry to memories of parental favoritism (Ross & Milgram, 1982). In contrast, however, Bedford (1993a) found in a study of 30- to 85-year-old adults, that perception of father's greater affection toward one's sibling in childhood predicted more, not less, positive feelings toward the sibling. Interestingly, in Bedford's sample, the nonfavored sibling had been more successful than the favored sibling in adulthood. This finding suggests that sibling comparison continues throughout life and adult sibling relations are enhanced if the siblings' total successes and favoritism are equal.

Many demographic variables have been found to predict sibling affect, but the underlying dynamics are yet to be determined. For instance, Allan (1977) reported that more working-class than middle-class respondents described at least one sibling, usually of the same gender and nearest in age, as a best friend. Similarly, Gold, Woodbury, and George (1990) suggested that adults in lower classes as compared to adults from upper classes may rely more on their siblings for support and closeness. Adams (1968) found high positive sibling affect among all socioeconomic groups except urban men in their late 20s to age 40 toward their age-near brother.

Johnson (1982) discovered that sibling solidarity varies by ethnicity. In her comparisons of intermarried and mixed Italian-American families, sibling solidarity was very strong among the intermarried, due to the hierarchical structure of the Italian-American family. In their investigation of late-life African Americans in the inner city of San Francisco, Johnson and Barer (1990) also found that the sibling relationship in many cases appeared to be the strongest bond for those who had a surviving sibling, most likely due to their chain migration to that city. Moreover, 75% of the respondents described the sibling relationship as emotionally rewarding. Similarly, Gold et al. (1990) found that whereas 85% of late-life White middle-class men and women reported their sibling relationships to be positive, 95% of the African American counterparts reported positive relations with siblings.

Gender has been the most common factor investigated in relation to sibling affect. Whereas studies first pointed to being female as predicting more positive sibling relationships, later studies focused on the gender makeup of the sibling dyad. Stocker et al. (1989) found closeness was equal for same-sex and less for cross-sex siblings in childhood. High levels of conflict between sisters have been attributed to the greater intensity of feeling in the relationship over all (Lowenthal et al., 1975) or to culture's devaluation of females' characteristics, which women themselves might incorporate (McGoldrick, 1989). Gold (1989b) and Suggs (1989) found a direct relation between the number of females in the dyad and the level of intimacy in the relationship. Thus, intimacy increases from brother–brother, brother–sister, to sister–sister. On the other hand, Connidis (1989) found that gender composition did not predict whether a sibling was a friend or a confidant. In contradiction, Lowenthal et al. (1975) found more positive evaluations of cross-sex siblings than same-sex ones, the latter relationship continuing a trend of rivalry into late life. Perhaps same-sex siblings engage in more comparisons than cross-sex dyads and, thus, are more subject to rivalry as was discussed earlier.

Sibling affect is also a function of social network composition. As the social network size decreases in late life, siblings may become relatively more important. Connidis and Davies (1990) found that siblings account for 33% of the confidant network of never married and childless older women. Middle-aged and late-life adults who have either lost their spouse or never married typically reported feeling closer and interacting more often with their siblings (Rosenberg & Anspach, 1973). For example, the never married and previously married turn to siblings more than do those who are married (Connidis & Davies, 1990; O'Bryant, 1988; Scott, 1990). O'Bryant's (1988) widows, however, turned more to their married than to their unmarried sisters, suggesting their brother-in-law is part of the attraction to this sister. Child status also seems to have repercussions for the relationship. Connidis and Davies (1990) found that sibling dyads with at least one childless member are more prone to mutual confiding and close friendship, provided they are geographically close.

Little is known about affect toward siblings-in-law, as mentioned earlier. One exploratory study found, however, that marital conflict and ambivalence on the part of both husband and wife were associated with greater contact by wives with their brother-in-law, but to a lesser extent this was true of wives' contact with kin generally (Burger & Milardo, 1995). Unfortunately, the association of feelings toward kin and contact frequency was not assessed.

Little is known about the influence of shared marital status on sibling affect. Adams (1968) suspected that commonalities based on shared marital status and child rearing accounted for the greater closeness between sisters in young adulthood compared to brothers. Perhaps feelings of closeness depend on whose perspective is considered. Bedford (1990b) found that respondents (all married) with unmarried siblings had more intensely bad feelings toward them and had more conflict themes in their sibling projective stories than did respondents with married siblings.

Some researchers have investigated the influence of family structure variables on sibling affect. Matthews, Delaney, and Adamek (1989) found, when investigating the sibling relationships of sisterless brothers, that age spacing was greatest between "disparate" brothers and smallest between "closely affiliated" brothers. Similarly, Furman and Buhrmester (1985) found that sisters (age 11 to 13) felt emotionally closer when they were close in age.

Just what instigates the increased value of siblings in later life? Earlier, perhaps having multiple roles lessened expectations or diluted the intensity of emotional involvement with them (Bedford, 1995). Both Bedford (1995) and Connidis and Davies (1992) proposed that leaving the child-rearing period and the labor force contribute to greater sibling significance. Connidis (1992) found that sibling ties are actualized, intensified, and deepened as key events of life are experienced and that siblings usually grow closer with the life transition of the arrival of children and the loss of family members through divorce, widowhood, or death. Connidis proposed that these life events have the effect of opening family subsystems to include more involvement with siblings, particularly in the form of greater emotional closeness and supportiveness. Additionally, Goetting (1986) proposed several implicit developmental tasks that drive the greater appreciation of siblings in life. Two of the late-life tasks speak directly to sibling affect. They are to provide companionship and emotional support and to resolve sibling rivalry.

Yet another instigator of sibling affect seems to be intergenerational transmission. Nagel (1995) found that there was a positive association between middle-aged parents' perceptions of their childhood sibling relationships and their parenting behaviors with their children. For fathers, the more conflict they perceived between themselves and their sibling when they were 8 to 12, the more partiality they, in turn, reported in the treatment of their children. For mothers, the greater the degree of closeness they experienced with their childhood siblings, the lower the degree of their differential treatment and the greater their involvement in fostering positive interactions between their children. Whether one's childhood experience of affect toward siblings influences the adult sibling relationships is not known except retrospectively. Long-term longitudinal data on the quality of adult sibling relationships are not yet available.

A unique study addresses the influence of level of closeness on the affects elicited during conversations using both physiological and event codes (Shortt, 1995). Closer siblings, compared to less close siblings, showed greater warmth during their conversation on enjoyable topics, whereas in less close dyads, the younger siblings showed less anger than the older siblings. During disagreeable topics of conversation, closer siblings, compared to less close siblings, displayed more affection and interest, and the older sibling in the closer dyads displayed more validation than the younger sibling.

4. DURATION AND VARIABILITY

Duration refers to length of time an instigated emotion persists; variability refers to frequency of affect shifts (Schultz, 1985). Technically, these dynamics have not been studied in relation to siblings due to a dearth of observational studies of sibling interaction. However, constancy and change in global ratings of positive and negative affect regarding siblings have been studied within the age intervals spanned by a few longitudinal studies. Carstensen (1992) found that emotional closeness to sibling declined from age 17 to 30 and then increased to age 40. Satisfaction with the relationship stayed constant until age 30 and then increased. Bedford (1990a) found that after 4 years, in a sample of 54 brother and sister pairs (37 to 72 years), negative feelings were likely to remain constant, especially for brothers, and when the degree of emotions changed they were as likely to increase as decrease. Positive feelings were more likely to change, again, especially in the case of brothers. But when they did change for sisters they were more likely to decrease. In general, though, the sibling relationship seems to increase in significance and become more positive in late life (Cicirelli, 1985).

III. SIBLING CONTRIBUTIONS TO AFFECT RESEARCH

Having organized research on feelings about siblings using concepts from affect research, we turn now to the question of whether sibling study has anything to contribute to the general study of affect. A nagging question is that there is something unique about sibling affect that cannot be understood using the existing concepts. The question this worry poses is whether the same affective experience differs according to the relationship category ("role type") of the people involved. If so, there is something unique about sibling affect simply due to the fact that the relational partner is a sibling. The evidence of sibling uniqueness derives from studies indicating psychological health (well-being) and social development as outcomes of sibling affect.

As part of a longitudinal study of sibling relationships in adulthood, Bedford (1993b) found that the positive affect state level was higher for men and women who nominated a sibling into their intimacy network (those "whose loss would be hard to bear") based on the PANAS short from (Watson, Clark, & Tellegen, 1988); nominating a friend, spouse, or child bore no such relation to affect. Two other predictions of positive affect state were simply being geographically near one's sibling and anticipating distress at separation from him or her. In contrast, predictors of negative affect state were negative feelings toward the sibling and anticipating negative feelings (such as anxiety, worry, or disappointment) at a sibling reunion. Cicirelli (1989) also demonstrated that the quality of the sibling relationship predicts well-being. Midwesterners aged 65 and older who had a positive relationship with a sister had fewer symptoms of depression than did those whose relationship with their sisters were unpleasant.

Another rather unique psychological outcome of sibling relationships is the finding that simply having a sibling in later life is beneficial to well-being (Cicirelli, 1977; McGhee, 1985). Similarly, contact frequency with siblings showed no relation whatsoever to morale in a large representative sample (Lee & Ihinger-Tallman, 1980). Research has repeatedly demonstrated that it is the perceived availability of siblings and not the actual interaction with siblings that predicts psychological well-being in late life (Blieszner, 1986; Scott, 1983).

Self-esteem is another psychological outcome that siblings influence. Specifically, siblings are the yardsticks by which social comparisons are made (Form & Geschwender, 1962), and the affective outcome of social comparison processes influence self-esteem (Schultz et al., 1994).

A wave of studies on child siblings are finding that sibling affect, in turn, bears on other relationships (McCoy, Brody, & Stoneman, 1995; Stocker & Dunn, 1990). It has been hypothesized that through interactions with siblings, young people develop social understanding skills that enable them to form peer relationships outside of the home (Stocker & Dunn, 1990). In their longitudinal analysis of sibling relationships, McCoy et al. (1995) found that sibling relationships mediated the association between youths' temperament and their close friendships. Specifically, youths whose sibling relationships were high in conflict and low in warmth also evinced poorer friendship quality.

Apparently, sibling influences on social relationships begin early. Youngblade and Dunn (1995) found dyadic conversations between kindergartners and their siblings about feeling states contributed to the child's participation in and sophistication about social pretense (specifically, pretend play). Positive sibling relationships foster social pretense as well, and the extent to which children pretend with their siblings is related to the development of the understanding of emotion, which informs social cognition.

What do findings on well-being and social outcomes contribute to general knowledge about affect? Findings on well-being offer an example of an affective experience with a particular role relation that has psychological consequences that are not as consistently found as the result of equivalent experiences of another role type. Perhaps the affective experience of siblings is qualitatively different. Perhaps role type influences one's affective responses to equivalent events in consistent, yet unique ways. Such unique responses to siblings might be explained by the especially long history of the relationship, by a primary effect due to its early origin, and/or by its original context in the highly charged nuclear family domain (in dominant Western societies, that is). These possible explanations imply that affects are attached to memories from various points in time that vary not only according to the intensity of the original experience, but when the experience occurred, and with whom.

Social outcomes of sibling interaction might relate to several factors. Easy access to siblings when living in the same home provides more opportunity structures for interaction compared to nonfamily members when very young, suggesting frequency contributes to the outcome early in life. Furthermore, the ascribed status of siblings allows greater experimentation throughout life than might be risked with friends (Kahn & Lewis, 1988). These formulations do not explain whether the outcomes with other role types under the same conditions would be the same. Perhaps norms and expectations transform the experience of sibling affect, which is originally equivalent across role types. Perhaps the affect associated with the memory of the experience rather than the experience itself makes a difference. For instance, given sibling norms and expectations, the consequences of sibling experiences might be more lasting or qualitatively different than the consequences of equivalent nonsibling experiences.

IV. FUTURE DIRECTIONS

In the review of the literature for this chapter, it was startling to realize just how much of the sibling literature directly pertains to affect. Future research will be enriched by capitalizing on the progress in both methods and theory of adult affect research.

By organizing feelings about siblings using concepts from adult affect research, the strengths and limitations of sibling affect research become apparent. Most notably missing from the sibling literature is an understanding at the more molecular level of processes that instigate and influence the variability and duration of feelings (Shortt's, 1995, study is a notable exception). Using observational techniques in conjunction with other data, such as personality inventories, is one approach to capture these processes. Additionally, the literature lacks longitudinal data tracking how sibling affect at different stages, transitions, and life events throughout the life course contribute to these same processes in memory. Tomkins's script theory would seem to be applicable for studying the latter, whether retrospectively or prospectively (see Carlson, 1981, for an example of such an application). Clearly, the study of sibling relationships is a fertile arena for research on adult affect processes. Adult sibling relationships, although varying in intensity and quality of feelings, constitute a consistent and typically important component in our lives. Moreover, due to the current trends of higher rates of divorce and childlessness, the salience of sibling ties is likely to increase in the future.

REFERENCES

Adams, B. (1968). *Kinship in an urban setting.* Chicago: Markham.

Allan, G. (1977). Sibling solidarity. *Journal of Marriage and the Family, 39.* 177–184.

Auhagen, A. E. (1990, July). *Friendship and sibling dyads in everyday life: A study with the new method of double diary.* Paper presented at the Fifth International Conference on Personal Relationships. Oxford, England.

Avioli, P. S. (1989). The social support functions of siblings in later life: A theoretical model. *The American Behavioral Scientist, 33,* 45–57.

Bank, S. P., & Kahn, M. D. (1982). *The sibling bond.* New York: Basic Books.

Bedford, V. H. (1989a). A comparison of thematic apperceptions of sibling affiliation, conflict, and separation at two periods of adulthood. *International Journal of Aging and Human Development, 28,* 53–65.

Bedford, V. H. (1989b). Sibling ambivalence in adulthood. *Journal of Family Issues, 10,* 211–224.

Bedford, V. H. (1989c). Understanding the value of siblings in old age: A proposed model. *The American Behavioral Scientist, 33,* 33–44.

Bedford, V. H. (1990a, July). *Changing affect toward siblings and the transition to old age.* Paper presented at the Second International Conference on The Future of Adult Life, Leeuwenhorst, The Netherlands.

Bedford, V. H. (1990b). Predictors of variation in positive and negative affect toward adult siblings. [Special Issue] *Family Perspectives on Aging, 24,* 245–262.

Bedford, V. H. (1993a, March). *Differential parental treatment in childhood and the quality of sibling relationships in adulthood.* Paper presented at the Biennial Scientific Meetings of the Society for Research in Child Development, New Orleans, LA.

Bedford, V. H. (1993b, August). *Attachment, intimacy and other relational links to well-being: Which apply to sibling relationship?* Paper presented at the 101st Annual Convention of the American Psychological Association, Toronto.

Bedford, V. H. (1995). Sibling relationships in middle and old age. In R. Blieszner & V. H. Bedford (Eds.), *Handbook of aging and the family* (pp. 201–222). Westport, CT: Greenwood Press.

Blieszner, R. (1986). Trends in family gerontological research. *Family Relations, 4,* 555–562.

Blieszner, R. (1988). Individual development and intimate relationships in middle and late adulthood. In R. M. Milardo (Ed.), *Families and social networks* (pp. 147–167). Newbury Park, NJ: Sage.

Boer, F., Goedhart, A. W., & Treffers, P. D. A. (1992). Siblings and their parents. In F. Boer & J. Dunn (Eds.), *Children's sibling relationships: Developmental and clinical issues* (pp. 139–152). Hillsdale, NJ: Erlbaum.

Brody, G. H., Stoneman, Z., & McCoy, J. K. (1994). Forecasting sibling relationships in early adolescence from child temperaments and family processes in middle childhood. *Child Development, 65,* 771–784.

Burger, E., & Milardo, R. M. (1995). Marital interdependence and social networks. *Journal of Social and Personal Relationships, 12,* 403–415.

Carlson, R. (1981). Studies in script theory: I. Adult analogs of a childhood nuclear scene. *Journal of Personality and Social Psychology, 40,* 501–510.

Carstensen, L. L. (1992). Social and emotional patterns in adulthood: Support for socioemotional selectivity theory. *Psychology and Aging, 7,* 331–338.

Cicirelli, V. G. (1977). Relationship of siblings to the elderly person's feelings and concerns. *Journal of Gerontology, 131,* 317–322.

Cicirelli, V. G. (1982). Sibling influence throughout the lifespan. In M. E. Lamb & B. Sutton-Smith (Eds.), *Sibling relationships: Their nature and significance across the lifespan* (pp. 267–284). Hillsdale, NJ: Erlbaum.

Cicirelli, V. G. (1985). Sibling relationships through the life cycle. In L. L'Abate (Ed.), *The handbook of family psychology and therapy* (Vol. 1, pp. 177–214). Homewood, IL: Dorsey Press.

Cicirelli, V. G. (1989). Feelings of attachment to siblings and well-being in later life. *Psychology and Aging, 4,* 211–216.

Cicirelli, V. G. (1995). *Sibling relationships across the life span.* New York: Plenum Press.

Connidis, I. A. (1989). Siblings as friends in later life. *American Behavioral Scientist, 33,* 81–93.

Connidis, I. A., & Davies, L. (1990). Confidants and companions in later life. The place of family and friends. *Journal of Gerontology, 45,* S141–149.

Connidis, I. A., & Davies, L. (1992). Confidants and companions: Choices in later life. *Journal of Gerontology, 47,* S115–122.

Cumming, E., & Schneider, D. M. (1961). Sibling solidarity: A property of American kinship. *American Anthropologist, 63,* 498–507.

Denham, S. A. (1986). Social cognition, prosocial behavior, and emotion in preschoolers: Contextual validation. *Child Development, 57,* 194–201.

Dunn, J. (1988). Connections between relationships: Implications of research on mothers and siblings. In R. A. Hinde & J. Stevenson-Hinde (Eds.), *Relationships within families: Mutual influences* (pp. 168–180). Oxford: Clarendon Press.

Form, W. H., & Geschwender, J. A. (1962). Social reference basis of job satisfaction: The case of manual workers. *American Sociological Review, 27,* 232–233.

Furman, W., & Buhrmester, D. (1985). Children's perceptions of the quality of sibling relationships. *Child Development, 56,* 448–461.

Goetting, A. (1986). The developmental tasks of siblingship over the life cycle. *Journal of Marriage and the Family, 48,* 703–714.

Gold, D. T. (1989a). Sibling relationships in old age: a typology. *International Journal of Aging and Human Development, 28,* 37–51.

Gold, D. T. (1989b). Generational solidarity: Conceptual antecedents and consequences. *American Behavioral Scientist, 33,* 19–32.

Gold, D. T., Woodbury, M. A., & George, L. K. (1990). Relationship classification
using grade of membership analysis: A typology of sibling relationships in
later life. *Journal of Gerontology, 45,* S43–S51.

Gutmann, D. L. (1987). *Reclaimed powers.* New York: Basic Books.

Hetherington, M. (1988). Parents, children, and siblings. Six years after divorce.
In R. A. Hinde & J. Stevenson-Hinde (Eds.), *Relationships within families: Mutual influences.* (pp. 311–331). Oxford: Clarendon Press.

Horney, K. (1945). *Our inner conflict.* New York: Norton.

Johnson, C. L. (1982). Sibling solidarity: Its origin and functioning in Italian-
American families. *Journal of Marriage and the Family, 2,* 155–165.

Johnson, C. L., & Barer, B. M. (1996). Childlessness and kinship organization:
Comparisons of very old Whites and Blacks. *Journal of Cross-cultural Gerontology, 10,* 289–306.

Johnson, C. L., & Troll, L. (1996). Family structure and the timing of transitions
from 70 to 103 years of age. *Journal of Marriage and the Family, 58* (1), 178–187.

Kahn, M. D., & Lewis, K. G. (Eds.). (1988). *Siblings in therapy: Life-span and clinical issues.* New York: Norton.

Labouvie-Vief, G., Hakim-Larson, J., DeVoe, M., & Schoeberlein, S. (1989). Emotions and self-regulations: A life span view. *Human Development, 32,* 279–299.

Lawton, M. P., Kleban, M. H., Rajagopal, C., & Dean, J. (1992). Dimensions of affective experience in three age groups. *Psychology and Aging, 7,* 171–184.

Lee, G. R., & Ihinger-Tallman, M. (1980). Sibling interaction and morale: The effects of family relations on older people. *Research on Aging, 2,* 367–391.

Lowenthal, M. F., Thurnher, M., & Chiriboga, D. (1975). *Four stages of life.* San
Francisco: Jossey-Bass.

Mancini, J. A., & Blieszner, R. (1989). Aging parents and adult children: Research themes in intergenerational relations. *Journal of Marriage and the Family, 51,* 275–290.

Matthews, S. H., Delaney, P. J., & Adamek, M. E. (1989). Male kinship ties: Bonds
between adult brothers. *American Behavioral Scientist, 33,* 58–69.

McCoy, J. K., Brody, G. H., & Stoneman, Z. (1995, March). *A longitudinal analysis
of sibling relationships as mediators and moderators of the link between individual
temperament, family processes and youths' best friendships.* Paper presented at the
biennial meeting of the Society for Research in Child Development, Indianapolis, IN.

McGhee, J. L. (1985). The effects of siblings on the life satisfaction of the rural elderly. *Journal of Marriage and the Family, 47,* 85–91.

McGoldrick, M. (1989). Sisters. In M. McGoldrick, C. M. Anderson, & F. Walsh
(Eds.), *Women in families* (pp. 244–266). New York: Norton.

Moss, S. Z., & Moss, M. S. (1989). The impact of the death of an elderly sibling:
Some considerations of a normative loss. *American Behavioral Scientist, 33,*
94–106.

Nagel, S. K. (1995, March). *The quality of parents' sibling interactions in relation to the quality of their children's sibling interactions.* Paper presented at the biennial meeting of the Society for Research in Child Development, Indianapolis, IN.

New York Times, September, 1993, (late edition). B1, B10.

O'Bryant, S. L. (1988). Sibling support and older widows' well-being. *Journal of Marriage and the Family, 50,* 173–184.

Rosenberg, G. S., & Anspach, D. F. (1973). Sibling solidarity in the working class. *Journal of Marriage and the Family, February,* 108–113.

Ross, H. G., & Milgram, J. I. (1982). Important variables in adult sibling relationships: A qualitative study. In M. E. Lamb & B. Sutton-Smith (Eds), *Sibling relationships: their nature and significance across the lifespan* (pp. 225–249). Hillsdale, NJ: Erlbaum.

Rubenstein, R. L., Alexander, B. B., Goodman, M., & Luborsky, M. (1991). Key relationships of never married, childless older women: A cultural analysis. *Journal of Gerontology: Social Sciences, 46,* S270–277.

Schneider, D. M. (1980). *American kinship: A cultural account.* Chicago: The University of Chicago Press.

Schultz, R. (1985). Emotion and affect. In J. E. Birren & K. W. Schaie (Eds.), *Handbook of the psychology of aging* (2nd ed., pp. 531–543). New York: Van Nostrand Reinhold.

Schultz, R., O'Brian, A. T., & Tompkins, C. (1994). The measurement of affect in the elderly. In M. P. Lawton & J. A. Terisi (Eds.), *Review of gerontology and geriatrics* (Vol. 14, pp. 210–344). New York: Springer.

Scott, J. P. (1983). Siblings and other kin. In T. Brubaker (Ed.), *Family relationships in later life* (pp. 47–62). Newbury Park, CA: Sage.

Scott, J. P. (1990). Siblings and other kin. In T. Brubaker (Ed.), *Family relationships in later life* (pp. 86–99). Newbury Park, CA: Sage.

Shortt, J. W. (1995, March). The ties that bind: Closeness in young adult sibling relationships. In M. Sommers (Chair), *Sibling relations in late adolescence and early adulthood.* Symposium conducted at the biennial meetings of the Society for Research in Child Development, Indianapolis, IN.

Stocker, C., & Dunn, J. (1990). Sibling relationships in childhood: Links with friendships and peer relationships. *British Journal of Developmental Psychology, 8*(3), 227–244.

Stocker, C., Dunn, J., & Plomin, R. (1989). Sibling relationships: links with temperament, maternal behavior and family structure. *Child Development, 60,* 715–727.

Suggs, P. K. (1989). Predictors of association among older siblings: A black/white comparison. *American Behavioral Scientist, 33,* 70–80.

Suitor, J. J., & Pillemer, K. (1993). Support and interpersonal stress in the social networks of married daughters caring for parents with dementia. *Journal of Gerontology: Social Sciences, 48,* S1–S8.

Sussman, M. B. (1985). The family of old people. In R. H. Binstock & E. Shanas (Eds.), *Handbook of aging and the social sciences,* 2nd ed. (pp. 415–449). New York: Van Nostrand Reinhold.

Tomkins (1963). *Affect, imagery, and consciousness. Vol. 2: The negative affects.* New York: Springer.

Vandell, D. L., Minnett, A. M., & Santrock, J. W. (1987). Age differences in sibling relationships during middle childhood. *Journal of Applied Developmental Psychology, 8,* 24–257.

Watson, D., Clark, L. A., & Tellegen, A. (1988). Development and validation of brief measures of positive and negative affect: The PANAS scales. *Journal of Personality and Social Psychology, 54*(6), 1063–1070.

Wellman, B., & Wortley, S. (1989). Brothers' keepers: Situating kinship relations in broader networks of social support. *Sociological Perspectives, 32,* 273–306.

White, L. K., & Riedmann, A. (1992a). When the Brady Bunch grows up: Step/half- and full-sibling relationships in adulthood. *Journal of Marriage and the Family, 54,* 197–208.

White, L. K., & Riedmann, A. (1992b). Ties among adult siblings. *Social Forces, 71,* 85–102.

Youngblade, L. M., & Dunn, J. (1995) Individual differences in young children's pretend play with mother and sibling: Links to relationships and understanding of other people's feelings and beliefs. *Child Development, 66,* 1472–1492.

CHAPTER 13

Affect in Intimate Relationships

The Developmental Course of Marriage

Laura L. Carstensen *and* Jeremy Graff
Department of Psychology
Stanford University
Stanford, California

Robert W. Levenson
University of California, Berkeley
Berkeley, California

John M. Gottman
University of Washington
Seattle, Washington

I. INTRODUCTION

The cardinal role that social relationships play in emotional development has been well established. Not only does social interaction serve to strengthen and refine links between feelings and environmental events early in life (deRivera, 1984), social interactions contribute importantly to the development of attachment (Ainsworth, 1982; Bowlby, 1973) and the acquisition of emotional knowledge (Shaver, 1984). Although the developmental course of social and emotional links in later stages of life has received far less attention, it is clear that the inextricable association between emotion and social contact never ceases. In all likelihood, emotional experience within the context of social relationships influences virtually all domains of human experience throughout the human life span.

In this chapter, we explore the role of emotion expression and experience within the context of intimate relationships in adulthood and old age. We focus on the marital relationship because in Western cultures it is the closest and most enduring relationship most adults experience. Over 95% of people in America marry at some point in their lives, and after 20 years more than half of these marriages are still intact; in cases of divorce, remarriage within two to three years is typical (U.S. Bureau of the Census, 1992b). Marriage also serves as a rite of passage that signals entry into adulthood and marks the beginning of a developmental path on which other emotionally charged life events, such as parenthood and widowhood, are likely to follow. Thus, the marital relationship serves as a principal context for emotional experiences and life events.

In the following pages, we argue that relationships characterized by heavy emotional investment have broad implications for individuals' mental and physical health. Next, we characterize at a more microscopic level emotional exchanges between husbands and wives at different points in the life cycle. And finally, we offer the beginnings of a theoretical framework within which to consider the developmental course of emotional experience during the second half of life.

II. LINKS AMONG MARRIAGE, EMOTION, AND HEALTH

Marriage in modern times is expected to serve as a principal resource for emotional support. Most married people count their spouses among the small circle of intimates who comprise the social convoy that accompanies them through life (Antonucci & Jackson, 1987). As people age, spouses exert direct and indirect influences on access to emotional closeness. In old age, for example, as the overall social network narrows, the spousal relationship comes to occupy an ever larger proportion of this social resource. Spouses contribute to the overall size of their partners' social networks, above and beyond their own presence, by introducing their own close friends and relatives to one another, thus expanding each other's social networks with social partners who might not otherwise be available (Lang & Carstensen, 1994).

In recent years a compelling case has been made for the link between social support and physical health. Married people are in better physical and mental health than their single counterparts (B. Hess & Soldo, 1985). At one level, support from a spouse or child can reduce high-risk health behaviors, such as alcohol consumption, smoking, and drug use (Costello, 1991). But even controlling for health practices and socioeconomic status, the increased presence of emotional confidants—which is clearly associated with marital status—predicts lower morbidity and lower mortality (Berkman & Syme, 1979; Blazer, 1982; Breslow & Engstrom, 1980).

The manner in which social relationships influence physical health remains elusive, however, and the health benefits of marriage require two important qualifiers related importantly to emotion: First, whereas married men appear to be healthier than single men irrespective of marital satisfaction, wives derive health benefits only when the marriage is happy (B. Hess & Soldo, 1985; Levenson, Carstensen, & Gottman, 1993), an issue to which we return later in this chapter. Second, the double-edged sword of emotional closeness is evident in marriage. When relationships are unhappy, the intimacy of marriage places spouses at risk for a number of deleterious outcomes. Unhappy marriages can entail physical violence, mental abuse (Markman, Renick, Floyd, & Stanley, 1993), and even murder (Tariq & Anila, 1993). Unhappy marriages are also strongly implicated in clinical depression. Among couples who seek marital therapy, half involve a depressed spouse (Beach, Jouriles, & O'Leary, 1985), and half of all women who seek treatment for depression report serious marital problems (Rounsaville, Weissman, Prusoff, & Herceg-Baron, 1979). Interestingly, the consequences of being in a good marriage are not all positive; when one spouse is depressed, the degree to which the couple is emotionally close is a risk factor for the other spouse also becoming depressed (Tower & Kasl, 1995).

III. THE DEVELOPMENTAL COURSE OF MARRIAGE

Most of the literature on marriage has focused on marital interaction and marital quality in relatively young couples (Krokoff, 1987) with the principle aim of identifying qualities in marriages that predict divorce (Gottman, 1993, 1994; Gottman & Levenson, 1992). When later stages of marriage have been studied, the emphasis most often has been on the influence that marital satisfaction has on other life domains, such as the extent to which happy marriages are associated with positive adjustment of offspring or productivity in the workplace. The bulk of the research on parenting, for example, examines the influence that parents have on their childrens' development as opposed to the influence that having children has on parental development (Seltzer & Ryff, 1994). Relatively little attention has been paid to potential changes in marital dynamics over time, as spouses come to know one another increasingly better, experience personal crises, pursue individual work trajectories, resolve identity issues, and coordinate their life goals. Subsequently, the nature of marriage as it unfolds across adulthood remains relatively uncharted territory. In this section, we briefly overview research findings that speak directly or indirectly to the developmental course of marriage.

The earliest empirical assessments of marital *satisfaction* over time suggest that satisfaction is highest among newlyweds and proceeds to decline steadily during the ensuing years (Blood & Wolfe, 1960; Pineo, 1961, 1969; White & Booth, 1985). More recent research also suggests that passionate love declines during the early years of marriage and after major life events such as childbirth (P. Tucker & Aaron, 1993). Studies of long-term marriages paint a more optimistic picture suggesting that although satisfaction with marriage does indeed decline during the first twenty years, it increases again in the later years (Burr, 1970; Guilford & Bengtson, 1979; Rollins & Cannon, 1974; Rollins & Feldman, 1970). One important longitudinal study of marriage, which asked spouses to describe both positive and negative aspects of their relationships, suggested that negative sentiment (e.g., disagreements about important issues, anger, and criticism) declines linearly over time, whereas positive interactions (e.g., laughing together, exchanging interesting ideas, etc.) follow a curvilinear pattern, reaching high points early and late in marriage (Guilford & Bengtson, 1979). Studies of marriage in old age, based on questionnaire and interview data, suggest that marriages that survive into the twilight years are often satisfying and emotionally close (Erikson, Erikson, & Kivnick, 1986; Levenson et al., 1993; Stinnett, Carter, & Montgomery, 1972).

There is emerging consensus in the literature that the reliable decline in satisfaction during the early years of marriage is associated, at least indirectly, with parenting. On average, the transition to parenthood holds negative consequences for marriage (Belsky & Pensky, 1988; Burr, 1970; P. Cowan & Cowan, 1988; C. Cowan et al., 1985; Rollins & Cannon, 1974). Although a significant minority of new parents report improved marital functioning following the birth of a child, most couples report a reduction in marital satisfaction (Belsky & Rovine, 1990; P. Cowan & Cowan, 1988) characterized by an increase in marital conflicts and a decrease in shared positive experiences (P. Cowan & Cowan, 1988). Both husbands and wives experience this drop in marital satisfaction. Wives, however, tend to feel the impact sooner. For wives the decline is experienced most strongly during the first six months after the birth of a child, whereas husbands experience a decline in marital satisfaction the following year (C. Cowan & Cowan, 1992).

Although social scientists initially attributed dissatisfaction to the demands of child rearing itself, the drop in marital satisfaction appears to be related more directly to the exacerbation of gender roles commonly experienced during the transition to parenthood (P. Cowan & Cowan,

1988) and from the challenge to parents to develop a coordinated approach to child rearing (Gable, Belsky, & Crnic, 1992). The division of labor appears to be particularly central to marital conflicts during this life stage (C. Cowan & Cowan, 1992). Most studies suggest that even with an increase in paternal involvement in child rearing observed over recent years, a disproportionate burden of parenting continues to be placed on wives, even in relationships that were previously equitable (C. Cowan & Cowan, 1992; Levant, Slattery, & Loiselle, 1987). Dissatisfaction is greatest when husbands' actual involvement in parenting is less than wives' expected it would be (Belsky, Ward, & Rovine, 1986; Garrett, 1983).

Marital satisfaction does not improve significantly until children leave home (Troll, 1985). However, as children grow older, child-related factors that influence marital satisfaction appear to change from issues related to the division of labor to qualitative aspects of parent–child relationships and parents' involvement in other life domains. Marital satisfaction in parents of adolescents, for example, is influenced by parental self-esteem and attitudes toward their own aging as well as characteristics of the teenager and the degree of closeness between parents and children (Steinberg & Silverberg, 1987). Parents who are highly work-oriented generally experience improvement in mental health as their children reach adolescence, whereas parents who are less work-oriented experience declines (Silverberg & Steinberg, 1990). Parenting of adolescents often co-occurs with the period in life that adults provide care to their aging parents. However, to the best of our knowledge, the potential influence of this additional external stressor on marital satisfaction has not been addressed in the marital or developmental literatures (see also George & Gold, 1991).

Despite the apparent challenge that children present to couples' satisfaction with their relationships, the effects of children on their parents' marriages are not uniformly negative. This becomes especially evident when one views parenting from a life course perspective. In retrospective accounts of marriages that had lasted for more than 50 years, the child-bearing years were viewed as both the most satisfying and least satisfying periods of marriages; and in old age, the presence of adult children is strongly predictive of emotional well-being (Lang & Carstensen, 1994). In our own research, children represent the greatest source of marital conflict among middle-aged couples but become the greatest source of pleasure older couples share (Levenson et al., 1993).

The effects of retirement on long-term relationships remain equivocal. Some studies show a positive effect of retirement on marriage, especially among middle- and upper-middle class couples who are in good health (Atchley, 1976), whereas other studies have documented negative effects of retirement on marital satisfaction, particularly on wives (John-ston, 1990; Lee & Shehan, 1989). Ekerdt and Vinick (1991) found that spouses adjusting to the retirement of their partners complained no more or less about their marriages than their nonretired counterparts. It is hard to imagine that a change as profound as retirement has no effect on the day-to-day lives of married couples, and couples who face retire-ment do report that they anticipate both positive and negative effects of the transition (Vinick & Ekerdt, 1991). However, the profile of find-ings in this literature suggests that the resiliency and continuity of long-term marriages probably precludes dramatic effects on the quality of the relationship.

The illness and eventual death of a spouse are also associated with marriage in the later years. The process and experience of widowhood can be emotionally devastating for husbands and wives. Gender, once again, makes a difference. Both caregiving and widowhood are far more com-mon experiences for women than men. Mens' shorter life expectancy, combined with the societal practice of women marrying older men, places women at greater risk for assuming the caregiver role and eventually be-coming widowed. By the age of 84, 62% of women but only 20% of men have lost spouses due to death (U.S. Bureau of the Census, 1992a).

The enormous burden of caregiving within the societal constraints imposed by the American health-care system is evidenced by the fact that 50% of caregivers become clinically depressed (Gallagher, Rose, Rivera, & Lovett, 1989). When a husband becomes ill, his wife typically assumes the primary caregiver role; when a wife becomes ill other female relatives are more likely to assume primary caregiving roles (Carstensen & Pasu-pathi, 1993). Moreover, when husbands do become caregivers, they are more likely than wives to receive assistance from other relatives and friends or to hire professional help (Zarit, Orr, & Zarit, 1982). Women, in contrast, are often reluctant to seek any help at all (Zarit et al., 1982). Subsequently, caregiving is typically more stressful for women than men (Barusch & Spaid, 1989).

Widowhood itself, however, appears to be particularly stressful for men. Among men, but not among women, widowhood is associated with increased mortality risk (Helsing, 1981; Longino & Lipman, 1981). Men are also four times more likely than women to remarry after the death of a spouse (Carstensen & Pasupathi, 1993). One can only speculate about the reasons for these gender differences in the experience of widowhood. One possibility involves emotional support. Married men are more likely to rely on their partner as their sole confidant, whereas women are more likely to have same-sex confidants outside of marriage (Komarovsky, 1976; Vaux, 1985). Because women have more emotional confidants than men, the death of a spouse is less likely to result in the loss of their entire emotional support network.

In addition, although widowhood is obviously negatively valenced for both women and men, for women in the current cohort of elderly people, it is also frequently associated with a newfound sense of autonomy and competence as women take over roles previously assumed by their husbands (e.g., managing finances) (George, 1981). Of course, practical issues also limit remarriage among older women, given the fewer available mates.

In closing, the literature suggests that the emotional climate of marriage changes across adulthood. The best documented change includes a general trend toward declining marital satisfaction following the birth of a child, which persists until children leave home. The normative developmental path along which couples become parents, "launch" children into the world, and return to a primarily dyadic unit inevitably entails emotionally taxing times. The experience of conflicts within marital relationships is arguably unavoidable. In the next section we review a literature that suggests that the ways in which couples resolve emotionally charged issues is centrally involved in the maintenance of satisfying, intimate relationships.

IV. THE EXPRESSION AND EXPERIENCE OF EMOTION IN MARRIAGE

A considerable literature on emotion expression and experience within the context of marriage provides ample evidence that the nature of emotional exchanges between spouses is related to marital satisfaction and marital dissolution (Gottman & Levenson, 1992; Levenson & Gottman, 1985; Storaasli & Markman, 1990). As noted above, the vast majority of the research on marriage has targeted relatively young couples. In this section, we briefly overview central findings from this literature and then compare and contrast these findings with those from an observational study of middle-aged and older couples that we have conducted over the last several years (Carstensen, Levenson, & Gottman, 1995; Levenson et al., 1993; Levenson, Carstensen, & Gottman, 1994).

For most people, the marital relationship entails the highest emotional highs and the lowest emotional lows experienced in adult life. Over the years couples share extremely intimate moments, marked by joy, hope, pride, feelings of accomplishment, and empathy. Yet the very intimacy that links two people also lays the groundwork for feelings of deep resentment, sadness, jealousy, and anger. Couples clearly differ along quantitative and qualitative dimensions in the degree to which they experience positive and negative emotions in their marriages as well as the strategies they enlist to cope with relationship conflicts. Most couples develop characteristic styles of dealing with conflict, from tacit agreements to avoid discussions of conflicts to the frequent and open airing of hostilities (Gottman, 1993). Because spouses' emotional well-being is so clearly linked to one another, in order for marriages to remain happy, a style must evolve that allows both partners to achieve satisfactory resolution of conflict. Indeed, couples' success in resolving negative issues in relationships predicts marital outcomes better than the frequency with which they share positive emotional experiences (Markman, 1992), and interventions that improve couples' effectiveness in resolving conflicts have been shown to strengthen troubled marriages (Jacobson & Addis, 1993).

The ability to handle emotional conflict in marriage relies, to a great extent, on the ability to deal simultaneously with one's own negative affect and the negative affect expressed by a partner (Markman, 1991). Issues that arouse strong feelings in both partners are very difficult to resolve when spouses rely on different coping strategies. For example, a particularly dissatisfying pattern occurs when one partner strives to resolve a conflict and the other partner withdraws in response to the negative emotions expressed by the first partner (Christensen & Heavey, 1990).

Discussions of relationship conflict clearly distinguish distressed from nondistressed couples. Compared to their happily married counterparts, unhappily married couples express more negative affect, are more likely to reciprocate negative affect expressed by their spouse and show greater physiological linkage to one another during a discussion of conflict (Levenson & Gottman, 1983). In addition, unhappily married couples tend to show a pattern in which one partner makes demands while the other partner withdraws (Christensen & Heavey, 1990; Levenson & Gottman, 1983).

Styles of conflict resolution are associated with gender. In general, men display attempts to end conflict discussions either through conciliation or withdrawal. Women, in contrast, are more likely to push toward resolution of conflicts. Gottman and Levenson (1992) attribute this male tendency to disengage verbally and emotionally, which they refer to as "stonewalling," to the relative intolerance of men for the physiological arousal that accompanies negative emotions. Christiansen and Heavey (1990) view the same pattern as a more general "demand/withdrawal" dynamic of interpersonal interaction. They argue that, regardless of gender, a person who desires change will make demands and a person who is being asked to change will withdraw. According to their view, the pattern becomes gendered because social structural factors that place women in subservient positions to men lead women to desire change more than men. In an experiment in which two conflictual topics were discussed, one in which wives wanted change and one in which husbands wanted change, they obtained partial support for their hypothesis. Wives showed more withdrawal behavior when their husbands asked for change and vice versa. Nevertheless, husbands remained more withdrawing and wives more demanding. Interestingly, Heavey, Layne, and Christensen (1993) observed that when husbands do make demands and wives withdraw, marital satisfaction increases over time. They speculated that wives interpret husbands' demands as evidence of interest in the relationship and/ or a willingness to break out of stereotyped gender roles in the service of improving marital relations (Heavey et al., 1993). It is also possible that a reversal of prototypical roles provides husbands and wives a way to soothe their partners. That is, when wives remove themselves from conflict discussions, they release their husbands from unpleasant feelings associated with conflictual interactions. When husbands push for conflict resolution, it suggests to their wives that they are invested in the relationship. Levenson and Gottman (1985) reported a similar pattern in predictors of future marital satisfaction. The greatest improvement in marital satisfaction over a 3-year period was found when husbands' negative affect was not reciprocated by their wives, and when wives' negative affect was reciprocated by their husbands.

As noted above, the vast majority of observational research on marriage has focused on relatively young couples. Several years ago three of us embarked on an observational study of middle-aged and older couples in order to see whether happy and unhappy couples who had been married for many years would show similar patterns as the younger couples described in the literature. Although it appeared from questionnaire research that marital satisfaction increases in old age, there was virtually no information on age differences in the dynamics of emotional exchange.

We anticipated that there might be differences in emotional interactions between older and younger couples for three primary reasons. One, there is some evidence in the literature that, with age, gendered roles soften (Hyde & Phillis, 1979) or even reverse (Guttmann, 1987). Because gendered patterns appear to underlie much marital conflict, a lessening of these roles could result in improved communication patterns between husbands and wives. Second, there is some suggestion in the literature that emotional understanding (Labouvie-Vief & DeVoe, 1991) and emotional regulation improve (Lawton, Kleban, Rajagopal, & Dean, 1992) and become more salient with age (Carstensen & Turk-Charles, 1994; Fredrickson & Carstensen, 1990). If so, there should be evidence of such improvement in the interactional dynamics of married couples. Third, although the subjective experience of specific emotions (Levenson, Carstensen,

Friesen, & Ekman, 1991; Malatesta & Kalnok, 1984) and the configuration of autonomic changes that accompanies basic emotions (Levenson et al., 1991) appear to remain unchanged with age, the magnitude of the associated physiological arousal appears to be somewhat reduced (Levenson, et al., 1991). We reasoned that such a reduction could reduce the toxicity of conflict discussions and facilitate conflict resolution.

In order to ensure that we were not studying exclusively happy couples, we actively recruited four subsamples of couples: unhappily married middle-aged couples, happily married middle-aged couples, unhappily married older couples, and happily married older couples (see Levenson et al., 1993 for a full description of sampling procedures). The experimental paradigm we used was identical to that used in Levenson and Gottman's (1983) research with younger couples. Following an initial telephone and mail screening which ensured appropriate cell assignment, couples arrived at the laboratory after an 8-hour period of separation. They were asked to engage in three conversations with one another while their behavior was videotaped and their physiological activity was recorded.

The three conversations included a discussion of the events of the day, a discussion of a conflict that was a source of continuing disagreement in their marriage; and a discussion of a mutually agreed upon pleasant topic. Each conversation lasted for 15 minutes, preceded by a 5-min silent period. For the events of the day conversation, couples were asked simply to discuss events that had happened during the day. Prior to initiating the problem area discussion, couples completed the Couple's Problem Inventory (Gottman, Markman, & Notarius, 1977) on which they rated the perceived severity of several marital issues. Prior to initiating the pleasant topic discussion, they completed a similar inventory, in which they rated the enjoyment derived from pleasant aspects of their relationships. An interviewer used these inventories to help couples select topics for conversations.

A day or two later, spouses returned separately to the laboratory to view the video recording of their interaction and provide a continuous report of their subjective affective experience during the interactions. This was accomplished by having spouses adjust a rating dial while they watched the videotape, which was anchored at one end by "extremely negative" and at the other end by "extremely positive" in order to indicate the degree of positivity or negativity they had experienced during the interaction.

Ratings of problem severity and enjoyment of pleasant events were analyzed. Videotapes were scored using the Specific Affect Coding System (Gottman & Krokoff, 1989) such that specific emotional behaviors expressed by spouses when they were speaking and listening could be quantified. Physiological activity as well as associated subjective states were also assessed.

As noted above, we were most interested in age and gender differences displayed by couples who had been married for many years. Because conflict resolution is so informative of younger couples' marriages, we were especially interested in potential age differences in the conflict arena.

Ratings of problems and pleasant topics suggested that older couples' conflicts were less severe than middle-aged couples' conflicts and centered around different issues (Levenson et al., 1993). Middle-aged couples disagreed more than older couples about children, money, religion, and recreation. None of the ten topics assessed were more conflictual for older couples than for middle-aged couples. Moreover, older couples derived more pleasure than middle-aged couples from four sources: talking about children and grandchildren, doing things together, dreams, and vacations. None of the topics assessed were more pleasurable for middle-aged couples than for older couples. Thus, it appears that older couples not only experience less conflict in their marriages, they also experience more pleasure.

There was direct evidence for improved emotion regulation in the observational data. Older couples, compared to middle-aged couples, expressed lower levels of anger, disgust, belligerence, and whining and higher levels of one important emotion, namely affection. This pattern of results holds even after controlling statistically for the severity of the problem discussed. Interestingly, the pattern is consistent with Guilford and Bengtson's (1979) longitudinal evidence for increasing positivity and decreasing negativity in marriage in late life.

By and large, we did not find evidence for a softening of gendered roles suggested in the literature. Older couples displayed the same gendered patterns as the middle-aged couples in our study and younger couples studied previously. Wives expressed more emotion, both positive and negative, than their husbands. Husbands displayed more stonewalling than wives.

However, there was one intriguing gender difference that offers a potential explanation for the apparent differences in health benefits marriage provides for husbands and wives. Recall that husbands appear to derive health benefits from marriage independent of marital quality, whereas wives derive health benefits only from happy marriages (Hess & Soldo, 1985). In our study as well unhappily married women were in poorer health than their happily married counterparts (Levenson et al., 1993). Recall also that Gottman and Levenson (1988) argue that stonewalling is due to the relative intolerance males have for the physiological arousal associated with negative emotions. Measures used in this study allowed us to examine the relationship between actual levels of physiological arousal and subjective distress (Levenson et al., 1994). We found significant correlations among six of the seven physiological indices and subjective distress in husbands. None of the physiological measures correlated significantly with subjective distress indicated by wives. In short, although mens' subjective distress was consistent with their level of physiological arousal, womens' was not.

Levenson et al. (1994) argue that this gender difference may account for the different effects bad marriages appear to have on women and men. Mens' sensitivity to physiological arousal may provide an internal "alarm system" that signals the need to reduce stimulation and produce the consequent withdrawal that is manifest as stonewalling behavior. Women, who are perhaps less aware of such signals, may persist in interactions characterized by extended periods of autonomic nervous system arousal. This persistence may be particularly distressing for women if their partner appears to be "sitting it out." Over the course of many years, these frequent unmitigated bouts of heightened physiological arousal on the part of women may contribute to the increase in physical symptoms experienced by unhappily married wives. In contrast, the withdrawal behavior on the part of men may be protective, thus accounting for the relative lack of negative impact of marital unhappiness on husbands' health.

Finally, the generalizability of these findings must be tested. Whereas there is considerable reliability of the findings we reported for younger couples, observational analysis of older couples' emotional patterns is limited largely to the study we described. Moreover, the vast majority of research on marriage—including ours—has focused predominantly on white, middle-class, and Judeo-Christian samples. We simply do not know the extent to which current research represents the experiences of minority couples. Clearly, regulatory styles are influenced by "emotion cultures" (Thompson, 1994). The extent to which subcultures vary in terms of the nature of intimate relationships very likely influences the degree to which our findings also characterize minority marriages. Examination of the relatively sparse literature on marriages among minorities in the United States suggests that there are important similarities to majority groups. Marital satisfaction, for example, is similar for African-American and Anglo couples (Tucker, Taylor, & Mitchell-Kernan, 1993) and spousal social support is similar for American and South Asian samples (Venkatraman, 1995). At the same time, however, differences have been reported that implicate conflict resolution styles. African-American couples describe both more positive and more negative aspects of marriage than Anglo couples (Oggins, Veroff, & Leber, 1993). Compared to Anglo couples, they also report more withdrawal from conflictual interactions (Oggins et al., 1993). The finding that African-American couples report that they are more likely than Anglo couples to withdraw from conflict, but fail to show lesser marital satisfaction suggests that interactions may be interpreted differently by different subgroups.

To recapitulate, the literature on emotional exchanges among married couples suggests that the manner in which couples resolve emotionally charged conflicts predicts marital satisfaction throughout adulthood. Spousal satisfaction with their marriages, even those that have lasted for decades, is related to the ways in which negative emotions are expressed and reciprocated. Emotional exchanges characterized by the expression of higher levels of negative than positive affect and the expression of high levels of specific affects, like contempt and disgust, are associated with unhappy marriages across the adult life span. There is also evidence for the consistency of gender differences across adulthood, characterized by emotional expressiveness and engagement on the part of females and relative inexpressiveness and withdrawal among males. These gendered patterns may relate importantly to physical health. Thus, there appears to be considerable consistency in interactional dynamics among married couples across adulthood.

Those age differences that were observed were quite positive. Although there are, of course, unhappy marriages in old age, by and large, couples that survive into the later years appear to derive from them more pleasure and less distress. At the interactive level it appears that older couples interweave expressions of affection into discussions of conflicts, which may serve an important emotional regulatory function. The extent to which these patterns are culture-bound remains to be seen.

V. A THEORETICAL FRAMEWORK FOR EMOTIONAL DEVELOPMENT AND INTIMACY IN ADULTHOOD

A consideration of emotional development within a life span perspective is only starting to take shape within the social sciences. The beginning of this line of research suggests that emotion may represent one psychological domain that is largely spared from the deleterious effects of the aging process. Certainly, early notions about emotional quiescence and disengagement in later life have not held up to empirical test (Carstensen, 1987; Malatesta & Izard, 1984). The integrity of the basic emotion system appears to be maintained. Older people experience emotions subjectively at levels of intensity comparable to younger adults

(Levenson, et al., 1991; Malatesta & Kalnok, 1984) and physiological signatures associated with specific emotions are also maintained into old age, even though the overall level of arousal is somewhat reduced (Levenson et al., 1991). Moreover, by self-report, older adults control their emotions better than young adults (Lawton et al., 1992) and show improved emotional understanding (Labouvie-Vief, DeVoe, & Bulka, 1989). The research we have reviewed herein on emotional intimacy in adulthood contributes to this relatively glowing picture.

Why might emotional functioning maintain or improve across the life course when functioning in other psychological arenas shows simultaneous decline? First, although cognitive processing of new information shows definite deterioration with age, knowledge-based performance is generally unaffected (Hess, 1994); that is, access to experience-based knowledge—also referred to as crystallized intelligence—does not lessen with age. On the contrary, in many people, this store of information about culture, language, people, and so on continues to increase well into very old age (Schaie, 1993). Because emotional functioning draws so heavily on cultivated knowledge structures, especially the regulation of emotional interaction with long-term friends and loved ones, age contributes to expertise. Self-knowledge and knowledge about other people (e.g., intimates) allows better situational control over emotion. Familiarity with thoughts and/or situations that have generated negative emotions in the past can enhance control over similar situations in the future, just as knowledge about topics or situations that have triggered particular emotions in mates can point to ways to improve further discussions.

Second, compared to younger adults, older adults show lower levels of physiological arousal associated with emotion whether emotions are induced via memories (Levenson et al., 1991) or during emotionally charged interactions between spouses (Levenson et al., 1994). The source of this age-related difference in autonomic nervous system arousal is not known. Although it is conceivable that less arousal is a consequence of improved emotion control, more likely it reflects a more generalized depression of the central or autonomic nervous systems that accompanies late-life aging. Regardless of its source, lower levels of arousal may facilitate the regulation of emotion. The absence of a racing heart or sweaty palms may circumvent a positive feedback system whereby emotions are exacerbated and instead allow for calmer, more reasoned consideration of the emotional experience.

Third, according to socioemotional selectivity theory (Carstensen, 1993, 1995)—a life span theory of social motivation—the motivation to seek emotionally meaningful experience and to regulate emotion increases with age. The theory contends that the hierarchy of social motives that instigates social behavior across life is reorganized when people consciously or subconsciously take account of the time that they left in their lives and conclude that time is limited. The recognition of limited time results in a prioritizing of short-term goals over long-term goals. Whereas future-oriented goals center around long-term payoffs, such as information acquisition, present-oriented goals involve current feeling states.

According to the theory, the construal of the future is inextricably associated with place in the life cycle. Early in adulthood, when time is perceived as largely open-ended, future-oriented goals, such as information seeking and self-development, are prioritized over short-term goals, whereas later in adulthood, goals such as self-verification and affect regulation become more salient. Socioemotional selectivity theory does not predict that exclusively positive emotional experience is sought in later adulthood. Rather, it contends that emotionally meaningful goals assume higher priority than goals that are relatively absent emotional meaning. Very likely emotionally rewarding experience involves both negative and positive emotions. Ideally, the experience is managed such that a optimal balance of emotions is achieved.

Analogies can be made between the individual life course and the life course of a relationship. Early in a relationship, when the future is looming large, the resolution of conflicts may be extremely important and adaptive. Even if negative emotions are experienced intensely during conflictual discussion, the potential long-term benefits of resolving conflicts are considerable. As couples move through life, three things happen. First, some conflicts get resolved, either because partners change their behavior or the problems go away. Grown children leaving home, for example, appears to remove one potential source of marital conflict. Second, habituation to old conflicts that have not been resolved may make some conflicts less toxic. Long-standing conflicts, minimally, become more predictable over time. In addition, a conflictual topic raised repeatedly over many decades is unlikely to retain the same threatening quality it had when first raised simply due to the perspective that time and shared history provide.

Third, the motivation to resolve some conflicts may subside over time. Socioemotional selectivity theory suggests that the motivation to regulate the immediate emotional climate of intimate relationships increases in later life. Especially if endings are primed, through the illness of a spouse or even the illness of age mates, couples may attempt increasingly to optimize the emotional climate. It is not that conflicts do not exist in old age; rather, heated debate about certain issues may be viewed as serving little purpose during this penultimate phase of life.

In sum, emotionally close social relationships offer many benefits to older adults. Intimate emotional relationships in later life appear to buffer individuals from mental and physical health problems. The closeness and predictability of long-term relationships provides an important context for achieving emotionally meaningful experience. It may be within this context that, ideally, people master an art of emotion regulation in which understanding a loved ones' emotions and even soothing that persons' emotions can occur simultaneous to the regulation of one's own emotional state.

REFERENCES

Ainsworth, M. D. S. (1982). Attachment: Retrospect and prospect. In C. M. Parkes & J. Sevenson-Hinde (Eds.), *The place of attachment in human behavior* (p. 457). New York: Basic Books.

Antonucci, T. C., & Jackson, J. S. (1987). Social support, interpersonal efficacy, and health: A life course perspective. In L. L. Carstensen & B. A. Edelstein (Eds.), *Handbook of clinical gerontology* (pp. 291–311). New York: Pergamon Press.

Atchley, R. C. (1976). *The sociology of retirement*. Cambridge, MA: Schenkman Publishing.

Barusch, A. S., & Spaid, W. M. (1989). Gender differences in caregiving: Why do wives report greater burden? *The Gerontologist, 29,* 667–676.

Beach, S. R. H., Jouriles, E. N., & O'Leary, K. D. (1985). Extramarital sex: Impact on depression and commitment in couples marital therapy. *Journal of Sex and Marital Therapy, 11,* 99–108.

Belsky, J., Crnic, K., & Gable, S. (1995). The determinants of coparenting in families with toddler boys: Spousal differences and daily hassles. *Child Development, 66,* 629–642.

Belsky, J., & Pensky, E. (1988). Marital change across the transition to parenthood. *Marriage and Family Review, 12,* 133–156.

Belsky, J., & Rovine, M. (1990). Patterns of marital change across the transition to parenthood. *Journal of Marriage and the Family, 52,* 109–123.

Belsky, J., Ward, H., & Rovine, M. (1986). Prenatal expectations, post-natal experiences and the transition to parenthood. In R. Ashmore & D. Brodzinsky (Eds.), *Perspectives on the family* (pp. 119–146). Hillsdale, NJ: Lawrence Erlbaum Associates.

Berkman, L. F., & Syme, S. L. (1979). Social networks, host resistance, and mortality: A nine-year follow-up study of Alameda County residents. *American Journal of Epidemiology, 109,* 186–204.

Blazer, D. G. (1982). Social support and mortality in an elderly community population. *American Journal of Epidemiology, 115,* 684–694.

Blood, R. O., & Wolfe, D. M. (1960). *Husbands and wives: The dynamics of married living*. Glencoe, IL: Free Press.

Bowlby, J. (1973). Affectional bonds: Their nature and origin. In R. S. Weiss (Ed.), *Loneliness: The experience of emotional and social isolation* (pp. 38–52). Cambridge, MA: MIT Press.

Breslow, L., & Engstrom, E. (1980). Persistence of health habits and relationship to mortality. *Preventative Medicine, 9,* 469–483.

Burr, W. R. (1970). Satisfaction with various aspects of marriage over the life cycle. *Journal of Marriage and the Family, 32,* 29–37.

Carstensen, L. L. (1987). Age-related changes in social activity. In L. L. Carstensen & B. A. Edelstein (Eds.), *Handbook of clinical gerontology* (pp. 222–237). New York: Pergamon Press.

Carstensen, L. L. (1993). Motivation for social contact across the life span: A theory of socioemotional selectivity. In J. Jacobs (Ed.), *Nebraska symposium on motivation* (pp. 209–254). Lincoln, NE: University of Nebraska Press.

Carstensen, L. L. (1995). Evidence for a life-span theory of socioemotional selectivity. *Current Directions in Psychological Science, 4,* 151–156.

Carstensen, L. L., Levenson, R. W., & Gottman, J. M. (1995). Emotional behavior in long-term marriage. *Psychology and Aging, 10,* 140–149.

Carstensen, L. L., & Pasupathi, M. (1993). Women of a certain age. In S. Matteo (Ed.), *Critical issues facing women in the '90s* (pp. 66–78). Boston: Northeastern University Press.

Carstensen, L. L., & Turk-Charles, S. (1994). The salience of emotion across the adult life span. *Psychology and Aging, 9,* 259–264.

Christensen, A., & Heavey, C. L. (1990). Gender and social structure in the demand/withdraw pattern of marital conflict. *Journal of Personality and Social Psychology, 59,* 73–81.

Costello, E. J. (1991). Married with children: Predictors of mental and physical health in middle-aged women. *Psychiatry, 54,* 292–305.

Cowan, C. P., & Cowan, P. A. (1992). *When partners become parents: The big life change for couples.* New York: Basic Books.

Cowan, C. P., Cowan, P. A., Heming, G., Garrett, E., Coysh, W. S., Curtis-Boles, H., & Boles, A. J. (1985). Transitions to parenthood: His, hers, and theirs. *Journal of Family Issues, 6*(4), 451–481.

Cowan, P., & Pape-Cowan, C. (1988). Changes in marriage during the transition to parenthood. In G. Y. Michaels & W. A. Goldberg (Eds.), *The transition to parenthood: Current theory and research* (pp. 114–154). Cambridge, UK: Cambridge University Press.

deRivera, J. (1984). The structure of emotional relationships. In P. Shaver (Ed.), *Review of personality and social psychology: Emotion, relationships, and health* (Vol. 5, pp. 116–145). Beverly Hills, CA: Sage.

Ekerdt, D. J., & Vinick, B. H. (1991). Marital complaints in husband-working and husband-retired couples. *Research on Aging, 13,* 364–382.

Erikson, E. H., Erikson, J., & Kivnick, H. (1986). *Vital involvement in old age.* New York: Norton.

Fredrickson, B. L., & Carstensen, L. L. (1990). Choosing social partners: How age and anticipated endings make people more selective. *Psychology and Aging, 5,* 335–347.

Gable, S., Belsky, J., & Crnic, K. (1992). Marriage, parenting and child development: Progress and prospects. *Journal of Family Psychology, 5,* 276–294.

Gallagher, D., Rose, J., Rivera, P., Lovett, S. (1989) Prevalence of depression in family caregivers. *Gerontologist, 29,* 449–456.

Garrett, E. T. (1983, August). *Women's experiences of early parenthood: Expectation vs.*

reality. Presented at 91st Annual Convention of the American Psychological Association, Anaheim, CA.

George, L. (1981). *Role transitions in later life*. Monterey: Wadsworth.

George, L., & Gold, D. (1991). Life course perspectives on intergenerational and generational connections. *Marriage and Family Review, 16*, 67–88.

Gottman, J. M. (1993). The roles of conflict engagement, escalation, and avoidance in marital interaction: A longitudinal view of five types of couples. *Journal of Consulting and Clinical Psychology, 61*, 6–15.

Gottman, J. M. (1994). *What predicts divorce?: The relationship between marital processes and marital outcomes*. Hillsdale, NJ: Lawrence Erlbaum.

Gottman, J. M., & Krokoff, L. J. (1989). The relationship between marital interaction and marital satisfaction: A longitudinal view. *Journal of Consulting and Clinical Psychology, 57*, 47–52.

Gottman, J. M., & Levenson, R. W. (1992). Marital processes predictive of later dissolution: Behavior, physiology, and health. *Journal of Personality and Social Psychology, 63*, 221–233.

Gottman, J. M., & Levenson, R. W. (1988). The social psychophysiology of marriage. In P. Notter & M. A. Fitzpatrick (Eds.), *Perspectives on marital interaction* (pp. 182–200). Cleredon, England. Multilingual Matters, Ltd.

Gottman, J. M., Markman, H., & Notarius, C. (1977). The topography of marital conflict: A sequential analysis of verbal and nonverbal behavior. *Journal of Marriage and the Family, 39*, 461–477.

Guilford, R., & Bengtson, V. (1979). Measuring marital satisfaction in three generations: Positive and negative dimensions. *Journal of Marriage and the Family, 41*, 387–398.

Guttmann, D. (1987). *Reclaimed powers: Toward a new psychology of men and women in later life*. New York: Basic Books.

Heavey, C. L., Layne, C., Christensen, A. (1993). Gender and conflict structure in marital interaction: A replication and extension. *Journal of Consulting and Clinical Psychology, 61*, 16–27.

Helsing, K. J. (1981). Factors associated with mortality after widowhood. *American Journal of Public Health, 71*, 802–809.

Hess, B., & Soldo, B. (1985). Husband and wife networks. In W. J. Sauer & R. T. Coward (Eds.), *Social support networks and the care of the elderly: Theory, research, and practice* (pp. 67–92). New York: Springer.

Hess, T. M. (1994). Social cognition in adulthood: Aging related changes in knowledge and processing mechanisms. *Developmental Review, 14*, 373–412.

Hyde, J. S., & Phillis, D. (1979). Androgyny across the life span. *Developmental Psychology, 15*, 334–336.

Jacobson, N. S., & Addis, M. E. (1993). Research on couples and couples therapy: What do we know? Where are we going? *Journal of Consulting and Clinical Psychology, 61*, 85–93.

Johnston, T. (1990). Retirement: What happens to marriage. *Issues in Mental Health Nursing, 11*, 347–359.

Komarovsky, M. (1976). *Dilemmas of masculinity*. New York: W. W. Norton.

Krokoff, L. J. (1987). Recruiting representative samples for marital research. *Journal of social and personal relationships, 4*, 317–328.

Labouvie-Vief, G., & DeVoe, M. (1991). Emotional regulation in adulthood and later life: A developmental view. In K. W. Schaie (Ed.), *Annual review of gerontology and geriatrics* (pp. 172–194). New York: Springer.

Labouvie-Vief, G., DeVoe, M., & Bulka, D. (1989). Speaking about feelings: Conceptions of emotion across the life span. *Psychology and Aging, 4*, 425–437.

Lang, F. R., & Carstensen, L. L. (1994). Close emotional relationships in late life: Further support for proactive aging in the social domain. *Psychology and Aging, 9*, 315–324.

Lawton, M. P., Kleban, M. H., Rajagopal, D., & Dean, J. (1992). Dimensions of affective experience in three age groups. *Psychology and Aging, 7*, 171–184.

Lee, G. R., & Shehan, C. L. (1989). Retirement and marital satisfaction. *Journal of Gerontology, 44*, S226–S230.

Levant, R. F., Slattery, S. C., & Loiselle, J. E. (1987). Fathers' involvement in housework and child care with school-age daughters. *Family relations: Journal of applied family and child studies, 36*, 152–157.

Levenson, R. W., Carstensen, L. L., Friesen, W. V., & Ekman, P. (1991). Emotion, physiology, and expression in old age. *Psychology and Aging, 6*, 28–35.

Levenson, R. W., Carstensen, L. L., & Gottman, J. M. (1993). Long-term marriage: Age, gender, and satisfaction. *Psychology and Aging, 8*, 301–313.

Levenson, R. W., Carstensen, L. L., & Gottman, J. M. (1994). The influence of age and gender on affect, physiology, and their interrelations: A study of long-term marriage. *Journal of Personality and Social Psychology, 67*, 56–68.

Levenson, R. W., & Gottman, J. M. (1983). Marital interaction: Physiological linkage and affective exchange. *Journal of Social and Personality Psychology, 45*, 587–597

Levenson, R. W., & Gottman, J. M. (1985). Physiological and affective predictors of change in relationship satisfaction. *Journal of Personality and Social Psychology, 49*, 85–94.

Longino, C. F., & Lipman, A. (1981). Married and spouseless men and women in planned retirement communities: Support network differentials. *Journal of Marriage and the Family, 43*, 169–177.

Malatesta, C. Z., & Kalnok, M. (1984). Emotional experience in younger and old adults. *Journal of Gerontology, 39*, 302–308.

Malatesta, C. Z., & Izard, C. E. (1984). Facial expression of emotion in young, middle-aged, and older adults. In C. Z. Malatesta & C. E. Izard (Eds.), *Emotion in adult development* (pp. 253–274). Beverly Hills: Sage

Markman, H. J. (1991). Backwards into the future of couples therapy and couples therapy research: A comment on Jacobson. *Journal of Family Psychology, 4*, 416–425.

Markman, H. J. (1992). Marital and family psychology: Burning issues. *Journal of Family Psychology, 5*, 256–275.

Markman, H. J., Renick, M. J., Floyd, F. J., & Stanley, S. M. (1993). Preventing marital distress through communication and conflict management training: A 4- and 5-year follow-up. *Journal of Consulting and Clinical Psychology, 61*, 70–77.

Oggins, J., Veroff, J., & Leber, D. (1993). Perceptions of marital interaction among black and white newlyweds. *Journal of Personality and Social Psychology, 65*, 494–511.

Pineo, P. C. (1961). Disenchantment in the later years of marriage. *Marriage and Family Living, 23,* 3–11.

Pineo, P. C. (1969). Developmental patterns in marriage. *Family Coordinator, 18,* 135–140.

Powell, W. E. (1988). The "ties that bind": Relationships in life transitions. Social Casework: *The Journal of Contemporary Social Work, 69,*(9) 556–562.

Rollins, B. C., & Cannon, K. L. (1974). Marital satisfaction over the family life cycle: A reevaluation. *Journal of Marriage and the Family, 36,* 271–282.

Rollins, B. C., & Feldman, H. (1970). Marital satisfaction over the family life cycle. *Journal of Marriage and the Family, 32,* 20–28.

Rounsaville, B. J., Weissman, M. M., Prusoff, B. A., & Herceg-Baron, R. L. (1979). Marital disputes and treatment outcome in depressed women. *Comprehensive Psychiatry, 20,* 483–490.

Schaie, K. W. (1993). The Seattle Longitudinal Studies of Adult intelligence. *Current Directions in Psychological Science, 2,* 171–175.

Seltzer, M. M., & Ryff, C. D. (1994). Parenting across the life-span: The normative and nonnormative cases. In D. Featherman, R. M. Lerner, & M. Perlmutter (Eds.), *Life-span development and behavior* (Vol. 11, pp. 1–40). Hillsdale, NJ: Lawrence Erlbaum.

Shaver, P. (Ed.). (1984). *Review of personality and social psychology: Emotion, relationships, and health* (Vol. 5). Beverly Hills, CA: Sage.

Silverberg, S. B., & Steinberg, L. (1990). Psychological well-being of parents with early adolescent children. *Developmental Psychology, 26,* 658–666.

Steinberg, S. B., & Silverberg, L. (1987). Influences on marital satisfaction during the middle years of the family life cycle. *Journal of Marriage and the Family, 49,* 751–760.

Stinnett, N., Carter, L. M., & Montgomery, J. E. (1972). Older persons' perceptions of their marriages. *Journal of Marriage and the Family, 32,* 428–434.

Storaasli, R. D., & Markman, H. J. (1990). Relationship problems in the early stages of marriage: A longitudinal investigation. *Journal of Family Psychology, 4,* 80–98.

Sporakowski, M. J., & Hughston, G. A. (1978). Prescriptions for happy marriage: Adjustments and satisfactions of couples married for 50 or more years. *The Family Coordinator, 27,* 321–327.

Tariq, P. N., & Anila, (1993). Marital maladjustment and the crime of murder among Pakistani female criminals. *International Journal of Psychology, 28,* 809–819.

Thompson, R. A. (1994). Emotion regulation: A theme in search of definition. In N. A. Fox (Ed.), The development of emotion regulation: Biological and Behavioral considerations (pp. 25–52). *Monographs of the Society for Research in Child Development, 59,* 2–3.

Tower, R. B., & Kasl, S. V. (1995). Depressive symptoms across older spouses and the moderating effect of marital closeness. *Psychology and Aging, 10,* 625–638.

Troll, L. (1985). *Early and middle adulthood* (2nd ed.). Monterey, CA: Brooks/Cole Publishers.

Tucker, M. B., Taylor, R. J., & Mitchell-Kernan, C. (1993). Marriage and romantic involvement among aged African Americans. *Journal of Gerontology, 48,* S123–S132.

Tucker, P., & Aron, A. (1993). Passionate love and marital satisfaction at key transition points in the family life cycle. *Journal of Social and Clinical Psychology, 12,* 135–147.

U.S. Bureau of the Census (1992a). *Current population reports, special studies, P23-178RV, sixty-five plus in America.* Washington, DC: U.S. Government Printing Office.

U.S. Bureau of the Census (1992b). *Current population reports, P23-180, Marriage, divorce, and remarriage in the 1990's.* Washington, DC: U.S. Government Printing Office.

Vaux, A. (1985). Variations in social support associated with gender, ethnicity, and age. *Journal of Social Issues, 41,* 89–110.

Venkatraman, M. M. (1995). A cross-cultural study of the subjective well-being of married elderly persons in the United States and India. *Journal of Gerontology, 50B,* S35–S44.

Vinick, B. H., & Ekerdt, D. J. (1991). Retirement: What happens to husband–wife relationships? *Journal of Geriatric Psychiatry, 24,* 23–40.

White, L. K., & Booth, A. V. (1985). The transition to parenthood and marital quality. *Journal of Family Issues, 6,* 435–449.

Zarit, S. H., Orr, N. K., & Zarit, J. M. (1982). *The hidden victims of Alzheimer's disease: Families under stress.* New York: New York University Press.

CHAPTER 14

The Understanding
of Friendship

An Adult Life Course Perspective

Brian de Vries

School of Family and Nutritional Sciences
University of British Columbia
Vancouver, British Columbia, Canada
and
Department of Medical Anthropology
University of California, San Francisco
San Francisco, California

I. INTRODUCTION

A sizable body of literature attests to the pivotal role played by friends in the social, psychological, and physical health of individuals of all ages (e.g., Antonucci & Akiyama, 1987). Friends also are believed to enable the smooth and orderly functioning of society (Paine, 1974). Pogrebin (1987) has written that "we've always valued our friends, but never before have we prized them as we do today" (p. 126). Standing in contrast to these accolades and impressive credentials is the modest attention directed to the ways in which such friendships are understood and experienced by the individuals (and societies) whose lives they influence, and how such understanding and experience varies over the life course (e.g., Matthews, 1986).

This chapter is a selective yet representative review of the friendship literature, focusing mainly on the meaning of friendship and the concomitant emotional experience. The review that follows is necessarily compromised and framed by four significant limitations of the existing literature amply reviewed elsewhere (e.g., Adams, 1989; Adams & Blieszner, 1994; Blieszner & Adams, 1992; Dickens & Perlman, 1981; Matthews, 1986): inadequate operationalizations, variability and inconsistency in target or referent stimulus, a predominantly nonrelational research focus, and the absence of a life course perspective. This chapter is organized around four topical areas or primary themes of the friendship research: one, friends vis-à-vis family (the primary constituents of social networks): two, dimensions of friendship; three, gender differences; and four, life events and life circumstances. The life course is highlighted in each of these areas, although the literature has been inconsistent in its focus on this aspect; that is, the life course is explicitly represented in analyses of friends and family and life events, and infrequently represented in analyses of gender differences and friendship dimensions. Understanding *the effects of friendship* has been the focus of much of this research; the *understanding of friendship* itself (upon which the emotional experience is predicated) has been implicit in these accounts (paradoxically better elaborated in the areas of gender differences and friendship dimensions, those same areas that are weaker in life course explorations). This chapter concludes with an attempt to make explicit such understanding, including a brief examination of friendship bereavement (i.e., an appreciation of what can be learned about experience from reports of what has been lost).

II. FRIENDS VIS-À-VIS FAMILY

Friends and family are the primary occupants of the convoys (e.g., Kahn & Antonucci, 1980) or the protective layers of social space surrounding individuals and assisting in adaptation to life (de Vries, Jacoby, & Davis, 1996). Relations with the family representatives of this space has been fertile ground for research and theory (e.g., Aldous, 1978; Duvall, 1977) although Johnson (1983) has cautioned that without "studying the two types of relationships in conjunction, the importance of either kinship or friendship can be overestimated or, on the contrary, overlooked" (p. 120). Included in the distinctions made by individuals between their friends and family is the meaning of both by inference.

The nature and structure of friendships in adulthood are believed to have their roots in the psychological changes that accompany adolescence (Dickens & Perlman, 1981). Early research on late adolescent friendships (Douvan & Adelson, 1966), for example, described an Eriksonian shift away from a focus on activity and toward interactions in the service of ego identity cohesion (e.g., self-confirming and self-validating functions) enhancing self-esteem. Shulman (1975) has written that the importance of the peer group increases dramatically in adolescence, often in the context of social evaluation and social comparison, with a concomitant and often conflictual shift away from family of origin and kin relations (Bell, 1981). Adolescents and young adults tend to be absorbed with such extrafamilial pursuits as education, career, and mate selection (Marcia, 1980).

With marriage or new committed relationships, kin involvement increases in importance. "Ideal marriages" often include bestowed best friend statuses for husbands and wives (Lopata, 1975). New kin members are added to the couples' repertoire of social relations; friendship numbers and involvement decrease (de Vries, 1991). Such changes are intensified with the introduction of children. The notion of family is reconceptualized as an individual finds him- or herself in the roles of both parent and child (e.g., de Vries, Dalla Lana, & Falck, 1994). With the additional responsibilities of parenthood and the concomitant familial constraints on leisure time, friendship contacts and friendship intimacy decline; a greater number and variety of needs are met by kin (Shulman, 1975). The cultural norms surrounding marriage and parenthood promote extended family relations, and may shape adult personality and interpersonal style (e.g., Gutmann, 1975).

The middle years of adulthood may be characterized by transitions in family phases: the "full house" through the "launching of children" to the "empty nest" (e.g., Aldous, 1978). Family issues have particular salience as midlife adults respond to their aging parents and adult children and grandchildren (e.g., Brim, 1976). Farrell and Rosenberg (1981), for example, found that midlife friendships were less intense than friendships during other periods of adulthood. These interpersonal priorities may underlie the dearth of empirical interest in and evidence on the nature, meaning, and form of friendship in the middle years (Blieszner, 1988).

Contributions to the understanding of friends (in contrast to family) are probably best elaborated in relation to later life. In general, friendship numbers decrease in the later years (de Vries, 1991) as does friendship contact (e.g., Adams, 1986a; Blieszner, 1989), although contact with kin increases (Dickens & Perlman, 1981). Such findings have led to a more focused analysis of the role of friend and family in later life. On the one hand, Blau (1973) has maintained that an older individual with a single good friend is better able to respond to the challenges of old age than one with a dozen grandchildren but no peer-group friend. Peer-group friends provide, for individuals, appropriate reference groups and opportunities for interaction unencumbered by family role responsibilities. Riley and Foner (1968), on the other hand, have suggested that although friends play an important role, they are generally less important to older people than are children and other family; friends serve as more of a complement than substitution for kinship associations.

Rosow (1970) and Wood and Robertson (1978) have suggested that the difference between friend and family is essentially the difference between choice and obligation and hold that the obligatory nature of the parent–child relationships, in particular, may detract from its quality. Family members provide generative connections with the past (and links to the future) and offer support (e.g., financial) less likely to come from other informal sources. In fact, Felton and Berry (1992) reported that older people feel better when their instrumental needs are satisfied through kin relations and their emotional needs through friend relations. Such friend relations maintain role continuity (Blau, 1973) and contribute to self-esteem and morale in the reciprocal exchange of assistance. The more particular dimensions implicit in these characteristics are elaborated below.

III. DIMENSIONS OF FRIENDSHIP

Friendship is a multidimensional experience. Although few would dispute this statement, there have been only modest attempts to systemize this multidimensional complexity. The empirical efforts in this area have been either (a) scalar and inductive, in which respondents complete standardized questionnaires representing theoretically and empirically derived key friendship constructs (e.g., Davis & Todd, 1985; Parker & de Vries, 1993) or (b) narrative and deductive, in which respondents describe their friends in more open-ended formats (e.g., Goldman, Cooper, Ahern, & Corsini, 1981; Weiss & Lowenthal, 1975).

Analyses of these sorts have revealed between 14 and 20 dimensions that may be distilled into three broad themes. The largest theme comprises the most frequently identified dimensions and represents the *affective* nature of friendship. This includes reference to the sharing of personal thoughts and feelings (i.e., self-disclosure) and other, related expressions of intimacy, appreciation, and affection (including respect and feelings of warmth, care, and love). Additionally, friends are described as providing encouragement, emotional support, empathy, and bolstering one's self-concept, all of which are made possible by an underlying sense of trust, loyalty, and commitment. A second theme reflects the *shared or communal* nature of friendship, in which individuals assist each other or participate in activities of mutual interest; shared or similar experience appears fundamental in this context. The third theme reflects *sociability* and compatibility; friends are sources of amusement, fun, and recreation.

The few results available concerning variations in the presence and strength of these dimensions over the life course have been equivocal. Weiss and Lowenthal (1975) commented on the surprising similarity of the dimensional profiles of friendship across the four early adulthood and midlife stages they studied. They suggested that the functions and perceptions of friends may be established at an early age and maintained throughout life. Candy, Troll, and Levy (1981) and Goldman et al. (1981) found evidence of both stability and change in their research on the friendships of women ranging in ages from early adolescence to later life. They suggested that developmental tasks, some of which have been reviewed above, help structure friendship.

In contrast to this content dimensionalization of the friendship construct, Roberto and Kimboko (1989) found three main categories in the definition of friend for older individuals: the *likeables* (characterizing friends in terms of sociability and similarity), the *confiders* (defining friends in terms of acceptance and self-disclosure), and the *trustables* (where friends were described as trusting, loyal, honest, and dependable), not unlike the themes characterized above. Matthews (1983, 1986) has also distilled broader categories used by older individuals to characterize the relational context of their friendships. One focuses on particular individuals and the other on relationships per se. In the former case, a definition of friend is reserved for specific persons who alone could qualify; in the latter case, the focus is on the relationship rather than the person involved so that the number of people who might qualify is greater. de Vries, Dustan, and Wiebe (1994) found that older respondents were more likely to include individual references in their definitions than were any other age category; as Matthews (1983) suggested, the use of individual definitions may be associated with precarious social support; as friends leave the network (through immobility, relocation, death), they are unlikely to be replaced (as other individuals cannot substitute) and respondents may feel isolated and lonely.

Such is more likely to be the case with those in late, late life. The common refrain of those aged 85 and older was, "I've outlived everyone" (Johnson & Troll, 1994, p. 82). Poor health and restricted access to friends (and hence asymmetry in the relationship) formed additional constraints on their friendships. Respondents reacted to such constraints by changing the criteria for friendship to no longer require propinquity or face-to-face contact, or to extend the friendship label to acquaintances or "hired help" or even to minimize the expressive content of friendship

(Johnson & Troll, 1994). This study in particular draws attention to the perimeters of the life course and the malleability of friendship definitions.

The intersection of a life course perspective with the multifaceted friendship construct holds great promise for researchers interested in studying either or both age and social relations. With greater frequency, researchers have explored the boundaries of friendship along gender lines, an account of which is found in the next section.

IV. THE GENDERED CONTEXT OF FRIENDSHIP

A common finding of the friendship literature, replicated with samples from across the life course, is what Lipman-Bluman (1976) called homosociality (similar to what Lazarsfeld and Merton, 1954, called homophily): the tendency of individuals to nominate as friends a greater proportion of members of their own sex (and ethnicity, race, or culture as well as age, marital status, etc). The influence of gender in particular, however, extends well beyond these nominating procedures; both popular wisdom and psychological research suggest that there are differences in how men and women understand and behave in their close friendships (e.g., Aries & Johnson, 1983; Bell, 1981; Caldwell & Peplau, 1982; Hacker, 1981).

For example, the friendships of women have been described as "face-to-face" with an affective and personalized focus on the other, in contrast to men's "side-by-side" friendships oriented to some external activity or task (Wright, 1982). Parker and de Vries (1993) reported that men and women differ in what they give, receive, and appreciate in their friendships. Women describe themselves as doing more of the "emotional work" in their close friendships, whereas men report assuming more control and initiating shared activity of a more emotionally detached nature. Dickens and Perlman (1981) cited a number of factors related to traditional male roles (e.g., competition, homophobia, aversion to vulnerability) that produce barriers to emotional intimacy in men (see also Lewis, 1978; and Miller, 1983).

Gilligan (1982) claimed that women and men differ in their basic life orientations and hence self-definitions and social perspectives. She has hypothesized that women construe their social worlds in terms of care, responsibility, and interdependence and see the self as connected and attached in relation to others; men, in contrast, construe their worlds in terms of justice, rights, and independence and see the self as separate and detached. de Vries, Blando, and Walker (1995) noted a greater connectedness and reference to others in the recalled life events of women and suggested that men may live lives that are less involved with the emotional concerns of others in general. Birren (personal communication, March 1992) has considered men as role specialists in their friendships having work friends, sports friends, and so on, and women as role generalists, sharing more of themselves perhaps with fewer individuals.

These foregoing differences tend to be gender-of-respondent "main effects"; the influence of gender also derives from the gender composition of the relationship (Reis, 1986). That is, women and men show significant differences in their understanding of and behavior in friendships based on whether they are same- or cross-sex relationships. Men's same-sex friendships are described as ones of solidarity of comradeship (Arnold & Chartier, 1986), emphasizing an activity orientation (Bell, 1981) and commonality (Weiss & Lowenthal, 1975), whereas women's same-sex friendships tend to be affectively richer (Booth, 1972), self-disclosing, and holistic (Wright, 1982) and more meaningful (Reis, 1986). Daly (1978) postulated that sex-role socialization influences such typologies of same-sex friendship, wherein male comradeship thrives on shared activity and the loss of personal identity, and female friendship thrives on the enhancement of personal identity and on heightened self-disclosure and self-awareness.

Outside of courtship and marriage, there is little research on the nature of close cross-sex friendships for women and men (O'Meara, 1989). In a study of self-disclosure, Hacker (1981) found that in cross-sex relationships, men tend to disclose strengths and women tend to disclose weaknesses, suggesting that "both sexes feel more constrained to fulfill gender role expectations in their relationships with the other sex" (p. 396). When men do self-disclose or experience emotional intimacy, it tends to be with women (Reis, 1986). Parker and de Vries (1993) found that the differences between women and men appeared to be moderated when men interact with women. Friendships appeared to be more reciprocal and to have higher levels of the dimensions that make friendships close when there was at least one woman in the relationship. Bernard (1976) referred to this effect as a "relational deficit" (p. 230) in which friendships with men do not, in general, provide as much support, affiliation, and attachment as do friendships with women.

As was previously the case, limited empirical attention has been directed toward life course gender variations in friendship, particularly with respect to meaning. Although in general, same-sex friendships tend to be of longer duration than cross-sex ones (e.g., Barth & Kinder, 1988)—perhaps best serving in the clarification, correction, and confirmation of one's self-perceptions (Aries & Johnson, 1983)—men tend to have friendships of shorter duration (Parker & de Vries, 1993). This latter finding in particular may reflect the more side-by-side, role specialist nature of male friendship and the extent to which it falters or fails in the absence of an agenda or a task. Not surprisingly, duration of friendship has also been found to be related to the reported intimacy of the relationship (Jackson, Fischer, & Jones, 1977), which may favor the friendships of women.

Wright (1982) observed that as the duration increases, so does the similarity between men's and women's friendships, perhaps in both a cause and effect approach. At the limits of another sort, Johnson and Troll (1994) reported that the gender differences common in samples of younger adults are noticeably absent when disability increases; in general, "the differences in life style between younger men and women that contribute to gender differences in friendships are much less apparent in the life styles of the oldest old" (p. 85).

The sex composition of the friendship has particular importance in the context of the life course, and widowhood is a striking example. Just as marriage creates "couples" out of individuals, widowhood creates individuals out of couples: the basis of the ways in which an individual responds to his or her friendship circle (e.g., McCall & Simmons, 1966), and the ways in which they respond to him or her. Given the combined facts that women have a longer life expectancy and that women tend to marry men older than themselves, a far greater proportion of older men are married and living with their spouses than women (e.g., de Vries, 1991). A widower, then, is disadvantaged relative to his married peers in that such differentiation of interest and experience "reduces the mutual bonds that serve as the basis for the formation and persistence of friendships" (Blau, 1961, p. 432). Alternatively, "widow" is a more normative later life role for women with a consequent "society of widows" (Lopata, 1993). This common experience often translates into less isolation and greater adaptation for women in their widowhood (Barer, 1994).

The role of gender in the beliefs about and values and behaviors in friendship is a currently debated issue with positions ranging from one describing "enormous consequences in areas of critical human interactions" (Surrey, 1985, p. 7) through "much commonality . . . regardless of . . . gender" (Peplau, 1983, p. 246) to gender differences that are "not great and, in many cases, . . . so obscure that they are hard to demonstrate" (Wright, 1982, p. 19). Nevertheless, several insights into friendship understanding are offered, some of which adhere to a pattern initiated above. That is, friends serve to validate identities and both are predicated upon and inform gender roles and life orientations. As an extension of the above, the two genders offer and expect different aspects from each other in friend relations. Although rarely studied, cross-sex friendships challenge these expectations (O'Meara, 1989) and may help define some of the parameters of friendship. The events and circumstances of life similarly challenge the construction of friend as discussed below.

V. LIFE EVENTS AND CIRCUMSTANCES

The events and circumstances of life create and/or delimit opportunities for the initiation, maintenance, and termination of friendships. Recall that the life course represents more than a concern with chronological age (e.g., Baltes, 1979): There is explicit attention directed toward the processes and events that occur throughout life, many of which take place in the family setting (Aldous, 1978; White, 1991). Some of the ways in which family events and circumstances influence friendship have been briefly characterized above. Marriage and the introduction of children occasion changes in friendship contact and interaction, perhaps filtered through a changing self-image and shaped by the tasks of parenting (e.g., Gutmann, 1975). Widowhood often changes the personnel of friendships (Allan & Adams, 1989) and the context within which friendships have been enacted. Over the course of adaptation to widowhood (see Bankoff, 1981), friends may become primary sources of support and particularly those who are themselves widowed (Lopata, 1993), whose emotional experiences most clearly resemble the recently bereft.

Later life is a time during which there is relatively dense spacing of those significant life events likely to influence friendship, including retirement as well as relocation and illness (Allan & Adams, 1989; Johnson & Troll, 1994). Retirement may bring about a change in financial resources sufficient to limit social interactions and access to friends. For men, work-based friendships are prone to erosion with the loss of the context through which these associations were forged and maintained (Allan, 1979). For women whose relationships have tended to be more broadly based, retirement may exert little influence, although it may also bring about (or be mandated by) greater caregiving responsibilities (e.g., Brody, 1985) and restrictions on access to friends. The cohort nature of these claims remains to be seen as does the long-term emotional toll exacted by these later life changes.

Relocation may also affect friendship contact and maintenance. For example, older individuals may move to be nearer to their friends (e.g., Gutman, 1986) enhancing contact, or they may move to be nearer to kin (e.g., for future or immediate caregiving services and either their own or their child's initiative) restricting friend access and contact (e.g., Johnson & Troll, 1994). Daily or even frequent contact is not necessarily a prerequisite for friendship, however. Matthews (1986) described individuals whose friends were seen rarely: "I haven't seen him in years" (p. 147). Choice of housing environment may additionally affect friendship activity, as may be seen in research on nursing homes (e.g., Gubrium, 1975), public housing (Hochschild, 1973), retirement communities (Shea, Thompson, & Blieszner, 1988), and single-room occupancy hotels (e.g., Cohen, 1989).

Johnson (1983) reported that "illness and infirmity impose[s] impressive hurdles for sociability among age peers" (p. 111). Johnson conducted interviews with older individuals hospitalized in an acute-care facility and follow-up interviews 9 months later; she found that following hospitalization, those individuals who experienced improvements in health and functional status reported decreased contact with family and increased contact with friends. In contrast, those who remained impaired reported continued contact with family and reduced contact with friends. "This finding suggests that friendships have difficulty in standing the test of time if the relationship is also tested by the demands of illness and dependency" (Johnson, 1983, p. 113). Johnson and Troll (1994) also reported that increased disability had a major and negative effect on friendship involvement among the oldest old. The imbalanced reciprocity and instrumental demands of disability obfuscates the inherently expressive nature of the relationship; many respondents reported that they did not want to see their friends until their health improved. It may also be that the disability of a friend elicits negative emotion in the relatively healthier friend ("There but for the grace of God go I"), who in response seeks some distance. Friendship and negative affectivity or conflict has rarely been studied and merits further consideration (e.g., Blieszner & Adams, 1995).

The effects of disability, when crossed with residential location, however, offer a somewhat different perspective. For example, Rosow (1967) reported that older people in poor health in residential retirement hotels had more contact with local friends than their relatively healthier neighbors. Adams (1986b) found that those with some disability in age-segregated buildings had more local friends. She hypothesized that esteem is bestowed upon those in relatively (and visibly) better health in such an age-segregated environment, whereas the reverse is evident in age-integrated environments where friendship opportunities are less numerous and disability is less visible.

As implied by the above, not all later life friendships are long-term friendships. Johnson and Troll (1994), for example, found that over one-half of their sample of the oldest old had formed friendship in adult life or after age 65, and 45% had made new friends after age 85. These friendships originated in community organizations or associations (such as church), particularly for men, or in the neighborhood, particularly for women. Previous work settings or family connections were less common sources. In partial contrast, de Vries et al. (1996) reported that the home setting was a primary source of friendship for their national sample of persons aged 65 and over. Friends through school, work, clubs, and family were the next most common sources (in descending order of frequency). Church groups, through other friends, and vacation activities were infrequently mentioned. The origins of these friendships may help shed light on the functions served by such friends and the meanings that such relationships hold.

Several authors have suggested that ethnic factors influence the nature of friendships and the extent and use of informal support, particularly among older persons (e.g., de Vries et al., 1996; Penning & Chappell, 1987). Ethnicity represents a subjective and shared sense of culture, heritage, and peoplehood (Penning & Chappell, 1987) and, as such, may influence the nature (and definition) of social networks, in general, and friendships in particular. Johnson and Barer (1990) have similarly noted race effects in which older African Americans created fictive kin relations (also identified as "play" or "foster" kin) through redefining their relationships with friends.

Parallels have been made between the literatures on gender and friendship and ethnicity (and race) and friendship. For example, the prevailing norms of homosociality and homophily along gender lines are more modestly reproduced along ethnic and racial lines. Additionally, Strain and Chappell (1989) reported ethnic differences in the numbers of friends and neighbors identified in comparisons of urban native elders with nonnatives (the former identifying about six times the number of friends). de Vries et al. (1996) compared British, French, European, and multiethnic older Canadians (the most prevalent groups among older Canadians). They found that the French identified fewer friends than did the other groups (and particularly the British) and that they lived closer to their friends and had more frequent contact. These authors, as Strain and Chappell (1989) and Creecy and Wright (1979) before them, interpreted these group differences as suggestive of cultural differences in the meaning of friend and neighbor (primarily centering on differing expressions and levels of intimacy).

The importance of including ethnicity in studies of friendship in later life or over the life course is often noted yet rarely manifested (de Vries et al., 1996). In conjunction with the events of life, such life circumstances offer the opportunity to explore variations in friendship understanding and a preliminary inventory of these meanings (in a life course context), elaborating upon the foregoing review, forms the basis of the section that follows.

VI. THE MEANING OF FRIENDSHIP

From the foregoing review, an awareness of friendship is uncovered evocative of its meaning in the lives of individuals. For example, notwithstanding the ambivalent relationship that may exist between friend and family (Johnson, 1983), friends serve as a complement, contrast, and sometimes substitute for family (e.g., Shanas, 1979). Their significance, in this light, emerges from what they are not—they are not (conventionally) family and hence they are free of many of the more formal role prescriptions that govern family relations. In fact, friendships are notable for their nonascribed and socially unregulated quality (Aries & Johnson, 1983), negotiated (including terminated) by the friend participants, and maintained on the basis of mutual preferences (Johnson, 1983); they represent the free expression of affect. They sustain role continuity and underwrite the formation and development of the ego; they provide appropriate yardsticks against which self-development, behavior, and thoughts may be evaluated. As Sullivan (1953) articulated, friends serve to clarify, correct, and confirm one's self-perceptions and provide "consensual validation of all components of personal worth" (Aries & Johnson, 1983, p. 1184). Friendships arise through the choices and unique voluntary commitments of participants (Adams & Blieszner, 1994), further enhancing self-esteem and self-awareness.

A survey of the most prominent dimensions by which friendships are characterized similarly reveals that friendships have their (voluntary) base in compatibility or shared and similar activities, interests, and experiences (i.e., homophily, Lazarsfeld & Merton, 1954), some of which are the grounds of status and esteem. Friends also serve as sources of support and encouragement and trust. Through interactions with friends, individuals also report increased self-respect, self-awareness, and the freedom to act in authentic ways, perhaps unencumbered by the roles and prescribed boundaries inherent in family interactions. As such, friend interaction is a source of satisfaction, and belongingness and even empowerment. Friends also function significantly in the affective domain (Johnson, 1983), in which members receive and offer affection, appreciation, and empathy or assist in other ways, enjoy themselves in recreation, and tell and hear secrets and confidences and hence maintain the essentially private nature of the content and organization of friendship (Allan & Adams, 1989).

Analyses of the role of gender reveals further nuances in friendship meaning and address the social context within which friendship takes place. Homosociality prevails in the friendship networks of women and men (e.g., Parker & de Vries, 1993): same-sex friends particularly validate self-perceptions and provide models of what the self can and cannot be and what the self should and should not be. Friendship identification and selection are influenced in a dynamic interplay by both self-definitions (e.g., Gilligan, 1982) and sex-role socialization (Daly, 1978). Women and men give and receive differently in their friendships with each other (Parker & de Vries, 1993); perhaps the "having a friend, being a friend" distinction (Davis & Todd, 1985) previously mentioned may parallel the "side-by-side" and "face-to-face" distinction (Wright, 1982) characteristic of men and women, respectively. The underlying assumption is that the definition of friend derives from and informs basic characteristics of the constructed self as influenced by gender and society.

Ethnic differences in friendship patterns are often interpreted along similar lines (i.e., reflecting differences in levels of intimacy, shared experiences, and peoplehood—e.g., de Vries et al., 1996). Furthermore, as the conditions and situations of life change, so too do friendships as seen in relation to relocation and changes in marital status, for example (Allan & Adams, 1989). Physical presence is not a prerequisite for friendship; if we cannot be with the ones we love, we can love the ones we are with. The stability and persistence of friendship, however, is severely challenged by some life situations such as illness, particularly those in which the norm of reciprocity cannot be fulfilled.

The foregoing summary offers several recurrent themes and features of the meaning and experience of friendship (see also Blau, 1973; Johnson, 1983). Friends are not family and, perhaps similar to the role of the father in the attachment process, friends represent *a point of contrast,* drawing individuals into worlds unlike those inhabited by family (similar to the role of mother as the primary attachment figure). This is a world that is largely *affective* and normed on *reciprocity* and *choice.* This contrast point may be seen to be one in which individuals explore and construct themselves in less socially structured ways. This exploration and construction process fosters *self-awareness, self-respect,* and *self-esteem,* in addition to facets of *self-definition* and *peoplehood.* As such, friends also represent yardsticks against which *self-development* may be assessed, addressing tasks of *socialization,* maintaining *role continuity,* and assisting in the *management of life's challenges.*

The life course variations in these themes and features as superordinate factors await extensive empirical attention. Are these themes manifested differently at various life course junctures? Are certain features more characteristic of certain age ranges than others? For example, the family members against which friends are contrasted vary as a function of family development (i.e., family of orientation, family of procreation); perhaps different contrasts reveal different images. Sociability and affective interactions would appear to be more prominent in earlier life, at least as attested to by frequency of contact. Alternatively, the constituents of sociability may vary, such as the stereotypic and popularized images of the shared laments of "Generation X" and the group discussions of stocks and bonds among "Yuppies" of the Baby Boom. The self-clearinghouse functions of friendship appear to maintain their strength over the life course as individuals look to their friends as a measure of their own respect, awareness, definition, and development. For example, individuals may "bask in the reflected glory" (e.g., Tesser & Campbell, 1982) of the accomplishment of their friends, hear reports of their own achievements and/or shortcomings, and learn that someone is always either in a more or a less desirable position than they are (e.g., "downward social comparison," Taylor, 1989). Such functions are also served during periods of transition where friends (either directly or indirectly) may facilitate the negotiation of life's challenges, appear to remain stable and consistent when all else appears to crumble, and help identify relevant tasks to complete. As previously reported, limits to these features may emerge in late, late life. The oldest-old speak of outliving their friends ("My friends just don't live as long as I do," Johnson & Troll, 1994, p. 84) and of relinquishing friendship, almost with an attitude of "good riddance" (Lowenthal & Robinson, 1976).

Surprisingly embedded in the accounts of experiences of loss are clear and poignant messages of meaning. Grief, after all, "is the study of people and their most intimate relationships" (Deck & Folta, 1989, p. 80). Previous research with bereaved parents (de Vries et al., 1994) and bereaved spouses (Arbuckle & de Vries, 1995) have charted this direction, revealing a depth of understanding not well represented by, for example, standard depression scores. The loss of a friend in later life—an occurrence for one-third of a large, representative sample of older Canadians (de Vries, Lehman, & Arbuckle, 1995) and for almost one-half of the oldest-old (as reported in Johnson & Troll, 1994)—offers a similar avenue for future research.

This avenue, however, has remained relatively untapped: few reports exist detailing the experiences of loss of a friend. In part, this void exists because of a family-centered society in which virtually no rights are granted to surviving friends (Sklar, 1991–92). In fact, Deck and Folta (1989) reported that interest in the bereaved by nonkin is considered "an infringement upon family rights and perogatives . . . an intrusion on the sanctity of the family" (p. 82). As such "friend-grievers" (Deck & Folta, 1989) or "survivor-friends" (Sklar & Hartley, 1990) are a hidden population experiencing "the social and emotional transformation of bereavement, while they are forced to suffer the lack of institutional outlets that act as support" (Sklar & Hartley, 1990, p. 105).

Roberto and Stanis (1994) examined the death of a friend for women in later life and found that the majority reported some sense of loss. The women reported an increased awareness of their own aging and mortality and a greater appreciation of their own lives. They "missed doing things and just being together" as well as "talking and sharing" (p. 41). Sklar and Hartley (1990) similarly found considerable unresolved feelings of despair, anger, guilt, emptiness, and fear of one's own mortality. Deck and Folta (1989) suggested that these feelings have, as their origins, the strong identification that individuals have with their friends such that the threat to the self, the essence of the loss, is very intense. "There is both the fear that 'it could have been me' and the relief that 'it wasn't me' " (p. 84). The death creates a loss of identity and a threat to self-esteem.

The key features of friendship appear amply demonstrated in these few accounts (i.e., point of contrast, affective domain, self-awareness, self-development, and management of life transitions and challenges). They further highlight some of the topical areas previously targeted, in particular the friend–family contrast, the multidimensionality of friendship, and life events. The study of friendship bereavement offers a window onto both the meaning and experience of friendship and the meaning of its loss.

REFERENCES

Adams, R. G. (1986a). A look at friendship and aging. *Generations, 10,* 40–43.

Adams, R. G. (1986b). Emotional closeness and physical distance between friends: Implications for elderly women living in age-segregated and age-integrated settings. *International Journal of Aging and Human Development, 22,* 55–76.

Adams, R. G. (1989). Conceptual and methodological issues in studying friendships of older adults. In R. G. Adams & R. Blieszner (Eds.), *Older adult friendship: Structure and process* (pp. 17–44). Newbury Park, CA: Sage.

Adams, R. G., & Blieszner, R. (1994). An integrative conceptual framework for friendship research. *Journal of Social and Personal Relationships, 11,* 163–184.

Aldous, J. (1978). *Family careers.* New York: Wiley.

Allan, G. A. (1979). *A sociology of friendship and kinship.* London: Allen & Unwin.

Allan, G. A., & Adams, R. G. (1989). Aging and the structure of friendship. In R. G. Adams & R. Blieszner (Eds.), *Older adult friendship: Structure and process* (pp. 45–64). Newbury Park, CA: Sage.

Antonucci, T. C., & Akiyama, H. (1987). Social networks in adult life and a preliminary examination of the convoy model. *The Gerontologist, 42*, 519–527.

Arbuckle, N., & de Vries, B. (1995). The long-term effects of later life spousal and parental bereavement on personal functioning. *The Gerontologist, 35*, 637–647.

Aries, E. J., & Johnson, F. L. (1983). Close friendship in adulthood: Conversational content between same-sex friends. *Sex Roles, 9*, 1183–1196.

Arnold, W. J., & Chartier, B. M. (1986, June). *Intimacy and solidarity in men's relationships*. Paper presented at the 47th annual convention of the Canadian Psychological Association, Toronto, Canada.

Baltes, P. B. (1979). Life-span developmental psychology: Some converging observations on history and theory. In P. B. Baltes & O. G. Brim (Eds.), *Life-span development and behavior* (Vol. 2, pp. 255–279). New York: Academic Press.

Bankoff, E. A. (1981). Effects of friendship support on the psychological well-being of widows. In H. Z. Lopata & D. Maines (Eds.), *Research in the interweave of social roles: Friendship* (pp. 109–139). Greenwich, CT: JAI.

Barer, B. M. (1994). Men and women aging differently. *International Journal of Aging and Human Development, 38*, 29–40.

Barth, R. J., & Kinder, B. N. (1988). A theoretical analysis of sex differences in same-sex friendships. *Sex Roles, 19*, 349–363.

Bell, R. R. (1981). Friendships of women and men. *Psychology of Women Quarterly, 32*, 402–417.

Bernard, J. (1976). Homosociality and female depression. *Journal of Social Issues, 32*, 213–238.

Blau, Z. S. (1961). Structural constraints on friendship in old age. *American Sociological Review, 26*, 429–439.

Blau, Z. S. (1973). *Old age in a changing society*. New York: New Viewpoints.

Blieszner, R. (1988). Individual development and intimate relationships in middle and late adulthood. In R. M. Milardo (Ed.), *Families and social networks* (pp. 147–167). Newbury Park, CA: Sage.

Blieszner, R. (1989). An agenda for future research on friendships of older adults. In R. G. Adams & R. Blieszner (Eds.), *Older adult friendship: Structure and process* (pp. 245–252). Newbury Park, CA: Sage.

Blieszner, R., & Adams, R. G. (1992). *Adult friendship*. Newbury Park, CA: Sage.

Blieszner, R., & Adams, R. G. (1995, November). *The causes and consequences of problems with friends in old age*. Paper presented at the 48th annual scientific meeting of the Gerontological Society of America, Los Angeles.

Booth, A. (1972). Sex and social participation. *American Sociological Review, 37*, 183–192.

Brim, O. G. (1976). Theories of the male mid-life crisis. *The Counseling Psychologist, 6*, 2–9.

Brody, E. (1985). Parent care as a normative family stress. *The Gerontologist, 25*, 19–29.

Caldwell, M. A., & Peplau, L. A. (1982). Sex differences in same-sex friendship. *Sex Roles, 8*, 721–732.

Candy, S. G., Troll, L. E., & Levy, S. G. (1981). A developmental exploration of friendship functions in women. *Psychology of Women Quarterly, 5,* 456–472.

Cohen, C. I. (1989). Social ties and friendship patterns of old homeless men. In R. G. Adams & R. Blieszner (Eds.), *Older adult friendships: Structure and process* (pp. 222–244). Newbury Park, CA: Sage.

Creecy, R. F., & Wright, R. (1979). Morale and informal activity with friends among black and white elderly. *The Gerontologist, 19,* 544–547.

Daly, M. (1978). *Gyn/Ecology.* Boston: Beacon Press.

Davis, K. E., & Todd, M. J. (1985). Assessing friendship: Prototypes, paradigm cases, and relationship description. In S. Duck & D. Perlman (Eds.), *Understanding personal relationships: An interdisciplinary approach* (pp. 17–38). Newbury Park, CA: Sage.

de Vries, B. (1991). Friendship and kinship patterns over the life course: A family stage perspective. In L. Stone (Ed.), *Caring communities: Proceedings of the Symposium on Social Supports* (pp. 99–107). Ottawa: Industry, Science and Technology.

de Vries, B., Blando, J. A., & Walker, L. J. (1995). The review of life's events: Analyses of content and structure. In B. Haight & J. Webster (Eds.), *The art and science of reminiscing: Theory, research, methods, and applications* (pp. 123–137). Washington: Taylor and Francis.

de Vries, B., Dalla Lana, R., & Falck, V. T. (1994). Parental bereavement over the life course: A theoretical integration and empirical review. *Omega: Journal of Death and Dying, 29,* 47–69.

de Vries, B., Dustan, L. A., & Wiebe, R. E. (1994, November). *The understanding of friendship over the life course.* Paper presented at the 47th annual scientific meeting of the Gerontological Society of America, Atlanta.

de Vries, B., Jacoby, C., & Davis, C. G. (1996). Ethnic differences in later life friendship. *Canadian Journal on Aging, 15,* 226–244.

de Vries, B., Lehman, A. J., & Arbuckle, N. (1995, November). *Reactions to the death of a close friend in later life.* Paper presented at the 48th annual scientific meeting of the Gerontological Society of America, Los Angeles, CA.

Deck, E. S., & Folta, J. R. (1989). The friend-griever. In J. K. Doka (Ed.), *Disenfranchised grief: Recognizing hidden sorrow* (pp. 77–89). Lexington, MA: Lexington Books.

Dickens, W. J., & Perlman, D. (1981). Friendship over the life-cycle. In S. Duck & R. Gilmore (Eds.), *Personal relationships: 2* (pp. 91–122). New York: Academic Press.

Douvan, E., & Adelson, J. (1966). *The adolescent experience.* New York: Wiley.

Duvall, E. (1977). *Family development.* Philadelphia: Lippincott.

Farrell, M. P., & Rosenberg, S. D. (1981). *Men at midlife.* Boston: Auburn House.

Felton, B. J., & Berry, C. A. (1992). Do the sources of urban elderly's support determine psychological consequences? *Psychology and Aging, 7,* 89–97.

Gilligan, C. (1982). *In a different voice: Psychological theory and women's development.* Cambridge, MA: Harvard University Press.

Goldman, J. A., Cooper, P. E., Ahern, K., & Corsini, D. (1981). Continuities and discontinuities in the friendship descriptions of women at six stages in the life cycle. *Genetic Psychology Monographs, 103,* 153–167.

Gubrium, J. F. (1975). *Living and dying at Murray Manor.* New York: St. Martin's.

Gutman, G. (1986). Migration of the elderly: An overview. In G. Gutman & N. Blackie (Eds.), *Aging in place: Housing adaptations and options for remaining in the community* (pp. 71–90). Burnaby, BC: Gerontology Research Centre, Simon Fraser University.

Guttmann, D. (1975). Parenthood: A key to the comparative psychology of the life cycle. In N. Datan & L. H. Ginsberg (Eds.), *Life-span developmental psychology: Normative life crises* (pp. 167–184). New York: Academic Press.

Hacker, H. M. (1981). Blabbermouths and clams: Sex differences in self-disclosure in same-sex and cross-sex friendship dyads. *Psychology of Women Quarterly, 5,* 385–401.

Hochschild, A. R. (1973). *The unexpected community.* Englewood Cliffs, NJ: Prentice-Hall.

Jackson, R. M., Fischer, C. S., & Jones, L. M. (1977). The dimensions of social networks. In C. S. Fischer (Ed.), *Networks and places: Social relations in the urban setting* (pp. 39–58). New York: Free Press.

Johnson, C. L. (1983). Fairweather friends and rainy day kin: An anthropological analysis of old age friendships in the United States. *Urban Anthropology, 12,* 103–123.

Johnson, C. L., & Barer, B. M. (1990). Families and networks among older inner-city Blacks. *The Gerontologist, 30,* 726–733.

Johnson, C. L., & Troll, L. E. (1994). Constraints and facilitators to friendship in late late life. *The Gerontologist, 34,* 79–87.

Kahn, R. L., & Antonucci, T. C. (1980). Convoys over the life course: Attachments, roles and social supports. In P. B. Baltes & O. G. Brim (Eds.), *Life-span development and behavior* (pp. 253–286). New York: Academic Press.

Lazarsfeld, P. F., & Merton, R. K. (1954). Friendship as social process: A substantive and methodological analysis. In M. Berger, T. Abel, & C. Page (Eds.), *Freedom and control in modern society* (pp. 18–66). New York: Van Nostrand.

Lewis, R. A. (1978). Emotional intimacy among men. *Journal of Social Issues, 34,* 108–121.

Lipman-Blumen, J. (1976). Toward a homosocial theory of sex roles: An explanation of the sex segregation of social institutions. In M. Blaxall & B. Reagan (Eds.), *Women and the workplace: The implications of occupational segregation* (pp. 15–31). Chicago: University of Chicago Press.

Lopata, H. Z. (1975). Support systems of the elderly: Chicago of the 1970's. *The Gerontologist, 15,* 34–41.

Lopata, H. Z. (1993). The support systems of the American urban widows. In M. S. Stroebe, W. Stroebe, & R. O. Hansson (Eds.), *Handbook of bereavement: Theory, research and intervention* (pp. 381–396). New York: Cambridge University Press.

Lowenthal, M., & Robinson, B. (1976). Social networks and isolation. In R. Binstock & E. Shanas (Eds.), *Handbook of aging and the social sciences* (pp. 432–456). New York: Van Nostrand Reinhold.

McCall, G., & Simmons, J. L. (1966). *Identities and interactions.* New York: Free Press.

Marcia, J. (1980). Identity in adolescence. In J. Adelson (Ed.), *Handbook of adolescent psychology* (pp. 159–187). New York: Wiley.

Matthews, S. H. (1983). Definitions of friendship and their consequences in old age. *Ageing and Society, 3,* 141–155.

Matthews, S. H. (1986). *Friendships through the life course.* Newbury Park, CA: Sage.

Miller, S. (1983). *Men and friendship.* San Leandro, CA: Gateway Books.

O'Meara, J. D. (1989). Cross-sex friendship: Four basic challenges of an ignored relationship. *Sex Roles, 21,* 525–543.

Paine, R. (1974). Anthropological approaches to friendship. In E. Leyton (Ed.), *The social compact: Selected dimensions of friendship* (pp. 1–14). Newfoundland: Memorial University of Newfoundland.

Parker, S., & de Vries, B. (1993). Patterns of friendship for women and men in same and cross-sex friendships. *Journal of Social and Personal Relations, 10,* 617–626.

Penning, M. J., & Chappell, N. L. (1987). Ethnicity and informal supports among older adults. *Journal of Aging Studies, 1,* 145–160.

Peplau, L. A. (1983). Roles and gender. In H. Kelley, E. Berscheid, A. Christensen, J. Harvey, T. Huston, G. Levinger, E. McClintock, L. Peplau, & D. Peterson (Eds.), *Close relationships* (pp. 220–264). New York: Freeman.

Pogrebin, L. C. (1987). *Among friends.* New York: McGraw-Hill.

Reis, H. T. (1986). Gender effects in social participation: Intimacy, loneliness, and the conduct of social interaction. In R. Gilmore & S. Duck (Eds.), *The emerging field of personal relationships* (pp. 91–105). Hillsdale, NJ: Lawrence Erlbaum.

Riley, M. W., & Foner, A. (1968). *Aging and society: An inventory of research findings.* New York: Russell Sage Foundation.

Roberto, K. A., & Kimboko, P. J. (1989). Friendships in later life: Definitions and maintenance patterns. *International Journal of Aging and Human Development, 28,* 9–19.

Roberto, K. A., & Stanis, P. I. (1994). Reactions of older women to the death of their close friends. *Omega: Journal of Death and Dying, 29,* 33–43.

Rosow, I. (1967). *Social integration of the aged.* New York: Free Press.

Rosow, I. (1970). Old people: Their friends and neighbors. *American Behavioral Scientist, 14,* 59–69.

Shanas, E. (1979). The family as a social support system in old age. *The Gerontologist, 19,* 169–174.

Shea, L., Thompson, L., & Blieszner, R. (1988). Resources in older adults' old and new friendships. *Journal of Social and Personal Relationships, 5,* 83–96.

Shulman, N. (1975). Life-cycle variations in patterns of close relationships. *Journal of Marriage and the Family, 37,* 813–821.

Sklar, F. (1991–92). Grief as a family affair: Property rights, grief rights, and the exclusion of close friends as survivors. *Omega: Journal of Death and Dying, 24,* 109–121.

Sklar, F., & Hartley, S. F. (1990). Close friends as survivors: Bereavement patterns in a "hidden" population. *Omega: Journal of Death and Dying, 21,* 103–112.

Strain, L. A., & Chappell, N. L. (1989). Social networks or urban native elders: A comparison with non-natives. *Canadian Ethnic Studies, 21,* 104–117.

Sullivan, H. S. (1953). *The interpersonal theory of psychiatry.* New York: Norton.

Surrey, J. L. (1985). Self-in-relation: A theory of women's development. *Work in Progress, No. 13.* Wellesley, MA: Stone Center Working Papers Series.

Taylor, S. (1989). *Positive illusions: Creative self-deception and the healthy mind.* New York: Basic Books.

Tesser, A., & Campbell, J. (1982). Self evaluation maintenance and the perception of friends and strangers. *Journal of Personality, 50,* 261–279.

Weiss, L., & Lowenthal, M. F. (1975). Life-course perspectives on friendship. In M. F. Lowenthal, M. Thurnher, D. Chiriboga, & Associates (Eds.), *Four stages of life* (pp. 48–61). San Francisco: Jossey-Bass.

White, J. M. (1991). *The dynamics of family development: The theory of family development.* New York: Guilford Press.

Wood, V., & Robertson, J. F. (1978). Friendship and kinship interaction: Differential effect on the morale of the elderly. *Journal of Marriage and the Family, 40,* 367–375.

Wright, P. H. (1982). Men's friendship, women's friendships and the alleged inferiority of the latter. *Sex Roles, 8,* 1–20.

CHAPTER 15

Emotional Reactions to Interpersonal Losses over the Life Span

An Attachment Theoretical Perspective

Mario Mikulincer *and* Victor Florian
Department of Psychology
Bar-Ilan University
Ramat Gan, Israel

I. INTRODUCTION

The human encounter with loss is one of the most expected and natural phenomena during the life span. However, at the same time, this encounter is a core emotion-arousing event, which is usually accompanied by painful affects and the need to cope with the new reality. Although many theoretical attempts have been made to understand the encounter with loss, there is general agreement that attachment theory (Bowlby, 1973, 1980) seems to present the most comprehensive conceptualization. According to Bowlby, loss should be understood in the context of the relationship that was lost, and reactions to loss might depend on the attachment functions that the lost person accomplished, such as the provision of love, support, and caring. Moreover, Bowlby contends that the main loss-related emotion, grief, reflects the frustration of the basic attachment need of maintaining proximity to a significant figure as well as the disruption of a sense of security in life (Bowlby's "secure base").

In the present chapter, we focus on three basic issues related to the encounter with loss. The first issue concerns Bowlby's hypothesis that the quality of the relationship with the lost person shapes the individual's reactions to the loss. In this context, we adopt Bowlby's view that (a) the quality of close relationships during the life span is related to early attachment experiences, and (b) this association is mediated by the formation of generalized attachment styles. In light of this view, we review data on the extent to which the quality of the lost relationship, the quality of early attachment experiences, and the person's attachment style may shape his or her reactions to loss.

The second issue deals with a complementary hypothesis that the experience of loss during the life span is an important shaping factor of the individual's attachment style. In this context, we review evidence from the literature and from our laboratory on the impact that early and current losses have on the way people relate to others. Finally, the third issue deals with a new attachment conceptualization of functional and dysfunctional responses to loss. We attempt to propose a theoretical framework in which adaptation to loss is the result of the dialectical interplay of two opposite attachment-related forces: the need to maintain proximity to the lost person and the need to detach from him or her in order to form new relationships.

II. THE IMPACT OF ATTACHMENT QUALITY ON REACTIONS TO LOSS

The basic premise of attachment theory is that the experience of grief should be expected only in response to the loss of an attachment relationship because these relationships foster security like that of child–parent attachment (Weiss, 1993). In adulthood, this attachment relationship can be found in marital ties, parental–child bonds, and sibling relationships. According to Weiss (1993), when people feel that their attachment figures are lost, they may experience an upsurge of attachment feelings and needs that cannot be further satisfied by the lost figure. Grief appears to be the emotional product of this arousal of attachment needs together with their frustration.

The attachment–loss link is already present in the fact that reactions to loss appear to differ according to the type of the lost relationship.

There is a wide consensus in the literature (e.g., Owen, Fulton, & Markusen, 1982) that the loss of a child has the most devastating effect on well-being. This loss may symbolically reflect the loss of one's being and the loss of meaning in life, overwhelming parents with feelings of helplessness and emptiness (Florian, 1989). Loss of a spouse is also considered a stressful event due to the loss of the social identity related to marital status. Major responses to this loss are loneliness and the shift of identity to that of a single person. Loss of a parent by an adult child is not expected to produce serious levels of distress. However, it may foster the emergence of childhood memories of unresolved attachment issues.

Both theory and research emphasize that reactions to loss are also related to the attachment-related qualities of the lost relationship. In their classic writing, Parkes and Weiss (1983) proposed that clinging, dependent relationships may have negative effects on grief reactions. They suggested that persons who lose the one on whom they depend are vulnerable to anxiety and worry simply because they are deprived of the strong, reliable support they once had. For them, security can only be found through desperate efforts to maintain the attachment relationship, and thereby the acceptance of the loss may produce unbearable anxiety. Indeed, Maddison and Viola (1968) and Parkes and Weiss (1983) found more pathological grief reactions among widows who described themselves as dependent on their husbands. This effect was replicated in a study of adult women who had experienced the death of a parent 1–5 years previously (Scharlach, 1991).

A related piece of evidence is found in the study of Futterman, Gallagher, Thompson, and Lovett (1990), who interviewed elders 2, 12, and 30 months after the loss of their spouses and compared their responses with those of nonbereaved elders. Whereas higher levels of depression were associated with lower ratings of love and dependency in the nonbereaved subjects, the opposite was found in the bereaved subjects. That is, more severe ratings of depression after the spouse's death were related to retrospective reports of higher levels of love before the loss. These findings may reflect the emotional pain and suffering of those persons who lost a positive attachment relationship.

Another component of close relationships that may hinder the resolution of the grief process is the presence of ambivalent feelings toward the lost person, a classic indicator of anxious attachment (Bowlby, 1973). Freud (1917) already theorized that ambivalent feelings in a relationship may result in distress and "obsessive reproaches" during bereavement, a constant form of self-denigration. Weiss (1993) suggested that ambivalence toward the attachment figure can impede emotional acceptance of the loss because there will be confusion regarding the nature of feelings, and because self-blame, guilt, and remorse may compound the pain of loss. In support of this view, Parkes and Weiss (1983) reported that bereaved persons who experienced higher levels of conflict with their spouses had more anxiety, depression, and guilt after the spouse's death.

In reviewing the above studies, we note that two opposite patterns of relationship, clinging-loving versus ambivalent-conflictual, have similar disrupting effects on the grief process. This paradox was examined by Stroebe and Stroebe (1993) in their study of adjustment to bereavement in young widows and widowers. They found that gender plays an important role in resolving the above contradiction. Whereas widows reported higher levels of distress after the loss of a happy rather than an unhappy marriage, widowers reported more distress if they had been less happy and close to their spouse. However, when observing the correlations between marital quality and distress, the authors reported weaker correlations for widowers than for widows. Stroebe and Stroebe (1993) speculated that "because marital quality seemed to be less important for the men in our sample while they were married, they might have suffered more guilt feelings after the loss" (p. 220).

Beyond examining the impact of the quality of the lost relationship, the most relevant test of Bowlby's hypothesis should involve the association between early experiences with attachment figures and responses to loss in adulthood. This association was empirically supported by Brown (1982), who found that early separation and loss experiences were apt to lead to anxious attachment and to increase the risk of women's depression after the loss of a spouse. Accordingly, Douglas (1990) reported that even many years after the death of parent, adults who recollected negative childhood memories about their interactions with parents reported more pathological grief reactions.

Stoll (1993) also found that the quality of early attachment experiences was related to middle-aged women's reactions to the death of their husbands. Findings support attachment theory that early disruptions of the attachment system may increase the risk of maladjustment to loss in adulthood. Widows who reported more satisfying relationships with greater number of attachment figures during childhood, and experienced fewer actual separations as well as fewer threats of loss of primary caregivers, reported lesser amounts of depression and psychosomatic symptoms between 6 and 24 months after the death of their husbands. Similar findings were reported by Goidel (1993) in an additional sample of widows and widowers and by Sable (1989) in a study of aged widows.

A careful analysis of attachment theory indicates that the association between early attachment experiences and subsequent grief reactions might be mediated by the individual's attachment style, the major hypothesized source of continuity during the life span. However, an extensive review of the literature we conducted reveals no published empirical data on this issue. Therefore, we can only present some indirect evidence from our study on the ways in which adult persons differing in attachment style cope with and adjust to a major loss: the process of marital separation and divorce (Birnbaum, Orr, Mikulincer, & Florian, in press). A sample of 123 subjects who were involved in a long process of divorce were classified according to their attachment style (secure, avoidant, anxious-ambivalent) and compared to a matched group of married subjects in a measure of mental health. In addition, they also reported on the way they appraise and cope with the divorce.

The results indicate that attachment style moderates emotional reactions to the breaking of the marital relationship. As expected, divorcing individuals reported more distress than married individuals. But this effect was found only among the two insecurely attached groups, avoidant and anxious-ambivalent, but not among the secure group. Differences among attachment groups were also found in the appraisal of, and coping with, the divorce crisis. Both secure and avoidant persons appraised themselves as more capable of coping with the loss than anxious-ambivalent persons. Avoidant and ambivalent persons appraised the divorce as more threatening and reported having used more maladaptive coping strategies than secure persons.

The relatively weak negative emotions of securely attached persons may reflect the conviction in their ability to cope with emotions and the beliefs in the availability of supportive others (Bowlby, 1973). Moreover, as secure persons constructively handled the childhood separation from attachment figures and learned that separation is a resolvable episode with which they have the resources to cope, the reconstruction of this experience, as it reappears in divorce, might be appraised as less threatening and might elicit less distress. For an anxious-ambivalent person, the loss of marital relationship may shake their fragile equilibrium and further increase the level of distress they habitually experience. Moreover, they may lack constructive ways of coping and may be unable to deal with the resulting distress.

The observed reactions of avoidant persons may reflect that the habitual working model of these persons (detachment, self-reliance) proves to be ineffective in dealing with a major loss. In this case, the pseudosafe world of avoidant persons is shattered, due to the break of their defensive dam, and they may find themselves helpless in the face of the loss.

This may be particularly true in the midst of a crisis and when there is a clear connection between the loss and the attachment system. The divorce may reactivate early unresolved separations from attachment figures, and therefore lead to a flood of negative feelings, which avoidant persons find it difficult to repress.

An overview of the studies presented above suggests two different patterns of associations between attachment and loss. On the one hand, it seems that securely attached persons, who experience warm and loving early relationships with caregivers, would suffer a lot of distress after the loss of a loved person, but, at the same time, would have sufficient inner resources to cope effectively with the loss. This conclusion is based on the finding that loss-related distress is higher among individuals who report a more positive relationship with the lost person, which is a prominent characteristic of secure individuals (Hazan & Shaver, 1987). However, this distress may be buffered by the presence of inner resources and abilities that help secure persons to overcome the painful experience of loss.

On the other hand, insecurely attached persons, who experience rejecting or unstable early relationships with caregivers, would experience overwhelming levels of distress following the breaking of a significant relationship, with which they are unable to cope. In these cases, the distress is related to the experience of conflictual and ambivalent feelings toward the lost person, which characterizes insecurely attached individuals (Hazan & Shaver, 1987). This distress may be compounded by the fact that insecure persons tend to adopt maladaptive coping strategies that hinder the resolution of the grief process and have a deleterious effect on psychological well-being.

III. THE IMPLICATIONS OF LOSSES TO THE ATTACHMENT SYSTEM

In this section, we follow Bowlby's theoretical proposition that loss and attachment may mutually influence each other. That is, the experience of loss is not only a product of the quality of early or current relationships, but it also may be an antecedent of the quality of future attachment relationships. Specifically, we examine existing data on the potential impact of separation and loss during the life span on the way people will relate to significant others.

Several studies, not based on an attachment perspective, have studied the impact of early loss on interpersonal relationships for persons who have lost a parent to death while they were adolescents (e.g., Jacobson & Ryder, 1968; Meshot & Leitner, 1994; Silverman, 1987; Taylor, 1983). Although Silverman (1987) reported no significant association between parental death and intimate relationships, Taylor (1983) found that people who had had a parent die viewed relationships as threatening, and Jacobson and Ryder (1968) found that intimate relationships may be terrifying and in jeopardy for those who had a parent die. In a recent study, Meshot and Leitner (1994) found that young adults who had experienced parental death showed an insecure interpersonal style that is marked by a strong desire that others take interest in them. Moreover, while males tended to be socially anxious (they seek close ties with everyone), females tended to be avoidant of close ties. These findings emphasize the deleterious impact that parental death may have on the way people relate to others.

A direct piece of evidence on the long-term impact of early loss on the attachment system was provided by Brennan and Shaver (1993), who assessed attachment style and quality of personal relationships among a sample of college students as a function of parental divorce. Contrary to the expectations, findings indicate that parental divorce was not significantly related to offspring's attachment styles or relationship outcomes. Brennan and Shaver suggested that this lack of association may reflect the fact that some intact marriages are distressing and have insecurity-producing effects on children's attachment styles, whereas some positive postdivorce arrangements could promote security in offsprings. In addition, it seems to us that the finding may be due to the lack of information on two factors that may moderate the impact of parental divorce on the offspring's attachment style: (a) the age of the child at the time of the divorce; and (b) whether the custodial parent remarried and therefore reconstructed the family environment.

In order to overcome the above limitations, we recently conducted an unpublished study in which we compared the current attachment styles of adolescents (age 17–18) who experienced parental divorce in different periods in their childhood to those of a matched control group of adolescents from intact families. The study group was divided into three according to their age at the time of divorce (0–4, 5–9, 10–14). Our data showed that parental divorce had a significant impact on the offspring's attachment style only when it occurred in infancy and early childhood (see Table 1). In these cases, there was an overrepresentation of the anxious-ambivalent attachment style and underrepresentation of the secure style. No such effect was found when the divorce occurred later in childhood. In addition, the detrimental effect of parental divorce vanished when the custodial parent remarried.

Table 1

Distribution of Attachment Styles across Different Study Groups

	Secure		Avoidant		Anxious-ambivalent	
	N	%	N	%	N	%
Parental divorce study						
Divorce at age 0–4	15	31	17	35	16	34
Divorce at age 5–9	19	47	14	35	7	18
Divorce at age 10–14	27	60	13	29	5	11
Control group	38	63	16	27	6	10
Father's death study						
Study group	18	36	15	30	17	34
Control group	30	60	13	26	7	14
Early losses study						
Study group	29	34	24	28	33	38
Control group	52	60	20	23	14	17

Overall, it seems that an early loss of attachment figures may play a crucial role in the construction of a "secure base" later in life. However, one should be careful and take into account the positive impact of the restoration of security due to the reconstruction of new alternative family relationships. The findings are conceptually similar to Murphy's (1991) report on more feelings of loneliness among adults who had experienced parental divorce earlier in their lives.

Additional empirical support for the contention that the experience of early losses may disturb the development of secure attachment was uncovered in another study conducted by our team. In this study, we examined whether the death of a father during the critical period of the first 3 years of his children's life influences the building of the offspring's attachment style 20 years later. We collected data on attachment styles of 50 young adults who lost their fathers 20 years before, during the Israel–Egypt attrition war (1969), and compared them to a matched control group of young adults from intact families. The results presented in Table 1 reveal that the early loss of an attachment figure may lead later in life to the development of insecure attachment styles. As compared to the control group, which showed the typical distribution of attachment styles, our study group showed an overrepresentation of the anxious-ambivalent style and an underrepresentation of the secure style.

A step forward in expanding the above findings was taken in another research project conducted in our laboratory. Using a community sample of young adults, we asked subjects to report on the experiences of different kinds of losses (e.g., mother's death, father's death, sibling's death, parental divorce) during their childhood (until age 17) as well as on their current attachment style. As can be seen in Table 1, the distribution of subjects who reported at least one early loss was significantly different from that of subjects who reported no loss. As in the above-mentioned studies, the experience of early losses was again related to an overrepresentation of the anxious-ambivalent style and to an underrepresentation of the secure style. In addition, it was found that among those subjects who reported early loss, the higher the number of losses and the earlier the age in which these losses occur, the higher the level of anxious-ambivalent attachment.

Beyond its impact on the formation of attachment style, early loss of a parent seems to also have long-term effects on the way adults fulfill their parental role (Zall, 1994). Although a large proportion of adults were found to function well as parents despite their experience with early parental loss, there is indication that in some cases, particularly when the same-sex parent was lost, difficulties and anxieties related to parenthood may develop.

In reviewing the literature on attachment and loss, we observe that the experience of current losses may also play an important role in the way adults form new relationships. Such an effect was reported by Shuchter and Sizook (1993) after the death of a spouse. They found that many bereaved persons had difficulties in becoming involved in new romantic relationships due to their devotion to the deceased, societal sanctions, or fear of recurrent loss. One possible explanation of this finding is that contact with others in the early phases of bereavement is painful because such an interaction may remind one of the lost person. In addition, Shuschter and Sizook (1993) found that when bereaved persons form new relationships, they reported problems related to the place of the lost person within the new relationship. Some persons reported feelings of disloyalty to the deceased spouse, painful comparisons, and problems of adaptation to the new marital role. The authors concluded that "even where successful remarriages occur, grief does not end but becomes incorporated into this new relationship" (p. 40).

Current losses may also have extended impact on the way people behave in their remaining close relationships. This effect was observed in the changes occurring in the marital relationship of spouses who lost a child. In a longitudinal study, Bohannon (1990) interviewed 33 couples who lost a child 2 months to 5 years before and found signs of marital disruption related to grief responses. However, negative feelings that spouses had about their marriages following the child's death declined as time progressed, suggesting a process of marital reorganization related to the mourning process. A similar disruption of the marital relationship was also observed after the death of a parent (Guttman, 1991).

A comprehensive examination of the effects of loss in adulthood on social relationships was provided by Scharlach and Fredriksen (1993). In reaction to parent death, most of the subjects reported changes in their relationships with spouses, children, friends, and the surviving parent. The authors concluded that "following the death of a parent, many respondents described a process of assessing and restructuring their personal relationships, often yielding closer, more meaningful interpersonal bonds. . . . For some respondents, the death of a parent led to problems in relationships with spouses and partners" (p. 316).

An overall view of the presented material supports the idea that the experience of losses during the life span may have a deleterious effect on the attachment system. However, one should clearly differentiate between early loss and the experience of loss in adulthood. On the one hand, findings indicate that people who experience early loss of primary attachment figures are more inclined to develop insecure attachment and to exhibit long-term difficulties in their interpersonal relationships. On the other hand, the experience of losses in adulthood is more complex. In some cases, the loss may impair the way people relate to others. In other cases, it may lead to a positive rebuilding of interpersonal ties. Unfortunately, there are no data on the possible factors that could determine these differential effects. At this point, we only can speculate that attachment style may be one of these factors. Whereas secure persons, who rely on adaptive ways of coping, may be able to positively reorganize their ties after the encounter with loss, insecure persons, who lack effective coping skills, may experience difficulties in their relationships after the loss.

IV. COPING WITH LOSS AS AN ATTACHMENT–DETACHMENT PROCESS

In this section, we attempt to incorporate the existing knowledge about adaptation to loss into the framework of attachment theory. From our perspective, adaptation to loss is the result of the interplay of two major attachment-related forces, each representing opposite poles in an attachment–detachment continuum. Specifically, we suggest that adaptation to loss requires the integrative accomplishment of two main psychological tasks: (a) the maintenance of attachment ties to the lost person, and (b) the relocation of psychological energy and the displacement of interpersonal needs toward new attachment figures.

On both theoretical and clinical grounds, one cannot expect bereaved individuals to forget memories of the lost person, to break psychological ties with him or her, and to dismiss the meaning and importance of the lost relationship, which is a source of security, comfort, and identity. Instead, people should be encouraged to express their feelings bout the lost person, to explore the meaning of the lost relationship, and to find new internal and external avenues of maintaining the lost bond despite the pain and grief caused by this work. In this way, bereaved persons can undergo the healthy process of incorporating the past into the present without splitting important segments of their personal and social identity related to the lost attachment. However, the accomplishment of the above task should be at the same time accompanied by the gradual reorganization of the attachment system, which will allow the individual to satisfy his or her attachment needs through new social contacts. Without this gradual detachment process from the lost figure, people would be stacked in their past relationship and unable to appraise and cope with the new reality. This process will allow the individual to work through the lost relationship not at the expense of the formation of present and future social ties.

The review of the literature provides extensive support to the data that the maintainance of ongoing attachment to the lost person is an important task in the process of adaptation to loss. In his theoretical formulation of the two-track model of bereavement, Rubin (1991) proposed that responses to loss include not only overt behavioral and personality modifications, but also changes related to the internalized relationship with the deceased. On one track, the loss is viewed as a stressor or trauma that affects somatic, psychological, and behavioral functioning. On the second track, the most relevant to our discussion, the loss is appraised as an attack upon a significant attachment bond requiring the individual to undergo a psychological reorganization of the lost relationship. This reorganization includes the construction of new psychological, symbolic links to the deceased that may perpetuate the emotional investment in the lost relationship.

In a validation study, Rubin (1991) interviewed a sample of Israeli parents who lost their young adult son during the war 4 or 13 years earlier. The findings support the idea of ongoing attachment and showed that these bereaved parents tended to be overinvolved with their lost sons. In Rubin's own terms,

The son's image is intensely bound up with the covert emotional life of the parents. As the son representation becomes more central to the parent's psychological world, it becomes more difficult for the parent to move away from intense involvement with this private relationship. (p. 198)

The task of maintaining ongoing attachment to the lost figure was also documented by Silverman, Nickman, and Worden (1992) in a study of children who were interviewed at 4 months and 1 year after the death of a parent. Five main responses were identified in children's reactions that reflect a continuous effort to maintain the bond to the deceased parent: (1) locating the deceased in heaven, (2) reaching out to the deceased, (3) experiencing the deceased as watching their actions, (4) waking memories, and (5) cherishing linking objects to the deceased. Silverman et al. (1992) concluded that bereavement in children should be understood as the establishment of a set of memories, feelings, and actions attempting to maintain their attachment to the deceased.

In another study, Silverman and Worden (1993) reported a similar pattern of behavior among college-age women who lost a parent to death. The results suggest that these women were constantly renegotiating their relationship with the deceased and trying to find a way for the deceased to still live in some way within their lives. This sort of ongoing attachment was also reported by Hogan and DeSantis (1992) in a sample of adolescents who experienced a sibling death.

Interestingly, the task of maintaining ongoing attachment to the lost person is not only present in the breaking of parent–child relationships, but it also seems to be an integral part of the process of coping with the loss of a spouse. In a longitudinal study of grief reactions to the death of a spouse, Shuchter and Zisook (1993) found that although widows and widowers must adapt to a new reality without their spouses, they do not relinquish their previous attachment to the deceased 2, 7, and 13 months after the loss. In contrast, they appear to maintain this tie by transforming

what had been a relationship operating on several levels of actual, symbolic, internalized, and imagined relatedness to one in which the actual (living and breathing) relationship has been lost, but the other forms remain or may even develop in more elaborate forms. (p. 34)

Bereaved persons were found to report experiencing comfort that the spouse was in heaven, experiencing the spouse's presence in daily life and dreams, talking with the spouse regularly, keeping the deceased's belongings, identifying with the diverse features of the deceased, perpetuating the deceased's wishes, and exposing themselves to reminders of the deceased.

Further support for the maintainance of ongoing attachment to a

lost spouse can be found in Stroube and Stroube's (1991) Tubingen longitudinal study of bereavement. The results suggest that among a sample
of young widows and widowers, even after 2 years, most of the subjects
still tend to maintain their ties to the deceased. Moreover, the deceased
was found to continue to have strong influence over the way widows and
widowers organized and planned their lives. In this context, it is useful to
acknowledge Rosenblatt and Meyer's (1986) argument that the maintainance of an inner dialogue with the deceased serves the positive function of helping the bereaved clarify thoughts, deal with the unfinished
relationships, and prepare for the future.

At this point, it is important to emphasize that the analysis of the literature also presents some supporting evidence to the relevance of the
gradual detachment from the lost person as a means of adjusting to the
new reality. In his theoretical formulation, Bowlby (1980) suggested that
bonds with the deceased need to be broken from the bereaved to adjust
and recover. Accordingly, Raphael and Nunn (1988) reviewed the literature on counseling and therapy for the bereaved and concluded that most
of these interventions are guided by the view that bereaved persons should
break their ties to the deceased, give up their attachments, form a new
identity of which the deceased has no part, and relocate emotional investment in other relationships.

A recent illustration of the relocation of attachment bonds after loss
was provided by Roberto and Stanis (1994) in a study of reactions of
older women to the death of their friends. They found that most of the
women reported feeling closer to their other surviving friends after the
loss. Only a few subjects (10%) felt that they had distanced themselves
from their friends. However, this did not mean that the deceased was forgotten, as most of the women reported that they maintained alive their
memories of the times they shared with the deceased.

The material reviewed in this chapter raises the basic question of
whether the opposite tasks of ongoing attachment and gradual detachment can coexist in the process of coping with loss. An interesting and
challenging view is proposed by Stroebe, Gergen, Gergen, and Stroebe
(1992), who suggested that these tasks represent two different cultural
perspectives. On the one hand, the tendency to detach from the lost person seems to be the most dominant way in which Western modernistic
cultures approach bereavement. This perspective that emphasizes goal
directness, efficiency, and rationality, seems to encourage bereaved persons to break ties with the deceased and to reduce attention to the loss.
On the other hand, the tendency to maintain certain ties with the deceased represents the most prevalent way in which non-Western traditional cultures look upon bereavement. This perspective leads bereaved

persons to construct new ways of spiritual and emotional bonding with the deceased and to establish an ongoing inner dialog with him or her. This approach promises that one's attachments will not be completely and irrevocably broken during life and in the hereafter.

Although this social constructivistic approach seems to be fruitful and appealing, we believe that the tasks of ongoing attachment and gradual detachment may coexist together in the same person, whether in a Western culture or an Eastern culture, and may be a prerequisite for the resolution of the grief process. These two tasks are accomplished in a dialectical interplay, in which progress in one task facilitates rather than impedes the progress in the other task. This interplay may enhance the balance between past and future, the integration of identity segments related to the lost person within the new social identity, and the restoration of a sense of "secure base" constructed now on both the internalized lost bond and the established new ties.

The dialectical movement between attachment and detachment during the process of coping with loss can be also found in Rando's clinical conceptualization of the process of mourning. On the one hand, bereaved persons should be encouraged to recollect and reexperience the deceased and the lost relationships, remembering them realistically and reviving their feelings. On the other hand, bereaved persons should be encouraged to relinquish the old attachments to the deceased. In fact, Rando (1992) pointed out that readjustment after loss involves a movement into the new reality without forgetting the past relationship.

Although there are no available published data on this line of thought, we would like to present some indirect evidence from our laboratory that might shed some light on the conceptualization of the attachment–detachment process after loss. In this study, we examined whether middle-aged divorced adults ($N = 123$) differing in their attachment style would reveal different patterns of ongoing bonding to their ex-spouse. The rationale behind this study was that securely attached persons, who are viewed as possessing a healthy attitude toward relationships and their dissolution, would satisfy their attachment needs in new social ties without totally cutting off their previous bonding. This balance between attachment and detachment would be absent in both insecure types, either avoidant or anxious-ambivalent. In the case of avoidantly attached persons, their habitual ways of coping with distress (e.g., distancing from negative emotions, dismissing the importance of lost relationships) would lead them to look for total detachment from their ex-spouses. In the case of anxious-ambivalent persons, their unsatisfied need for dependency and protection would lead them to perpetuate their emotional investment in ex-spouses, impeding the acceptance of the loss and the formation of new relationships. The findings clearly support this expectation: Whereas anxious-ambivalent persons reported a strong on-going attachment to their ex-spouses (e.g., frequent contacts, high levels of perceived and expected intimacy, passion, and commitment) and avoidant persons reported a strong tendency toward forgetting and detachment, secure persons reported more balanced feelings toward their ex-spouses.

V. CONCLUSION

In concluding this chapter, one can note that our attachment–detachment model of coping with loss may serve as a useful explanation for the reciprocal influences between attachment and loss. If one of the tasks of coping with loss is the maintenance of ongoing attachment to the lost person, then one can better explain the finding that the existence of insecure, conflictual bond during the relationship hinders the resolution of the grief process. In fact, it seems that security in attachment underlies the development of a warm relationship before and after the loss. Furthermore, if the other task of coping with loss is the formation of new interpersonal relationships, then one can better explain the finding that the experience of loss alters the way people relate to others after the traumatic experience. Once again, security in attachment may facilitate the gradual detachment from the lost person and underlie the positive rebuilding of the individual's social life after the loss. In light of this conclusion, one should only acknowledge the contribution of Bowlby's "secure base" for understanding the human encounter with loss. We hope that our theoretical framework will inspire further empirical research and clinical applications.

REFERENCES

Birnbaum, G. E., Orr, I., Mikulincer, M., & Florian, V. (in press). When marriage breaks up—Does attachment style contribute to coping and mental health? *Journal of Social and Personal Relationships.*

Bohannon, J. R. (1990). Grief responses of spouses following the death of a child: A longitudinal study. *Omega, 22,* 109–121.

Bowlby, J. (1973). *Attachment and loss: Separation, anxiety and anger.* New York: Basic Books.

Bowlby, J. (1980). *Attachment and loss: Sadness and depression.* New York: Basic Books.

Brennan, K. A., & Shaver, P. R. (1993). Attachment styles and parental divorce. *Journal of Divorce and Remarriage, 21,* 161–175.

Brown, G. W. (1982). Early loss and depression. In C. W. Parkes & J. Stevenson-Hinde (Eds.), *The place of attachment in human social behavior* (pp. 161–183). New York: Basic Books.

Douglas, J. D. (1990). Patterns of change following parent death in midlife adults. *Omega, 22,* 123–137.

Florian, V. (1989). Meaning and purpose in life of bereaved parents whose son fell during active military service. *Omega, 20,* 91–102.

Freud, S. (1917). Mourning and melancholia. In J. Strachey (Ed.), *Standard edition of the complete psychological works of Sigmund Freud* (vol. 14, pp. 237–258). London: Hogarth Press.

Futterman, A., Gallagher, D., Thompson, L. W., & Lovett, S. (1990). Retrospective assessment of marital adjustment and depression during the first 2 years of spousal bereavement. *Psychology and Aging, 5,* 273–280.

Goidel, J. (1993). Social, situational, and psychological factors in the psychological adjustment of widows and widowers. In K. Pottharst (Ed.), *Research explorations in adult attachment* (pp. 257–268). New York: Lang.

Guttman, H. A. (1991). Parental death as a precipitant of marital conflict in middle age. *Journal of Marital and Family Therapy, 17,* 81–87.

Hazan, C., & Shaver, P. (1987). Romantic love conceptualized as an attachment process. *Journal of Personality and Social Psychology, 52,* 511-524.

Hogan, N., & DeSantis, L. (1992). Adolescent sibling bereavement: An ongoing attachment. *Qualitative Health Research, 2,* 159–177.

Jacobson, G., & Ryder, R. G. (1968). Parental loss and some characteristics of the early marriage relationship. *American Journal of Orthopsychiatry, 39,* 779–787.

Maddison, D., & Viola, A. (1968). The health of widows in the year following bereavement. *Journal of Psychoanalytic Research, 12,* 297–306.

Meshot, C. M., & Leitner, L. M. (1994). Death threat, parental loss, and interpersonal style: A personal construct investigation. In R. A. Neymeyer (Ed.), *Death anxiety handbook* (pp. 181–191). Washington, DC: Taylor & Francis.

Murphy, P. (1991). Parental divorce in childhood and loneliness in young adults. *Omega, 23,* 25–35.

Owen, G., Fulton, R., & Markusen, E. (1982). Death at a distance: A study of family survivors. *Omega, 13,* 191–225.

Parkes, C. M., & Weiss, R. S. (1983). *Recovery from bereavement.* New York: Basic Books.

Raphael, B., & Nunn, K. (1988). Counseling the bereaved. *Journal of Social Issues, 44,* 191–206.

Rando, T. A. (1992). The increased prevalence of complicated mourning: The onslaught is just beginning. *Omega, 26,* 43–60.

Roberto, K. A., & Stanis, P. I. (1994). Reactions of older women to the death of their close friends. *Omega, 29,* 17–28.

Rosenblatt, P., & Meyer, M. (1986). Imagined interactions and the family. *Family Relations, 35,* 319–324.

Rubin, S. S. (1991). Adult child loss and the two-track model of bereavement. *Omega, 24,* 183–202.

Sable, P. (1989). Attachment, anxiety, and loss of a husband. *American Journal of Orthopsychiatry, 59,* 550–556.

Scharlach, A. E. (1991). Factors associated with filial grief following the death of an elderly parent. *American Journal of Orthopsychiatry, 61,* 307–313.

Scharlach, A. E., & Fredriksen, K. I. (1993). Reactions to the death of a parent during midlife. *Omega, 27,* 307–320.

Shuchter, S. R., & Zisook, S. (1993). The course of normal grief. In M. S. Stroebe, W. Stroebe, & R. O. Hansson (Eds.), *Handbook of bereavement* (pp. 23–43). The impact of parental death on college-age women. *Psychiatric Clinics of North America, 10,* 387–404.

Silverman, P. R. (1987). The impact of parental death on college-age women. *Psychiatric Clinics of North America, 10,* 387–404.

Silverman, P. R., Nickman, S., & Worden, J. W. (1992). Detachment revisited: The child's reconstruction of a dead parent. *American Journal of Orthopsychiatry, 62,* 494–503.

Silverman, P. R., & Worden, J. W. (1993). Children's reaction to the death of a parent. In M. S. Stroebe, W. Stroebe, and R. O. Hansson (Eds.), *Handbook of bereavement* (pp. 300–316). New York: Cambridge University Press.

Stoll, M. (1993). Predictors of middle aged widows' psychological adjustment. In K. Pottharst (Ed.), *Research explorations in adult attachment* (pp. 219–255). New York: Peter Lang.

Stroebe, M. S., Gergen, M. M., Gergen, K. J., & Stroebe, W. (1992). Broken hearts or broken bonds. *American Psychologist, 47,* 1205–1212.

Stroebe, M. S., & Stroebe, W. (1991). Does "grief work" work? *Journal of Consulting and Clinical Psychology, 59,* 57–65.

Stroebe, M. S., & Stroebe, W. (1993). Determinants of adjustment to bereavement in younger widows and widowers. In M. S. Stroebe, W. Stroebe, & R. O. Hansson (Eds.), *Handbook of bereavement* (pp. 208–226). New York: Cambridge University Press.

Taylor, D. A. (1983). Views of death from sufferers of early loss. *Omega, 14,* 77–82.

Weiss, R. S. (1982). Attachment in adult life. In C. W. Parkes & J. Stevenson-Hinde (Eds.), *The place of attachment in human social behavior* (pp. 98–120). New York: Basic Books.

Weiss, R. S. (1993). Loss and recovery. In M. S. Stroebe, W. Stroebe, & R. O. Hansson (Eds.), *Handbook of bereavement* (pp. 271–284). New York: Cambridge University Press.

Zall, D. S. (1994). The long-term effects of childhood bereavement: Impact on roles as mothers. *Omega, 29,* 219–230.

PART IV

Stress, Health, and Psychological Well-Being

CHAPTER 16

The Role of Coping in the Emotions and How Coping Changes over the Life Course

Richard S. Lazarus
University of California, Berkeley
Berkeley, California

I. INTRODUCTION

When the extraordinary proliferation of interest in the emotions began to unfold in the 1980s, a new research literature emerged. This literature cut across fields, which included psychology, anthropology, sociology, and physiology. It was, to a large extent, powered by an outlook that emphasized cognitive mediation and centered on the concept of appraisal.

This outlook flowered in the field of psychological stress (Lazarus, 1966), and for the most part was later incorporated into the allied field of emotion (see Lazarus, 1991; and Ekman & Davidson, 1994, for a variety of versions of cognitive mediation). Although psychological stress could fruitfully be considered a subset of the concept of emotion (Lazarus, 1993a), the two literatures—one centered on stress, the other on emotion—have tended to remain separate.

Coping became an integral feature of stress theory in the 1960s and 1970s (Coelho, Hamburg, & Adams, 1974). It was apparent that the important issue was the way stress was managed rather than stress arousal, per se. Not only could stress be ameliorated by effective coping, but ineffective coping exacerbated stress with its potentially damaging consequences.

Ego psychology favored the idea that defenses were characterological—that is, traits or styles employed by the person when threatened. In contrast, my work with Folkman (Lazarus & Folkman, 1984) emphasized a process view of defense and, more broadly speaking, of coping. We defined coping as "constantly changing cognitive and behavioral efforts to manage specific external and/or internal demands that are appraised as taxing or exceeding the resources of the person" (p. 141).

More recently (Lazarus, 1993b), I qualified this position by observing that coping involved both style and process. The two approaches ask different but valid questions, process focusing on changes in coping over time and across transactions, style focusing on consistency in the person's coping strategies.

Coping must be regarded as an integral part of emotion when viewed as playing an essential role in adaptation, because it involves thinking, acting, and action tendencies or impulses. Emotions cannot be adequately understood without paying close attention to the coping process. The separation of the literatures of stress and emotion has contributed to a tendency to underemphasize coping as an essential feature of emotion.

This chapter is divided into two main parts. The first deals with the coping process itself, its importance in our emotional lives, and the misunderstandings that have plagued the theory and measurement of coping. This sets the stage for the second part, which deals with adult development and aging.

II. THE COPING PROCESS

There are three common misunderstandings about the coping process: (a) the tendency to treat the functions of coping as if they were distinctive types of action; (b) the tendency in measurement to divorce the coping process from the person who is doing the coping; and (c) the tendency to separate coping from the emotion process.

A. Treating Coping Functions as If They Were Distinctive Action Types

Coping serves a number of functions in human adaptation and the emotional life (Lazarus & Folkman, 1984, 1987; Folkman & Lazarus, 1988a). During the heyday of the Berkeley Stress and Coping Project, we singled out two functions as especially important. The first is to manage harms, threats, and challenges to a person's integrity in any transaction in which that person has a stake by trying to change the situation for the better. Stake refers to general goals and situational intentions in which the person is invested.

This function, which we referred to as *problem-focused,* is directed at the conditions of life that arouse stressful emotions. If a person has been harmed, coping is aimed at undoing or repairing the harm, keeping it from being made worse, or preventing it from happening again. If a person has been threatened rather than harmed, coping is focused on preventing the harm that might ensue. And when challenged, a person tries to do whatever is needed to actualize the goals being challenged by efforts to overcome obstacles.

The second function of coping is to manage the emotional reaction to a harm or threat by transforming it—that is, changing the meaning of the transaction—or by regulating its expression. We called this *emotion-focused coping* because the coping actions (which also include coping thoughts) are directed at the emotions themselves rather than the troubled person–environment relationship that aroused them. This function is favored by the coper in situations appraised as refractory to change.

Transforming or regulating our emotions is required, in part, because the emotion, and the information it provides about oneself, may be threatening. It may also seriously interfere with the ongoing behavioral requirements of a transaction, as when anxiety interferes with constructive thinking. And when an emotion, such as anger and its associated aggression, is displayed toward a loved one or a powerful other, it can damage social relationships that are important to the person.

I should say a word in passing about positive emotions, which I have not emphasized here. Some years ago, my colleagues and I (Lazarus, Kanner, & Folkman, 1980) suggested that coping is relevant even in positive circumstances, which can still be touchy, as when one's happiness could distress others, or when pride is overweening and could be resented. In addition, there is always the likelihood that the positive situation will not last. Therefore, coping in positive situations has the function of preventing the negative as well as sustaining the positive.

But to return to the coping functions, the distinction between problem- and emotion-focused coping has been widely endorsed and used in stress research, and to a lesser extent, in research on emotion. The coping thoughts and actions people reported in our research using the Ways of Coping Interview/Questionnaire (Folkman & Lazarus, 1988b) were analyzed into eight factors. Some of them, such as confrontive coping and planful problem solving, appeared, at least on the surface, to represent the problem-focused function, whereas others, such as distancing, escape-avoidance, and positive reappraisal, appeared to represent the emotion-focused function.

The expression, "on the surface" in the above sentence indicates a problem with what has become a standard view of the coping process. Distinguishing between the two functions, but treating them as if they were distinctive types of coping actions, has led to an oversimple conception of the way coping works and is measured in much research, including our own.

My own writings on the subject have sometimes inadvertently contributed to this problem by allowing the concept of functions to slip into the language of action types. It is difficult to talk about the two functions without speaking as though they were distinctive actions. When one researches coping, the task of measurement encourages the researcher to make an action typology to distinguish problem-focused from emotion-focused action. But functions do not refer clearly or consistently to actions; any action can have more than one function. And if one does not know the full context of coping, including what the person is trying to accomplish, the classification is often specious.

Consider, for example, the person who suffers from debilitating performance anxiety and faces an important upcoming presentation to a professional audience. In such a situation, the anxiety may become so severe that the person is unable to think clearly and experiences tremulousness and a dry mouth, two common symptoms of anxiety. The audience perceives the speaker's distress, reacts coldly or with its own distress, creating a downward spiral in which the speaker views what is happening as a personal failure. The performance may be seriously impaired and the performer feels helpless to reverse the debacle.

To cope with the debilitating anxiety, which can often be anticipated in advance, this person might take a Valium or a beta blocker, which helps to reduce the anxiety and its physical symptoms and thereby saves the day. Should we regard this coping action, and the anticipatory thoughts that underlie it, as emotion-focused or problem-focused? The answer is that it is clearly both. On the one hand, the drug is used to reduce the emotional distress—and so it is emotion-focused, but the user's intention is also to make possible an adequate performance, and so it is also problem-focused.

By the same token, should we consider escape-avoidance, which is one of the eight factors of the Ways of Coping Questionnaire, to be emotion-focused or problem-focused? When the person is seeking to avoid or escape a damaging situation, the action might be regarded as problem-focused. But it also serves to control the emotional distress of anxiety, fear, guilt, or shame, so the action might also be considered emotion-focused. The bottom line of this argument is that *any* thought or action can serve either problem- or emotion-focused functions, and frequently both.

Although it is useful to know which function is being emphasized in a given transaction, and to keep both in mind, it makes little sense to pit one against the other, especially when we have not examined the context of the transaction in enough depth to be sure. The two functions are interdependent. They work together as part of a total pattern in which a person struggles to manage a troubled person–environment relationship as well as the emotion itself. It is their relative balance and integration that contributes to overall coping efficacy.

When the two functions are contrasted, there is a common bias in the way psychologists think about them. Problem-focused coping is widely favored by psychologists as more efficacious or healthy, whereas emotion-focused coping is often viewed as a form of defense—tantamount to self-deception and pathology. Although this is not an accurate reading of what my colleagues and I meant by emotion-focused coping, changing a troubled relationship is valued in our society more than self-deception.

Most evidence points to an important role for emotion-focused coping in all stressful life situations. There is also insufficient recognition that people need to draw on both functions, emotion-focused as well as problem-focused. A number of research studies can be cited on this point, but I mention one here—namely, that of Collins, Baum, and Singer (1983). Its findings support the idea that in situations that cannot be changed, persistent problem-solving efforts may be counterproductive and lead to chronic distress and dysfunction.

Even in encounters in which people are all but powerless to overcome egregious circumstances, such as life-threatening or terminal diseases, there is usually a mix of problem-focused efforts to do something to change the situation for the better and emotion-focused efforts to sustain morale and feel better about what is happening.

Efforts to sustain positive emotions often provide a basis for trying to improve a situation despite the pain and suffering such efforts require. Without the conviction or hope that can come from emotion-focused coping, problem-solving efforts to ameliorate the negative conditions— even if only slightly—will not be undertaken or sustained, and despair and depression are apt to be their emotional legacy. An example is debilitating arthritis, which can, in the main, be only endured, but for which painful activity or the use of drugs to reduce the pain and remain active are valuable.

It is futile and misleading to ask which is more efficacious or psychologically healthy, problem-focused or emotion-focused coping. They are both part of the total coping effort, and each facilitates the other. However seductive it may be to do so, coping should never be thought of in either-or terms, but as a complex of actions aimed at improving the relationship with the environment and regulating or transforming the emotions experienced by reappraising their meaning.

Why are so many different coping actions endorsed by people on the Ways of Coping Questionnaire? I do not know for sure. To know the answer, one would have to examine the sequence of coping actions over time and to try to link each to a particular source of stress. One possibility is that people try things out. When an action fails to help, they shift to some other strategy in a search for the best way to deal with what is happening. In effect, coping involves a flux of many strategies, all functionally related to one another, to the changing circumstances, and to the general goals and situational intentions of the person who is coping.

Consider a man who has just learned he has prostate cancer. Shocked by the unexpected news, he struggles to grasp what is involved and what might be done, fighting off counterproductive ruminations, obtaining information, seeing several doctors, trying to decide whether to accept surgery or wait and see. He may seem to others to be highly controlled, even cheerful, though, even without realizing it, he has mobilized to deal with the problem in an effort to stay in control of his emotional state. His mood may rise and fall without seeming provocation, depending on whether he accepts what has happened, resents it, or is frightened by it. This is a complex, time-bound pattern of coping, which is not well described by a list of separate actions. The whole person is engaged in the struggle, which brings us to the second misunderstanding.

I suggest that the two functions of coping are never really separated. In much of our empirical research on coping (reviewed in Lazarus and Folkman, 1984, 1987, and Lazarus, 1991), people reported using a wide variety of coping thoughts and actions in all major stressful situations. Nearly all the eight coping factors were drawn upon by our subjects in each stressful transaction. It is only for analytic convenience that specific actions can be separated from the total coping configuration.

B. Divorcing Coping from the Person Who Is Doing the Coping

As valuable as they might be for certain types of research, factorial questionnaires that address a given context of stress run the risk of isolating coping from other life struggles to adapt. Not only will they produce an unrepresentative sample of how that person copes, but even more important, they may lead to a failure to appreciate what is the most and least important threat to that person. I recently suggested (Lazarus, 1993b) that more than one personal meaning can be generated in a complex stressful transaction, and if we are to understand the choice of coping strategy, it is necessary to identify their relative importance.

In the Ways of Coping Questionnaire, and any other comparable procedures for scaling coping strategies, coping tends to get divorced from the personal goals and belief systems that make us all distinctive individuals. In the early stages of theory development and research measurement, it was useful to develop a factorial method for studying the process of coping in particular stressful contexts, as the Berkeley Stress and Coping Project did in the 1980s. However, if coping measurement remains disembodied from the heart of the individual's life and personality, advances in our knowledge of the process could be retarded because our understanding would be too superficial. Unfortunately, because such scales are so easy to use, they have tended to become a false gold standard of coping measurement in much current research.

I (Lazarus, 1993b) cited two research programs that illustrate the need to sort out the personal meanings lying behind the psychological surface of a stressful transaction. In research reported by Folkman and Chesney (1994) on the coping processes employed by the caregivers of partners dying of AIDS, it was not environmental demands that made the experience so terrible, but rather, the existential significance of what was happening. The main sources of threat, identified by means of repeated, in-depth interviews, were twofold: first, coming to terms with the loved one's imminent loss, and second, recognizing one's own terrifying future as a consequence of having the HIV virus or being at risk to get it.

For the caregiver what was likely to happen was far more threatening than the enervating and often disgusting tasks of caring daily for the deteriorating partner. To the contrary, these onerous tasks were often emblematic of positive meanings, such as helping the suffering partner, expressing a loving commitment to him or her, and being able to exercise some control over an otherwise chaotic situation.

And in research reported by Laux and Weber (1991), the coping strategies used by individual partners in marital conflicts depended on the personal meanings attributed to what was happening. If, during an intense argument, one partner feared the breakup of the relationship, the expression of the anger by that partner was apt to be inhibited; the coping intent was to preserve the relationship. But if a partner experienced what happened in the argument as a deep wound to the ego, anger at the offending spouse was likely to be escalated and expressed harshly; the coping intent was to repair the wound, even if it was at the expense of the relationship.

In both these studies, the key to the choice of coping strategy was the situational intent that emerged from the personal meaning of the transaction. Meaning cannot usually be identified normatively—each partner may derive different meanings and generate different coping intentions—but it can only be known by exploring in depth the individual's goals, belief systems, and appraisals. Coping questionnaires, which are not usually designed to reveal the meanings underlying coping choices, cannot, therefore, provide the ideal methodology.

This point has also been expressed in a searching series of articles by Labouvie-Vief and her colleagues (Labouvie-Vief, DeVoe, & Bulka, 1989; Labouvie-Vief, Hakim-Larson, DeVoe, & Schoeberlein, 1989; Labouvie-Vief, Hakim-Larson, & Hobart, 1987), who suggested that the most important changes in coping may not be readily identified by questionnaires. Even when research participants endorsed similar coping actions, the motives underlying what they think and do still differed sharply as a function of age. These researchers suggest, wisely, I believe, that careful, in-depth interviews would provide a better understanding of individual and group differences in coping and what motivates them than relatively superficial questionnaires.

To speak more programmatically about the bases of coping choices, the personal meanings that underlie coping depend on two major factors, the immediate situation being faced by the person and the background.

The situation, as appraised, imposes all sorts of *provocations* to react with emotions, *social pressures* to react in certain ways, *social constraints* on action, and *opportunities* for the attainment of goals. The background includes person variables, such as *goal hierarchies* that define which of several goals are most pressing or important, and individual *views of the self and world*—for example, whether the environment is seen as benign and supportive or hostile and dangerous, and whether the self is adequate or inadequate to deal with that world.

These person variables arise, in part, from distinctive and embodied life experiences and, in part, from the internalization of cultural meanings and values. If we imbed the coping process in this larger arena of situational and background factors, we will understand it far better than if we look at isolated actions, and even patterns of action.

What I said previously about situational and background factors in coping has major implications for the study of how coping changes throughout life. Coping development and change are not merely about a set of skills or outlooks acquired and altered. Skills and outlooks are always in the service of goals and beliefs which, in turn, arise from life experiences, biological endowments, cultural values, and situational contingencies, aspects often ignored in theory and research.

C. Separating Coping from the Emotion Process

Most psychologists think of an emotion as one event or process, and coping as another, both separate but presumably connected by learning. This stems from the long tradition in psychology of separating stimulus and response, afferent and efferent, and perception and action. This is a consequence of the penchant of science to analyze everything into basic elements and to ignore the need to resynthesize the elements into a living system. The tradition was especially strong in the early decades of this century when academic psychology was centered heavily on conditioning. Learning psychologists spoke of separate drive stimuli and learned responses or habits, which is what connected them.

An alternative epistemology, transactionalism, as outlined by Dewey (1896) and Dewey and Bentley (1949/1989), recognizes that input and output are inherently connected. Perceptions always imply actions. More abstractly stated, stimuli cannot be dissociated from the responses that have been connected to them by nature and/or by nurture. This position has also been effectively argued by Gallistel (1985), von Hofsten (1985), Neisser (1985), and others, all in a volume dealing with goal-directed behavior—but not taken to heart by many psychologists.

As Dewey and Bentley pointed out, living cells, in vivo not in vitro, take on special characteristics when they are organized into organs. The cellular characteristics then derive from the structure and functions of the organ and are different from cells lying unconnected in a petri dish. To reduce a bit of tissue to a mere collection of cells without taking into account the operating context—that is, the organ in which they function— is to make a fundamental mistake about the nature of cells in larger biological units.

Those who draw on the concept of affordances (Baron & Boudreau, 1987; Gibson, 1966) also view mind in more synthetic terms. They speak of the perception of objects as infused with their functional significance. Depending on the species and specific context, an apple is something to eat, to throw and catch, to juggle, to use in striking another person aggressively, and so forth. The object cannot be divorced from its significance for the organism confronting it.

By the same token, coping is an integral part of the emotion process. When people react to their circumstances with, say, anger, shame, or anxiety, the defining secondary appraisal already contains the options for coping, whether acted on or not. Once an appraisal resulting in anger has occurred, the impulse to attack is also present, ready to be expressed. The impulse to act is part of the emotion. We can separate aspects of the emotion for analytic convenience, but the intimate connection between coping and emotion makes it a distortion to treat them as separate events.

Coping actions can also emerge slowly and deliberately, even planfully, and these may counter the impulse to action that is a part of the emotion process. One may see an apple as something to bite, but if it is for sale on the shelf of a store, we do not act on the impulse. And one may have the impulse to lash out in anger to retaliate for a slight, but this impulse, too, which is part of the anger, may never be acted on.

The point to bear in mind is that the emotion process, which is responsive to feedback from the environment, involves coping at every stage of its unfolding: at the initial determination of the emotion experienced, and at the response end of the process of whether and how it is to be expressed. Deliberate control can be exercised by inhibiting or shaping actions; or one can transform the meaning of transactions, and with it the emotion that is experienced. We must abandon the bad habit of thinking of an emotion as an event that leads to a coping response, and instead recognize that the emotion process includes coping.

Therefore, in addition to analyzing an emotion into its component elements, we need to reorganize these elements conceptually into a living whole. The personal significance of what is happening constitutes a higher level of abstraction than the component elements. I have used the concept of *core relational theme* to identify this meaning (Lazarus, 1991), which varies predictably with each emotion. Coping contributes to it importantly by indicating what can and cannot be done and, therefore, whether the emotion will be, say, anger and attack, anxiety (fear) and avoidance or flight, guilt and its impulse to atone, or shame and the tendency to hide, and so on for each of the emotions.

III. ISSUES OF COPING
AND EMOTIONAL DEVELOPMENT

Aldwin (1994) has already published a competent and up-to-date review of research on how coping changes over the life span, and there is no need to duplicate her substantial scholarship here. Instead, my objective is to examine the serviceability of a number of hypotheses about coping development in adulthood and aging. My central thesis is that there is a conflict between broad—mostly too broad—normative concepts about how coping changes as a function of age, and individual differences in the dynamics of coping. I believe that our penchant for simplifying generalizations should be abandoned in favor of a more complex, mutivariate approach, focused on the patterns of individual variation.

How have scholars and researchers tackled the question of coping change? Some have done cross-sectional studies on different age groups, whereas others have done longitudinal studies, which are necessary if one is to avoid the danger of finding merely cohort effects. Other researchers, influenced heavily by psychoanalytic ego psychology, have looked only at ego defenses using projective tests or in-depth interviews. And still others have drawn on standardized coping questionnaires, which focus on specific stresses and are used to compare different age groups.

The effect of this diversity of focus and method has been to create a body of work that is difficult to interpret because it provides only weak, often inconsistent normative trends, which are commonly overstated. Many of the findings have not been replicated. They manage to reach statistical significance—a properly criticized methodological shibboleth if there ever was one—but the huge individual variations that are always present have, in the main, been ignored.

Leaving aside the details, three main themes in research on coping in later life can be identified. Two of them are developmental or stage-related. The first sets up hypotheses about how *people in general* change in the ways they cope with problems of living from early adulthood to old age. The second is a complication on the first and suggests that *men and women* follow different trajectories over the life course—in effect, there is an interaction between age or stage of life and gender. The third is contextual in outlook—in effect, when coping changes, it is the result of changes in the demands, constraints, and opportunities available as the person ages. These have to do with social changes and losses in personal resources and roles, which force new forms of adaptation on the older person.

A. Stage-Related Themes

Early on, Jung (1933) speculated about normative transitions in coping—or more accurately, in the self, which he interpreted developmentally. Young people were described as energetic, impulsive, and passionate, focused on constructing a vocation, marrying, having a family, and establishing themselves in the community. In the late thirties and forties, youthful concerns are replaced by cultural and civic interests, and in middle age the self becomes more introverted, less impulsive, and more philosophical, spiritual, and wise.

Based on data from stories told about Thematic Apperception Test pictures, Guttmann (1974) suggested that young adults used a style of coping characterized by "active mastery," by which he meant confronting and solving problems. In middle age, subjects cope by means of "passive mastery," which means accepting one's problems without struggle. When old, they employ "magical mastery"; in effect, their conflicts magically resolve themselves, a process presumably akin to wishful thinking.

In a longitudinal study that followed Harvard men for 30 years, Vaillant (1977) made use of in-depth interviews and focused on patterns of ego defense. His analysis of the data was that as people grew older their defenses matured, shifting from immature ones, such as intellectualization, repression, reaction formation, and displacement to mature ones, such as sublimation, altruism, anticipation, and humor. Vaillant also suggested that mature defenses were associated with more effective functioning.

There have also been a number of cross-sectional studies of coping as measured by questionnaires, such as the Ways of Coping, and the use of in-depth interviews. Some of these have emphasized stages of development, whereas others adopted a more contextual view. Representative examples include studies by Aldwin, 1991; Aldwin & Revenson, 1985; Felton & Revenson, 1987; Folkman, Lazarus, Pimley, & Novacek, 1987; Irion & Blanchard-Fields, 1987; Labouvie-Vief, DeVoe, & Bulka, 1989; Labouvie-Vief, Hakim-Larson, DeVoe, & Schoeberlein, 1989; Labouvie-Vief et al., 1987; McCrae, 1982, 1989; and others cited by Aldwin, 1994.

B. *Different Trajectories for Men and Women*

A recent theme in stage approaches to aging is that men and women show different coping patterns as they age. In early adulthood, women have been described as nurturing, accepting, and loving, having subordinated any hostile and aggressive tendencies to the softer role of wife and mother. However, in later life such women become more aggressive and dominant. Men, on the other hand, show the reverse pattern, beginning adult life aggressively and competitively, but giving up this pattern later and becoming more passive and mild (see, for example, Haan, Milsap, & Hartka, 1986; Helson & Wink, 1987; and Lowenthal, Thurnher, & Chiribogo, 1975).

A problem with this theme is that it reflects the way men and women are socialized in most cultures and recent changes in these patterns in modern societies, rather than signifying inherent developmental stages. Clearly, the ideals of how men and women should behave and feel have been changing in the Western world, and even in less developed societies as a result of worldwide media influences.

One should be wary about generalizing about men and women, and humankind. What is observed is time- and culture-bound, and it is difficult to know to what extent the trends reflect biological universals, what is learned from the societal context, or both. We see here a failure to pay much attention to the huge individual differences that are always found and probably account for the largest proportion of the variance.

In my opinion, the stage approach is not truly developmental because the coping changes over the adult life course are based on changing social, physical, and psychological demands, constraints, and resources. To me, the most reasonable and useful way to see the problem is to consider, as I do below, the changing context of living rather than to assume a built-in, orthogenetic process.

C. *The Influence of the Changing Life Context on Coping*

Research by my colleagues and me in the 1980s (e.g., Folkman, Lazarus, Pimley, & Novacek, 1987; see also McCrae, 1982; and Folkman & Lazarus, 1980) found extensive normative differences in the *sources of stress* experienced by younger adults between the ages of 35 and 45 and older adults between the ages of 65 and 74. The younger sample consisted mostly of working parents with young children who were still living at home. The older sample was largely retired and their children had grown up and lived independently.

Their daily hassles differed too. For the younger sample, their hassles were found predominantly in certain life domains, such as financial problems, work, taking care of the household, and dealing with personal problems, family, and friends. The hassles of the older sample had to do much less with work and child rearing and much more with health issues and the lack of ability to carry out the maintenance tasks of living as easily as before.

The younger sample, not surprisingly, also appraised their encounters as more changeable than did the older sample. They felt a greater sense of control over their circumstances, which was reflected in comparable differences in the emphasis on problem- or emotion-focused strategies. The coping patterns of both groups reflected their circumstances of life and were closely related to the sources of stress experienced and the way they were appraised.

In our data, gender did not make much of a difference in coping, and any such difference was interpretable in terms of differences in the sources of stress. For example, if the stresses were work related, working women used problem-focused coping strategies as extensively as men, but if the stresses were about family well-being, female homemakers emphasized emotion-focused coping more than men. If the roles were reversed, one should expect the sources of stress to reverse, too, along with their coping patterns.

We also found that the younger sample used more active, inter-personal problem-focused forms of coping (confrontive, seeking social support, and planful problem solving) more than the older sample, as measured as a proportion of the total coping pattern. In contrast, the older sample used more passive, intrapersonal emotion-focused coping (distancing, acceptance of responsibility, and positive reappraisal) than the younger sample. This seems to overlap with McCrae's (1982) data and, if we interpret our findings metaphorically, is reminiscent of some of what Jung, Guttmann, and Vaillant suggested. However, given the possi-bilities of cohort effects, we could not prove that these changes were truly developmental.

It seems to me that most differences in the coping process in aging can be most simply explained by what younger and older adults have to cope with. As people age, more and more of them develop health prob-lems that sap their energy and time, generate pain, and increasingly limit what they can do. It takes longer to manage their daily hygiene and other routine tasks of living. Older people are also more likely to suffer loss of loved ones. As they reach their seventies and beyond, the odds of heart and circulatory problems also rise, along with the emergence of cancers that require surgery or other debilitating treatments. With retirement, they also experience the loss of occupational and social roles that have long defined who they are and how they live, which to some extent re-moves them from competitive struggles and requires substitute activities to overcome boredom and provide social contact.

Why would these changes in the sources of stress, and the coping processes directed at them, be thought of as developmental? It is true that the odds of such changes taking place increase with age. But they are re-ally not predictable; they occur at different ages and different ways in dif-ferent people, and are coped with in different ways. I am not convinced of the utility of thinking of these changes as mandated by life stage. It is not age, per se, that should be considered causal here, but the correlates of age—such as loss of health—which require alterations in the pattern of adaptation.

The same could be said about Vaillant's and Guttmann's observations, Jung's speculations, and observations of different trajectories for men and women. Older men retire and then experience different threats to defend against. Older women pass off their maternal care problems, are more free to actualize themselves, and so their sources of stress change. To cope with these changes, values and goals may have to be changed, too. Since there is such variety in the losses of aging and their timing, and in the coping process for dealing with them, a developmental stage conception is hardly the best way to understand what is going on.

In my discussion thus far, the picture of aging seems a bit too negative, and for many older persons there is much that could be viewed in more positive terms. Older people make much of a sardonic joke[1] that expresses a great deal about being a survivor; when someone complains about health problems, the listener, who has his or her own problems, enjoins them to consider the chilling alternative.

Aldwin (1994) ended her discussion of coping in aging with observations made by Johnson and Barer (1993), which provide chapter and verse to Baltes's (1987) encouraging thesis that successful aging involves the acquisition of strategies to compensate for inevitable social, physical, and psychological decay. Old people who can afford it are often able to organize their environments to maximize their capacities to remain involved in life—for example, by the use of safety bars in the bathtub area to minimize the danger of serious injury, use of walkers and canes to increase their mobility, choosing to live in communities with buses that can take them shopping, and limiting their driving to relatively safe areas within a community of older persons.

I remember a moving article, written by the distinguished psychologist B. F. Skinner (1983), by then quite old, in which he spoke of the many ways he compensated for memory losses. For example, on days it might rain, he said, he would hang an umbrella on the doorknob at the moment the thought occurred to him so as not to forget to take it with him when he went out. I suppose I was moved because I recognized that my wife and I, both aging, were increasingly doing the things he wrote about to maintain control over our lives and to sustain commitments of importance. In this article, Skinner also took the position I have in this chapter, that changes incident to aging should not be regarded developmentally.

---

[1] Two other amusing jokes are told by the elderly, most of whom can neither see, hear, or remember as they once did.

In one, a husband and his wife have been arguing about which one of them is most hard of hearing. He insists that his wife is, so without telling her, he puts her to the test. Standing fifteen feet from the kitchen while she is making dinner, he yells at the top of his voice, "What's for dinner?" There is no answer. Then he moves ten feet away and again yells, "What's for dinner?" Still no answer. On the third try, five feet from the kitchen he yells the same question. Now the answer comes back, "For God's sake, I'm telling you for the third time, Steak and potatoes."

In the second joke, two old men are on the golf course and one is about to drive the ball from the tee. He says to his partner, "I don't see so well, so please watch where the ball falls." After he hits the ball he asks his partner, "Did you see where it went? Where did it go?" The partner says ingenuously, "Yes, I did see it, but I can't for the life of me remember where it is."

IV. CONCLUSIONS

When all is said and done, the contextual argument I have emphasized above suggests that, although there are probably some common trends, we need to take a far more individualized and concrete approach to changes in coping as people age than has typically been the case. People age at different rates and have different physical and mental problems. Once they accept the reality of their situations, they deal with them as best they can, often in constructive and distinctive ways.

We must get away from emphasizing only broad common trends, from which we then make sweeping generalizations, most of which do not greatly advance our understanding. It would be more valuable instead to describe the rich variety of ways older people cope with their lot in life. If we carefully described coping as it occurs in each person we study from the standpoint of what is being coped with, and the meanings—including existential ones—inherent in what is being faced—we would be better able to find proximal causes of coping strategies and the principles underlying them.

In my view, the inescapable conclusion to draw is that our main research task is to identify the various forms of coping necessitated by changes in the conditions of life. We may find some of these to be widely shared because, if we are lucky, we all age, suffer losses, and die. We should get over the bad habit of promoting small differences into simplifying generalizations about people in general, the old, the young, or about men and women, or whomever. These generalizations stereotype large segments of the population, and give us little help in understanding the details of how coping changes over the life course.

REFERENCES

Aldwin, C. M. (1991). Does age affect the stress and coping process? Implications of age differences in perceived control. *Journal of Gerontology, 46,* 174–180.

Aldwin, C. M. (1994). *Stress, coping, and development: An integrative perspective.* New York: Guilford.

Aldwin, C. M., & Revenson, T. A. (1987). Does coping help? A reexamination of the relationship between coping and mental health. *Journal of Personality and Social Psychology, 53,* 337–348.

Baltes, P. B. (1987). Theoretical propositions of life-span developmental psychology: On the dynamics between growth and decline. *Developmental Psychology, 24,* 611-626.

Baron, R. M., & Boudreau, L. A. (1987). An ecological perspective on integrating personality and social psychology. *Journal of Personality and Social Psychology, 53,* 1222–1228.

Coelho, G. V., Hamburg, D. A., & Adams, J. F. (Eds.). (1974). *Coping and adaptation*. New York: Basic Books.

Collins, D. L., Baum, A., & Singer, J. E. (1983). Coping with chronic stress at Three Mile Island. *Health Psychology, 2,* 149–166.

Dewey, J. (1896). The reflex arc concept in psychology. *Psychological Review, 3,* 357–370.

Dewey, J., & Bentley, A. F. (1989). Knowing and the known. In J. A. Boydston (Ed.), *The later works of John Dewey, 1925–1953* (Vol. 16, pp. 96–130). Carbondale: Southern Illinois University Press. (Original work published in 1949)

Ekman, P., & Davidson, R. J. (1994). (Eds.) *The nature of emotion: Fundamental questions.* New York: Oxford University Press.

Felton, B. J., & Revenson, T. A. (1987). Age differences in coping with chronic illness. *Psychology and Aging, 2,* 164–170.

Folkman, S., & Chesney, M. A. (1994). Stress and coping in caregiving partners of men with AIDS. *Psychiatric Clinics in North America, 17,* 35–53.

Folkman, S., & Lazarus, R. S. (1980). An analysis of coping in a middle-aged community sample. *Journal of Health and Social Behavior, 21,* 219–239.

Folkman, S., & Lazarus, R. S. (1988a). The relationship between coping and emotion: Implications for theory and research. *Social Science and Medicine, 26,* 309–317.

Folkman, S., & Lazarus, R. S. (1988b). *Manual for the Ways of Coping Questionnaire.* Palo Alto, CA: Consulting Psychologists Press.

Folkman, S., Lazarus, R. S., Pimley, S., & Novacek, J. (1987). Age differences in stress and coping processes. *Psychology and Aging, 2,* 171-184.

Gallistel, C. R. (1985). Motivation, intention, and emotion: Goal directed behavior from a cognitive-neuroethological perspective. In M. Frese & J. Sabini (Eds.), *Goal directed behavior: The concept of action in psychology* (pp. 48–65). Hillsdale, NJ: Erlbaum.

Gibson, J. J. (1966). *The senses considered as perceptual systems.* Boston: Houghton Mifflin.

Guttmann, D. L. (1974). The country of old men: Cross-cultural studies in the psychology of later life. In R. I. LeVine (Ed.), *Culture and personality: Contemporary readings* (pp. 95–121). Chicago: Aldine.

Haan, N., Millsap, R., & Hartka, E. (1986). As time goes by: Change and stability in personality over fifty years. *Psychology and Aging, 1,* 220–232.

Helson, R., & Wink, P. (1987). Two conceptions of maturity examined in the findings of a longitudinal study. *Journal of Personality and Social Psychology, 53,* 531–541.

Irion, J. C., & Blanchard-Fields, F. (1987). A cross-sectional comparison of adaptive coping in adulthood. *Journal of Gerontology, 42,* 502–504.

Johnson, C. I., & Barer, B. M. (1993). Coping and a sense of control among the oldest old. *Journal of Aging Studies, 7,* 67–80.

Jung, C. G. (1933). *Modern man in search of a soul.* New York: Harcourt, Brace, & World.

Labouvie-Vief, G., DeVoe, M., & Bulka, D. (1989). Speaking about feelings: Conceptions of emotion across the life span. *Psychology and Aging, 4,* 425–437.

Labouvie-Vief, G., Hakim-Larson, J., DeVoe, M., & Schoeberlein, S. (1989). Emotions and self-regulation: A life span view. *Human Development, 32,* 279–299.

Labouvie, G., Hakim-Larson, J., Hobart, C. (1987). Age, ego level, and the life-span development of coping and defense processes. *Psychology and Aging, 2,* 286–293.

Laux, L., & Weber, H. (1991). Presentation of self in coping with anger and anxiety: An intentional approach. *Anxiety Research, 3,* 233–255.

Lazarus, R. S. (1966). *Psychological stress and the coping process.* New York: McGraw-Hill.

Lazarus, R. S. (1991). *Emotion and adaptation.* New York: Oxford University Press.

Lazarus, R. S. (1993a). *From psychological stress to the emotions: A history of changing outlooks. Annual Review of Psychology, 1993* (pp. 1–21). Palo Alto, CA: Annual Reviews, Inc.

Lazarus, R. S. (1993b). Coping theory and research: Past, present, and future. *Psychosomatic Medicine, 55,* 234–247.

Lazarus, R. S., & Folkman, S. (1984). *Stress, appraisal, and coping.* New York: Springer.

Lazarus, R. S., & Folkman, S. (1987). Transactional theory and research on emotions and coping. In L. Laux & G. Vossel (Eds.), Personality in biographical stress and coping research. *European Journal of Personality, 1,* 141–169.

Lazarus, R. S., Kanner, A., & Folkman, S. (1980). Emotions: A cognitive-phenomenological analysis. In R. Plutchik & H. Kellerman (Eds.), *Theories of emotion* (pp. 189–217). New York: Academic Press.

Lowenthal, M. F., Thurnher, M., & Chiriboga, D. (1975). *Four stages of life.* San Francisco: Jossey-Bass.

McCrae, R. R. (1982). Age differences in the use of coping mechanisms. *Journal of Gerontology, 37,* 454–460.

McCrae, R. R. (1989). Age differences and changes in the use of coping mechanisms. *Journal of Gerontology: Psychological Sciences, 44,* 161–169.

Neisser, U. (1985). The role of invariant structures in the control of movement. In M. Frese & J. Sabini (Eds.), *Goal directed behavior: The concept of action in psychology* (pp. 97–108). Hillsdale, NJ: Erlbaum.

Pfeiffer, E. (1977). Psychopathology and social pathology. In J. E. Birren & K. W. Schaie (Eds.), *Handbook of the psychology of aging* (pp. 39–58). New York: Van Nostrand Reinhold.

Skinner, B. F. (1983). Intellectual self-management in old age. *American Psychologist, 38,* 239–244.

Vaillant, G. E. (1977). *Adaptation to life.* Boston: Little, Brown.

von Hofsten, C. (1985). Perception and action. In M. Frese & J. Sabini (Eds.), *Goal directed behavior: The concept of action in psychology* (pp. 80–96). Hillsdale, NJ: Erlbaum.

CHAPTER 17

Emotion, Personality, and Health

Joan S. Tucker *and* Howard S. Friedman
Department of Psychology *Department of Psychology*
Brandeis University *University of California, Riverside*
Waltham, Massachusetts *Riverside, California*

I. INTRODUCTION

Can personality and associated emotional response patterns have important, long-term influences on physical health? As researchers continue in their efforts to identify risk factors for disease and premature death, as well as to focus on health promotion and wellness, this question is assuming increasing importance. Although the traditional focus on somatic risk factors such as cholesterol level and blood pressure has been somewhat useful in predicting disease development, these risk factors cannot fully explain why some individuals develop a particular disease and others do not. Furthermore, a focus on these traditional risk factors does not tell us what types of individuals tend to exhibit these risk factors. In an attempt to more fully understand disease development and resistance, efforts have now intensified on identifying psychosocial predictors of physical health, with personality and emotion at the forefront of this effort.

Although serious health problems are often not manifested until mid- to late-adulthood, the seeds of adult health status are planted much earlier. Was the hostile and aggressive middle-aged executive who recently had a heart attack a hostile and aggressive child who developed a maladaptive style of approaching the world? He may not have learned, for example, how to establish and nurture interpersonal relationships or how to cope effectively with stress. His hostile and aggressive disposition may have led to physiological, psychosocial, and behavioral difficulties that eventually contributed to his poor health. Thus, we are turning to the study of personality and emotional response patterns in childhood and early adulthood in an effort to expand our knowledge of how these personal characteristics influence health and longevity across the life span.

This chapter begins by providing an overview of the evidence linking personality and emotional response patterns to physical health. We will then describe behavioral and psychosocial mechanisms through which personality and emotion might have their effects on health. Although most of the past work has been limited to samples of middle-aged adults, we will review some recent research indicating that individuals who are likely to exhibit risk factors for disease and premature mortality can be identified as early as childhood. Lastly, we will provide an overview of our work with the Terman Life-Cycle Study archive, which explores the associations between childhood personality and longevity across the life span, testing specific models of how personality might have its long-term influence on health.

II. PERSONALITY AND EMOTION AS PREDICTORS OF PHYSICAL HEALTH

Hundreds of studies have investigated the associations among personality, emotional response patterns, and physical health. Although this area of research has its modern roots in the psychodynamic literature of the 1940s and 1950s (e.g., Alexander, 1950; Dunbar, 1943), it has received a resurgence of interest in recent years. Among the personality traits and emotional response patterns that have received the most empirical attention in terms of their associations with health and longevity are Type A, hostility, optimism, and neuroticism (including anxiety and depression).

A. Hostility

The strongest and most consistent evidence linking personality and emotional response patterns to physical health comes from studies of hostility and its associated emotional response style (including, but not limited to, anger expression). Interest in the study of hostility and its emotional correlates initially stemmed from research on the Type A Behavior

Pattern (TABP), which found that hostility is the pathogenic component of the TABP. This research also indicated that emotion-based measures of the TABP, such as coding nonverbal behaviors from a structured interview, were more strongly predictive of physical health than paper-and-pencil measures of the construct (Booth-Kewley & Friedman, 1987).

Although anger expression is often thought to be a necessary component of hostility, this is not the case. Hostility is multifaceted, and hostile individuals may or may not exhibit overt anger and aggression. Two main facets of hostility are experiential hostility and expressive hostility (Smith, 1992). Experiential hostility refers to hostile feelings, which may include cynicism, resentment, or suspiciousness. Expressive hostility, in contrast, refers to the more overt aspects of hostility such as assaultiveness or verbal aggressiveness.

The most convincing evidence of the link between hostility and physical health has come from prospective investigations in which hostility, initially assessed in a group of healthy individuals, is used to predict the incidence of disease (usually coronary heart disease) or mortality over a number of years. Both experiential hostility and expressive hostility have been prospectively associated with poorer health, although it is not clear whether these different aspects of hostility affect health through common mechanisms (see Smith, 1992, for a review of this literature). Numerous prospective studies convincingly point to hostility and anger expression as risk factors for death from coronary heart disease (Almada et al., 1991; Dembroski, MacDougall, Costa, & Grandits, 1989; Shekelle, Gale, Ostfeld, & Paul, 1983), although there have also been exceptions (e.g., McCranie, Watkins, Brandsma, & Sisson, 1986). Hostility has also been related to overall mortality risk (Almada et al., 1991; Barefoot, Dahlstrom, & Williams, 1983; Barefoot et al., 1987), as well as deaths from violence (Koskenvuo et al., 1988) and cancer (Shekelle et al., 1983).

B. Optimism

One might think that optimistic individuals would be physically healthier than pessimistic individuals due to their more positive outlook on life and their optimistic expectations for the future. However, the research to date has not been able to establish a firm link between optimism and physical health. The most commonly used measure of optimism is the Life Orientation Test (LOT; Scheier & Carver, 1985). Individuals scoring higher on the LOT tend to report fewer symptoms (Scheier & Carver, 1985) and enjoy quicker and better recovery after surgery (Chamberlain, Petrie, & Azariah, 1992; Scheier et al., 1989). The LOT is also correlated with the use of more adaptive coping strategies and with greater psychological well-being, both of which may enhance an individual's short-term ability to deal effectively with health problems or physical limitations (see Scheier & Carver, 1993, for a review of this literature). However, there is little evidence that the LOT predicts disease incidence or mortality risk. Only a few studies to date have investigated the association between aspects of optimism and mortality risk. One such study, focusing on sense of humor, failed to find such a relation (Rotton, 1992). Our own work, discussed below, indicates that children who were rated by their parents and teachers as being cheerful and having a sense of humor were at *higher* mortality risk across the life span than their less optimistic peers (Friedman et al., 1993; Martin et al., 1995). The discrepancy between our results and those that come from studies using the LOT may be due to several factors. It may be that our optimism scale and other measures of optimism such as the LOT are measuring qualitatively different constructs. Until the degree of overlap between these scales is determined, we cannot rule out this possibility. It might also be the case that the qualities that allow optimistic individuals to report fewer symptoms and to recover more quickly from acute health problems are also the qualities that put them at greater long-term risk for health problems. For example, smokers may optimistically believe that they will not be harmed by tobacco.

C. Neuroticism

Neuroticism, commonly defined as chronic negative affect, has been consistently associated with self-reported symptomatology, but sometimes not with more objectively measured health outcomes such as mortality risk (e.g., Almada et al., 1991; Costa, 1987). This has led many researchers to conclude that neurotic individuals are more likely to report experiencing aches and pains, but are not more susceptible to disease. Although it is true that certain measures of neuroticism seem to be more strongly related to symptom reporting than to disease development, there appear to be pathological components of neuroticism that are associated with more objectively defined health outcomes. For example, in their meta-analysis of this literature, Friedman and Booth-Kewley (1987) found that anxiety and depression, often conceptualized as components of neuroticism, are weakly but reliably associated with a number of diseases. In the case of coronary heart disease, their analysis indicated that anxiety and depression are associated with the incidence of this disease in both concurrent and prospective investigations. And following up that meta-analysis, depression is now seen as an important risk factor for coronary disease (Aromaa et al., 1994). Our own research has shown that males with more mood instability (a characteristic of neuroticism) have a higher mortality risk across the life span compared to males who are more emotionally stable (Friedman et al., 1993).

III. DISEASE-SPECIFIC ASSOCIATIONS

An important issue that has been the topic of debate in the personality–disease literature is the extent to which certain personality traits are exclusively associated with certain diseases or causes of death. Earlier work on personality predictors of disease would refer to individuals as having a "coronary-prone personality" or a "cancer-prone personality." These descriptors seem to imply, for example, that hostile individuals are exclusively at increased risk for heart disease, whereas depressed or repressed individuals are exclusively at increased risk for cancer. Might it not be the case that a number of personality traits and emotional response patterns have a more general deleterious effect on health, putting individuals at higher risk for a number of diseases? In a meta-analysis of the personality and disease literature, Friedman and Booth-Kewley (1987) addressed this question by reviewing the studies that had been conducted to date on the associations between the most widely studied personality traits and a number of diseases commonly thought to have a "psychosomatic" component. The personality traits they investigated were depression, anger/hostility/aggression, anxiety, and extroversion. They determined the extent to which these personality traits were associated with asthma, arthritis, ulcers, headaches, and coronary heart disease. Anxiety, depression, and anger/hostility/aggression were consistently associated with each of these diseases, although results for all but coronary heart disease were weak. These associations held even when the analyses were limited to only prospective studies. Friedman and Booth-Kewley used the term "disease-prone personality" to summarize their findings: that a certain constellation of personality traits puts one at higher risk for developing a number of different diseases. Subsequent research, which considers multiple predictors and multiple outcomes, has tended to confirm that there is at present little evidence for specific psychosocial patterns limited to single diseases.

There is now little doubt that certain personality traits and emotional response patterns should be considered risk factors for disease—just as elevated cholesterol and hypertension have traditionally been considered risk factors for disease. An important advantage of identifying personality- and emotion-based risk factors has to do with the stability of personality and emotional response patterns. Evidence from longitudinal studies, such as the Baltimore Longitudinal Study of Aging (Costa & McCrae, 1994), indicates that these personal characteristics are relatively stable across adulthood. Although the extent to which personality and emotional response patterns are stable from childhood to adulthood has not been fully investigated, it seems likely that hostile and angry characteristics in childhood, for example, will affect coping and health behaviors in adulthood. As discussed in the next section, we know that children with certain personal characteristics grow up to be adults who engage in health-compromising lifestyles. The implication of a possible stability in personality and emotional response patterns is that individuals at higher morbidity and mortality risk can be identified as early as childhood, when preventive measures would be most effective.

IV. MECHANISMS THROUGH WHICH PERSONALITY AND EMOTION MIGHT AFFECT HEALTH

Personality and emotional response patterns can impact health through a variety of psychosocial mechanisms. Unhealthy behaviors (such as smoking and excessive drinking), unstable social relationships, and negative or stressful life events are a few mechanisms that seem most promising in terms of understanding the links between personality, emotional response patterns, and health.

A. Behavioral Mechanisms

The two health behaviors which are most strongly and consistently associated with morbidity and mortality risk are smoking and alcohol consumption. It is estimated that one out of every six deaths in the United States is attributable to smoking (U.S. Department of Health and Human Services, 1989), and 3% of annual deaths in this country are directly attributable to alcohol consumption (U.S. Department of Health and Human Services, 1990). A vast literature has explored the associations between personality and each of these behaviors, with most of these studies being cross-sectional investigations of adults. However, prospective investigations in which personality, measured in childhood or adolescence, is used to predict future smoking and drinking are especially valuable for two reasons. First, because substance use can produce changes in personality and emotional response patterns, the best way to determine the causal linkages between personality and these health-related behaviors comes from prospective studies of substance-use initiation. In other words, what types of people are most likely to start smoking and drinking? Second, identifying the types of children who are most likely to start smoking and drinking allows for prevention programs to especially target those children at greater risk.

A number of longitudinal studies of children and adolescents have predicted smoking and/or drinking behavior from various personality characteristics. These studies show that several of the personality traits that predict long-term health outcomes, such as hostility and (discussed below) conscientiousness, also predict the initiation of smoking and alcohol use. For example, individuals at greatest risk for engaging in these behaviors include those who are rebellious or risk takers (Bauman, Fisher, Bryan, & Chenoweth, 1984; Collins et al., 1987; Lipkus, Barefoot, Williams, & Siegler, 1994; Sussman, Dent, Flay, Hansen, & Johnson, 1987; Teichman, Barnea, & Ravov, 1989), who are aggressive (Farrington, 1991; Kellam, Ensminger, & Simon, 1980), who have a higher tolerance of deviance (Chassin, Presson, Sherman, Corty, & Olshavsky, 1984; Webb, Baer, McLaughlin, McKelvey, & Caid, 1991), who feel alienated (Brunswick & Messeri, 1984), who have low self-esteem (Ahlgren, Norem, Hochhauser, & Garvin, 1982; Semmer, Cleary, Dwyer, Fuchs, & Lippert, 1987; Semmer et al., 1987; Sussman et al., 1987), and who have low personality stability (Bates & Pandina, 1991).

Most of the above-mentioned studies have followed individuals for only a few years. Thus, they could be investigating personality predictors of *experimentation,* rather than personality predictors of long-term substance use. However, there is some evidence that personality can predict substance use over several decades. In a study of over 4000 individuals, hostility measured in adolescence predicted smoking behavior approximately 20 years later (Siegler, Peterson, Barefoot, & Williams, 1992). Our own work with the Terman data set has similarly shown that cheerfulness, sociability, and lack of conscientiousness predict smoking and drinking behavior over a 30-year period (Tucker et al., 1995). (For a recent review of smoking studies see Conrad, Flay, & Hill, 1992, and for alcohol studies see Hawkins, Catalano, & Miller, 1992.)

In addition to smoking and alcohol consumption, personality characteristics and emotional response patterns have been linked with a number of other known risk factors for disease. To take the case of hostility, for example, individuals who report higher hostility have been found not only to smoke more (Musante, Treiber, Davis, Strong, & Levy, 1992; Raikkonen & Keltikangas-Jarvinen, 1991; Scherweitz & Rugulies, 1992) and to consume more alcohol (Raikkonen & Keltikangas-Jarvinen, 1991; Scherwitz & Rugulies, 1992), but also to have poorer dietary habits (Musante et al., 1992; Scherwitz & Rugulies, 1992) and to be less physically active (Raikkonen & Keltikangas-Jarvinen, 1991) than individuals who are less hostile (it should be noted that sex differences are sometimes found in these associations). Thus, individuals with certain personality characteristics and emotional response patterns tend to engage in unhealthy behaviors—very possibly beginning in childhood or adolescence—that set the stage for health problems later in life.

B. Psychosocial Mechanisms

A second way in which personality traits and emotional response patterns may impact physical health is through psychosocial mechanisms such as social support and the experience of negative or stressful life events. In the case of social support, a hostile or depressed individual, for example, may have trouble initiating and maintaining close relationships. Or such individuals may simply perceive that the quantity or quality of their relationships is inadequate. The link to physical health comes from the vast literature indicating the individuals who are socially isolated, experience social instability (such as through marital breakup), or perceive that they have poor social relations are at higher morbidity and mortality risk compared to individuals who have adequate and stable social relationships (e.g., House, Umberson, & Landis, 1988). These health effects in turn occur through a wide variety of mechanisms including stress, resources, and behavior.

To once again consider the case of hostility, several studies have found that hostile individuals report having less social support, and social support which is of poorer quality, compared to less hostile individuals (Hardy & Smith, 1988; Raikonen, Keskivaara, & Keltikangas-Jarvinen, 1992; Scherwitz, Perkins, Cheona, & Hughes, 1991; Smith & Frohm, 1985; Smith, Pope, Sanders, Allred, & O'Keeffe, 1988). Hostile individuals also tend to be less satisfied with their social relationships (Smith et al., 1988). At least two other large-scale studies of young adults have confirmed that hostile individuals report having less social support than individuals who are less hostile. Other evidence linking personality to the quality of close relationships comes from the divorce literature. The most interesting of these studies have used prospective designs to show that certain personality traits, measured either before marriage or at the beginning of the marriage, predict the occurrence of divorce several years later. These studies show that certain personality characteristics known to predict physical health outcomes are also predictive of marital instability. For example, individuals who are neurotic (Kelly & Conley, 1987; Kiernan, 1986), lack impulse control (Kelly & Conley, 1987), and have problems in coping or are ill-tempered (Caspi, Elder, & Bem, 1987; Rockwell, Elder, & Ross, 1979) are more likely to experience future divorce.

Personality and emotional response patterns may also be associated directly with physical health through stress and coping mechanisms. Certain types of people are more prone to experiencing stress in their lives. For example, hostile individuals tend to report experiencing more negative life events and daily hassles compared to individuals who are less hostile (Hardy & Smith, 1988; Scherwitz et al., 1991; Smith & Frohm, 1985; Smith et al., 1988). It would not be surprising if these hostile individuals often react physiologically to negative or stressful situations in ways that ultimately exacerbate the problem. More generally, individuals who are characterized by a high level of negative affect (hostility, anxiety, and depression), are more likely to report experiencing stressful life events (Brett, Brief, Burke, George, & Webster, 1990). Both the experience of negative or stressful life events and the inability to effectively cope with these events can contribute to health problems (Lazarus & Folkman, 1984).

V. TERMAN LIFE-CYCLE STUDY

For the past several years, our interdisciplinary research team has been exploring the long-term effects of personality on physical health. Specifically, we have used archival data from the Terman Life-Cycle Study (Terman & Oden, 1947) to investigate the relation between childhood personality (assessed in 1922, at approximately age 11) and longevity (as of 1991). Our focus on childhood personality as a predictor of longevity has allowed us to prospectively investigate the influence of personality on physical health across a 70-year period. Furthermore, it has allowed us to tease apart the causal links between personality, adult behavioral and psychosocial mediators, such as smoking and marital history, and physical health.

The Terman Life-Cycle Study participants are 1528 men and women who have been assessed at 5–10 year intervals from 1922–1991 (approximately age 11–80). This study was initiated by Lewis Terman, who was interested in studying the development of gifted children. As such, the sample is comprised of very bright individuals. Although the sample is homogeneous (I.Q. of at least 135, 99% white, and mostly middle class), the select nature of the sample allows for a more focused investigation of psychosocial influences on physical health. It is not the case, for example, that participants in this study had inadequate access to medical care, could not understand treatment recommendations, or experienced extreme poverty or inadequate housing. To the extent that childhood personality predicts longevity in this sample, it is most likely through psychosocial and behavioral mechanisms.

To develop measures of childhood personality, we used ratings that Terman asked each child's parent and teacher to make of the child in 1922 (Terman, 1925). There were two main considerations in constructing the personality measures. First, we wanted to develop measures that current theory suggests are related to physical health, such as optimism. Second, we wanted to develop measures that were relevant to current conceptualizations of personality, such as the so-called Big Five model of personality. Of course, we were also constrained by the information that Terman collected in 1922. Ultimately, we were able to develop the following six measures of childhood personality. Our *Sociability* scale corresponds to the Extroversion factor common to most personality theories (sample item: fondness for large groups). The *Conscientiousness / Social Dependability* scale corresponds to the Big Five dimension of Conscientiousness (sample item: prudence, conscientiousness, and truthfulness). Two of our measures are relevant to the Neuroticism factor that is included in many personality theories, although assessing different aspects of this dimension: the *Self-Esteem / High Motivation* scale is comprised of such items as "self-confidence" and "will power," and our *Permanency of Moods* (single item) measure assesses emotional stability. Corresponding to measures of optimism is our *Cheerfulness* scale (items: rated "optimism" and "sense of humor"). Last, we included a *High Energy / Activity* scale that assesses the child's vitality (sample item: rated physical energy) (see Friedman et al., 1993, for details on how these measures were constructed).

Our results indicate that children who were rated as more conscientious and those who were rated as *less* cheerful had a lower mortality risk in adulthood compared to their more impulsive and cheerful counterparts (Friedman et al., 1993). The magnitude of these associations was impressive. After adjusting for age, sex, and the other five personality dimensions, children who were in the 75th percentile on Conscientiousness had only 77% the risk of dying in any given year compared to children in the 25th percentile on Conscientiousness. Children in the 75th percentile on Cheerfulness had a 23% greater risk of dying in any given year compared to children in the 25th percentile. Thus, the risk associated with being an impulsive or cheerful child is comparable to more traditional risk factors for premature mortality such as blood pressure.

Our next step in this project was to gain a better understanding of the long-term health consequences of these impulsive and cheerful children. We took two approaches in addressing this issue. First, we examined cause of death to determine if these children were especially susceptible to certain causes of death. For example, perhaps children who lack conscientiousness tend to engage in impulsive and reckless behavior, putting themselves at higher risk for death from injury or accidents. Perhaps cheerful children have an unrealistically optimistic or Pollyanna out-look, leading them to ignore warnings against harmful behaviors such as smoking; this might put them at higher risk for death from cancer or cardiovascular disease. In investigating cause of death, a certified nosologist used death certificates (supplemented by other sources of information such as obituaries and letters from family members) to classify the deceased individuals into one of five broad cause of death categories: cardiovascular diseases, all cancers, injury (including suicides, accidents, and violence), other causes, and unknown causes.

Our second approach to gaining a better understanding of the relations between childhood personality and mortality was to identify adult mediators of these relations by testing two basic models. One plausible model suggested that impulsive or cheerful children were at higher mortality risk because they tended to engage in an unhealthy lifestyle which might include smoking, excessive alcohol consumption, overeating, or risky hobbies. A second model suggested that these children might be at higher mortality risk due to psychosocial difficulties; for example, perhaps they tended to have unstable social relationships (either in childhood or adulthood), lower educational/socioeconomic attainment, or lower adult psychological well-being.

In the case of impulsive children, they were not more likely to die only from cardiovascular disease or cancer or injury, suggesting that impulsivity affects longevity through more general physiological or behavioral mechanisms (Friedman et al., 1995a). There was some suggestion that impulsive children were more likely to die from injury, supporting the idea that these children grew up to be impulsive, reckless adults. However, the number of such deaths was small and could not fully account for the higher mortality risk of impulsive children.

Conscientious children tended to grow up to engage in a healthier lifestyle than impulsive children. Conscientious children were less likely to smoke and consumed less alcohol in adulthood, but conscientiousness was unrelated to obesity. This would suggest that the higher mortality risk of impulsive children might be due to engagement in these unhealthy behaviors. However, although smoking and alcohol consumption could account for some of the higher mortality risk of impulsive children (in separate analyses alcohol consumption accounted for 11% of the risk, whereas smoking accounted for 26% of the risk), conscientiousness remained a significant predictor of longevity after taking these health-related behaviors into account. Thus, the higher mortality risk of impulsive children cannot be fully explained by their engagement in these unhealthy behaviors.

We have found significant associations between conscientiousness and health-relevant variables on nearly every characteristic we have investigated. Conscientious children were less likely to have experienced parental divorce as children and were also less likely to have experienced a divorce by midlife (approximately age 40). Conscientious children were less likely to have experienced mental difficulties by midlife (a tendency toward nervousness, special anxieties, or nervous breakdown), although they were not more likely to report greater psychological well-being (measured by a scale comprised of six self-report items, the last three of which were reverse-coded: happiness of temperament, self-confidence, easy to get along with, moodiness, feelings of inferiority, and sensitive feelings). Conscientious children were also more likely to have completed more years of education by midlife than impulsive children. Each of these characteristics (parental divorce, adult divorce, mental difficulties, and lower cumulative education), in turn, were significant predictors of mortality.

In determining the extent to which these characteristics could account for the relation between childhood impulsivity (lack of conscientiousness) and longevity, we separately controlled for each variable. For the total sample, controlling for parental divorce reduced the risk of mortality associated with impulsivity by about 9%, controlling for adult divorce reduced the risk by about 9%, controlling for mental difficulties reduced the risk by about 13%, and controlling for cumulative education reduced the risk by about 13%. Controlling simultaneously for these four variables reduced the risk of mortality associated with impulsivity by about 33% for the total sample, although conscientiousness was still a significant predictor of longevity. This final analysis was done separately for men and women. In the case of women, conscientiousness was no longer a significant predictor of longevity in this smaller subsample. However, controlling for these four variables reduced the risk of mortality by 18% for women. Controlling for these variables reduced the risk of mortality by 40% for men, resulting in conscientiousness no longer being a significant predictor of mortality. Thus, these psychosocial characteristics could explain much, but not all, of the association between childhood conscientiousness and longevity.

Turning to cheerfulness, we found that cheerful children were not more susceptible to certain causes of death (Martin et al., 1995). As is the case for conscientiousness, this suggests that cheerfulness has its effects on mortality through general physiological or behavioral mechanisms. In terms of their health-related behaviors, cheerful children tended to smoke and drink more than their less cheerful counterparts, but there was no association with obesity. Interestingly, these health-related behaviors accounted for very little of the mortality risk of cheerful children (Martin et al., 1995).

We have been able to rule out a number of other plausible explanations for the inverse association between cheerfulness and mortality (see Martin et al., 1995). For example, it appears that the higher mortality of cheerful children is not due to lower goals that they set for themselves—at least as evidenced in terms of their socioeconomic status. Both cumulative education and income as of midlife were unrelated to childhood cheerfulness. It also appears that the higher mortality risk of cheerful children is not due to marital instability or the detrimental effects of parental divorce; both parental divorce and marital instability are unrelated to childhood cheerfulness in this sample. Although cheerfulness was not associated with experiencing mental difficulties by midlife, it was associated with *better* psychological adjustment and the tendency to have a more carefree attitude in adulthood. Although cheerful children grew up to have a more carefree attitude, this carefree attitude accounted for little of the association between cheerfulness and mortality.

Our study of the association between childhood cheerfulness and longevity leaves open many avenues for future research. It is likely that cheerfulness has its long-term impact on health through complex mechanisms that are not easily identifiable by focusing on a small number of behavioral or psychosocial mediators. For example, a constellation of health-related behaviors, in addition to smoking and alcohol consumption, may better explain the higher mortality risk of cheerful individuals. These health-related behaviors may interact with psychosocial variables, such as life stressors and coping mechanisms, to impact health across the life span.

We found some evidence that certain aspects of Neuroticism measured in childhood predicted longevity across the life span. Boys who had less permanent moods tended to have a higher mortality risk than boys who were more emotionally stable (Friedman et al., 1993). Interestingly, permanency of moods was not a significant predictor of longevity for females. We have not yet fully explored why having less permanent moods increases males' risk of mortality. However, we have been able to rule out several potential explanations for this relationship. It is possible that boys with unstable moods are more likely to smoke, consume alcohol, and overeat, resulting in a higher mortality risk. However, we have found that permanency of moods is not a significant predictor of smoking, alcohol consumption, or obesity for males (Tucker et al., 1995). It might also be the case that boys with unstable moods experience less stable social relationships. In terms of the variables we have been considering, boys with less permanent moods might have been more likely to have experienced parental divorce, and their mood instability might have contributed to their own divorce in adulthood. Contrary to expectations, permanency of moods in childhood is not a significant predictor of marital instability in this sample (Tucker, Friedman, Wingard, & Schwartz, 1996). Although children with less permanent moods are more likely to have experienced parental divorce compared to children with more stable moods, Permanency of Mood remained a significant predictor of mortality risk after controlling for parental divorce (Schwartz et al., 1995). To summarize, although Permanency of Mood is a significant predictor of longevity for males, the mechanisms through which this aspect of personality affects health remain unclear.

The other three personality scales we included in our investigation (Sociability, Self-Esteem/Motivation, and Energy/Activity) were not significant predictors of mortality risk. This was particularly surprising in the case of Sociability, given the vast literature showing that individuals who are socially integrated tend to have better health and live longer than those who are socially isolated. We further explored the association between sociability and mortality risk in adulthood by following up on an analysis that Terman had done in the 1950s. Terman was interested in how society could recruit more scholars to be scientists, and also how to foster greater cooperation between scientists and nonscientists. To better understand these issues, he compared men who were scientists versus nonscientists on a number of psychosocial dimensions (because there were few women scientists in the sample, he did not consider this group). One of the fundamental differences he found between scientists and nonscientists was that scientists tended to be unsociable; both in childhood and young adulthood, scientists tended to be more shy and less interested in social activities and relationships. We were able to re-create Terman's original classification of these men and to determine whether these unsociable scientists had a higher mortality risk than the more sociable nonscientists. Contrary to expectations, the nonscientists had a 23% greater risk of dying in any given year (marginally significant) compared to the scientists. Thus, although being socially integrated may have a beneficial effect on health, our results indicate that having a sociable, extroverted personality does not necessarily have a long-term beneficial effect on health.

VI. CONCLUSIONS

The Terman Life-Cycle Study, rich in psychosocial data, is the only cohort study to follow a substantial-sized sample from childhood across seven decades through old age and death. By gathering information about longevity and cause of death, and by developing numerous health-related indexes from the archives, we have been able to create a unique opportunity to trace the relations among personality, behavior, and health across the life span. Although the Terman participants are not representative of the general population, the homogeneous and intelligent nature of the sample provides for clear insights about likely psychosocial links.

Most basically, it is fascinating to discover that childhood personality is indeed predictive of longevity across the life span. Given the multiple random influences on longevity, the clear links to personality and emotional response patterns suggest that psychology may play a major role in physical health. Interestingly, it seems to be a certain social dependability and lack of impulsivity that most characterizes those who are destined to live long lives. Conscientious children go on to have a host of documentable health-relevant behaviors that go a long way towards preserving their health.

There does not seem to be any single mechanism (such as alcohol abuse) or any single disease (such as heart disease) that accounts for personality's relations to longevity. Rather, different children seem to set off down different health-relevant paths, with assorted relevant health implications. These include psychosocial influences (such as marital relationships and educational attainment), psychoemotional influences (i.e., stress), and behavioral influences (such as substance use) (Friedman et al., 1995b).

Other aspects of personality also seem relevant to longevity, though less important than the conscientious social dependability. Mood instability, at least for males, seems to be a health threat, but it is not yet clear why this may be. Cheerfulness is seen to be not necessarily health protective in the long term; although it may help short-term coping, it may not lead to optimal health habits. Surprisingly, although social stability seems to be relevant to good health, the personality trait of sociability does *not* seem so relevant.

It is interesting that personality tended to predict deaths from each of the broad cause-of-death categories we investigated (cardiovascular disease, cancer, and injury). This finding lends credence to models of homeostasis and health, in which individual problems and disruptions can impair health in a variety of ways. We do not find support for oversimplified ideas of coronary-prone or cancer-prone personalities.

How are our findings relevant to the often found detrimental influences of hostility on health? Perhaps hostility is a sign of rebellion or frustration or cynical relations with others. That is, hostility might be thought of as a key psychoemotional component of intraindividual or interpersonal stress. If so, then our Terman sample life span results are quite consistent: We find that it is the stable, well-adjusted, socially integrated life pattern that not only characterizes mental health, but leads to a substantially longer life as well.

ACKNOWLEDGMENTS

This chapter was supported by a research grant from the National Institute on Aging #AG08825, Howard S. Friedman, Principal Investigator. Part of the data for our research described in this chapter were made available from the Terman Life-Cycle Study, begun by Lewis Terman. Further assistance was provided by Eleanor Walker of the Terman project. We would like to acknowledge our collaborators on this research project (listed alphabetically): Michael H. Criqui, M.D., M.P.H., University of California, San Diego; Leslie Martin, M.A., University of California, Riverside; Joseph E. Schwartz, Ph.D., State University of New York, Stony Brook; Carol Tomlinson-Keasey, Ph.D., University of California, Davis; and Deborah L. Wingard, Ph.D., University of California, San Diego.

REFERENCES

Ahlgren, A., Norem, A. A., Hochhauser, M., & Garvin, J. (1982). Antecedents of smoking among pre-adolescents. *Journal of Drug Education, 12,* 325–340.

Alexander, F. (1950). *Psychosomatic medicine.* New York: Norton.

Almada, S. J., Zonderman, A. B., Shekelle, R. B., Dyer, A. R., Daviglus, M. L., & Costa, P. T., Jr. (1991). Neuroticism and cynicism and risk of death in middle-aged men: the Western Electric Study. *Psychosomatic Medicine, 53,* 165–175.

Aromaa, A., Raitasalo, R., Reunanen, A., Impivaara, O., Heliovaara, M., Knekt, P., Lehtinen, V., Joukamaa, M., & Maatela, J. (1994). Depression and cardiovascular diseases. *Acta Psychiatrica Scandinavica. Supplementum, 377,* 77–81.

Barefoot, J. C., Dahlstrom, W. G., & Williams, R. B., Jr. (1983). Hostility, CHD incidence, and total mortality: A 25-year follow-up study of 255 physicians. *Psychosomatic Medicine, 45,* 59–63.

Barefoot, J. C., Siegler, I. C., Nowlin, J. B., Peterson, B. L., Haney, T. L., & Williams, R. B., Jr. (1987). Suspiciousness, health, and mortality: A follow-up study of 500 older adults. *Psychosomatic Medicine, 49,* 450–457.

Bates, M. E., & Pandina, R. J. (1991). Personality, stability, and adolescent substance use behaviors. *Alcoholism, Clinical and Experimental Research, 15,* 471–477.

Bauman, K. E., Fisher, L. A., Bryan, E. S., & Chenoweth, R. L. (1984). Antecedents, subjective expected utility, and behaviors: A panel study of adolescent cigarette smoking. *Addictive Behaviors, 9,* 121–136.

Booth-Kewley, S., & Friedman, H. S. (1987). Psychological predictors of heart disease: A quantitative review. *Psychological Bulletin, 101,* 343–362.

Brett, J. F., Brief, A. P., Burke, M. J., George, J. M., & Webster, J. (1990). Negative affectivity and the reporting of stressful life events. *Health Psychology, 9,* 57–68.

Brunswick, A. F., & Messeri, P. (1984). Causal factors in onset of adolescents' cigarette smoking: A prospective study of urban black youth. *Advances in Alcohol and Substance Abuse, 3,* 35–52.

Caspi, A., Elder, G. H., Jr., & Bem, D. J. (1987). Moving against the world: Lifecourse patterns of explosive children. *Developmental Psychology, 23,* 308–313.

Chamberlain, K., Petrie, K., & Azariah, R. (1992). The role of optimism and sense of coherence in predicting recovery following surgery. *Psychology and Health, 7,* 301–310.

Chassin, L., Presson, C. C., Sherman, S. J., Corty, E., & Olshavsky, R. W. (1984). Predicting the onset of cigarette smoking in adolescents: A longitudinal study. *Journal of Applied Social Psychology, 14,* 224–243.

Collins, L. M., Sussman, S., Rauch, J. M., Dent, C. W., Johnson, C. A., Hansen, W. B., & Flay, B. R. (1987). Psychosocial predictors of young adolescent cigarette smoking: A sixteen-month, three-wave longitudinal study. *Journal of Applied Social Psychology, 17,* 554–573.

Conrad, K. M., Flay, B. R., & Hill, D. (1992). Why children start smoking cigarettes: Predictors of onset. *British Journal of Addiction, 87,* 1711–1724.

Costa, P. T., Jr. (1987). Influence of the normal personality dimension of neuroticism on chest pain symptoms and coronary artery disease. *American Journal of Cardiology, 60,* 20J–26J.

Costa, P. T., Jr., & McCrae, R. R. (1994). Set like plaster? Evidence for the stability of adult personality. In T. F. Heatherton & J. L. Weinberger (Eds.), *Can personality change?* (pp. 21–40). Washington, DC: American Psychological Association.

Dembroski, T. M., MacDougall, J. M., Costa, P. T., Jr., & Grandits, G. A. (1989). Components of hostility as predictors of sudden death and myocardial infarction in the Multiple Risk Factor Intervention Trial. *Psychosomatic Medicine, 51,* 514–522.

Dunbar, F. H. (1943). *Psychosomatic diagnosis.* New York: Harper.

Farrington, D. P. (1991). Childhood aggression and adult violence: Early precursors and later-life outcomes. In D. J. Pepler & K. H. Rubin (Eds.), *The development and treatment of childhood aggression* (pp. 5–29). Hillsdale, NJ: Lawrence Erlbaum Associates.

Friedman, H. S., & Booth-Kewley, S. (1987). The "disease-prone personality:" A meta-analytic view of the construct. *American Psychologist, 42,* 539–555.

Friedman, H. S., Tucker, J. S., Schwartz, J. E., Martin, L. R., Tomlinson-Keasey, C., Wingard, D. L., & Criqui, M. H. (1995a). Childhood conscientiousness and longevity: Health behaviors and cause of death. *Journal of Personality and Social Psychology, 68,* 696–703.

Friedman, H. S., Tucker, J. S., Schwartz, J. E., Tomlinson-Keasey, C., Martin, L. R., Wingard, D. L., & Criqui, M. H. (1995b). Psychosocial and behavioral predictors of longevity: The aging and death of the "Termites." *American Psychologist, 50,* 69–78.

Friedman, H. S., Tucker, J. S., Tomlinson-Keasey, C., Schwartz, J., Wingard, D., &

Criqui, M. (1993). Does childhood personality predict longevity? *Journal of Personality and Social Psychology, 65,* 176–185.

Hardy, J. D., & Smith, T. W. (1988). Cynical hostility and vulnerability to disease: Social support, life stress, and physiological response to conflict. *Health Psychology, 7,* 447–459.

Hawkins, J. D., Catalano, R. F., & Miller, J. Y. (1992). Risk and protective factors for alcohol and other drug problems in adolescence and early adulthood: Implications for substance abuse prevention. *Psychological Bulletin, 112,* 64–105.

House, J. S., Umberson, D., & Landis, K. R. (1988). Structures and processes of social support. *American Review of Sociology, 14,* 293–318.

Kellam, S. G., Ensminger, M. E., & Simon, M. B. (1980). Mental health in first grade and teenage drug, alcohol, and cigarette use. *Drug and Alcohol Dependence, 5,* 273–304.

Kelly, E. L., & Conley, J. J. (1987). Personality and compatibility: A prospective analysis of marital stability and marital satisfaction. *Journal of Personality and Social Psychology, 52,* 27–40.

Kiernan, K. E. (1986). Teenage marriage and marital breakdown: A longitudinal study. *Population Studies, 40,* 35–54.

Koskenvuo, M., Kapiro, J., Rose, R. J., Kesaniemi, A., Sarnaa, S., Heikkila, K., & Langinvanio, H. (1988). Hostility as a risk factor for mortality and ischemic heart disease in men. *Psychosomatic Medicine, 50,* 330–340.

Lazarus, R. S., & Folkman, S. (1984). *Stress, appraisal, and coping.* New York: Guilford.

Lipkus, I. M., Barefoot, J. C., Williams, R. B., & Siegler, I. C. (1994). Personality measures as predictors of smoking initiation and cessation in the UNC Alumni Heart study. *Health Psychology, 13,* 149–155.

Martin, L. R., Friedman, H. S., Tucker, J. S., Tomlinson-Keasey, C., Criqui, M. H., Wingard, D. L., & Schwartz, J. E. (1995). *Cheerfulness and longevity: A longitudinal examination of the inverse relationship.* Unpublished manuscript.

McCranie, E. W., Watkins, L. O., Brandsma, J. M., & Sisson, B. D. (1986). Hostility, coronary heart disease (CHD) incidence, and total mortality: Lack of association in a 25-year follow-up study of 478 physicians. *Journal of Behavioral Medicine, 9,* 119–125.

Musante, L., Treiber, F. A., Davis, H., Strong, W. B., & Levy, M. (1992). Hostility: Relationship to lifestyle behaviors and physical risk factors. *Behavioral Medicine, 18,* 21–26.

Raikkonen, K., & Keltikangas-Jarvinen, L. (1991). Hostility and its association with behaviorally induced and somatic coronary risk indicators in Finnish adolescents and young adults. *Social Science and Medicine, 33,* 1171–1178.

Raikkonen, K., Keskivaara, P., & Keltikangas-Jarvinen, L. (1992). Hostility and social support among type A individuals. *Psychology and Health, 7,* 289–299.

Rockwell, R. C., Elder, G. H., Jr., & Ross, D. J. (1979). Psychological patterns in marital timing and divorce. *Social Psychology Quarterly, 42,* 399–404.

Rotton, J. (1992). Trait humor and longevity: Do comics have the last laugh? *Health Psychology, 11,* 262–266.

Scheier, M., & Carver, C. (1985). Optimism, coping, and health: Assessment and implications of generalized outcome expectancies. *Health Psychology, 4,* 219–247.

Scheier, M., & Carver, C. (1993). On the power of positive thinking: The benefits of being optimistic. *Current Directions in Psychological Science, 2,* 26–30.

Scheier, M. F., Matthews, K. A., & Owens, J. F., Magovern, G. J., Lefebvre, R., Abbott, R. C., & Carver, C. S. (1989). Dispositional optimism and recovery from coronary artery bypass surgery: The beneficial effects on physical and psychological well-being. *Journal of Personality and Social Psychology, 57,* 1024–1040.

Scherwitz, L., Perkins, L., Chesney, M., & Hughes, G. (1991). Cook-Medley Hostility scale and subsets: Relationship to demographic and psychosocial characteristics in young adults in the CARDIA study. *Psychosomatic Medicine, 53,* 36–49.

Scherwitz, L., & Rugulies, R. (1992). Life-style and hostility. In H. S. Friedman (Ed.), *Hostility, coping, and health* (pp. 77–98). Washington, DC: American Psychological Association.

Schwartz, J. E., Friedman, H. S., Tucker, J. S., Tomlinson-Keasey, C., Wingard, D. L., & Criqui, M. H. (1995). Childhood sociodemographic and psychosocial factors as predictors of mortality across the life-span. *American Journal of Public Health, 85,* 1237–1245.

Semmer, N. K., Cleary, P. D., Dwyer, J. H., Fuchs, R., & Lippert, P. (1987). Psychosocial predictors of adolescent smoking in two German cities: The Berlin-Bremen study. *Morbidity and Mortality Weekly Reports, 36,* 3–10.

Semmer, N. K., Dwyer, J. H., Lippert, P., Fuchs, R., Cleary, P. D., & Schindler, A. (1987). Adolescent smoking from a functional perspective: The Berlin-Bremen Study. *European Journal of Psychology of Education, 11,* 387–402.

Shekelle, R. B., Gale, M., Ostfeld, A. M., & Paul, O. (1983). Hostility, risk of coronary heart disease, and mortality. *Psychosomatic Medicine, 45,* 109–114.

Siegler, I. C., Peterson, B. L., Barefoot, J. C., Williams, R. B. (1992). Hostility during late adolescence predicts coronary risk factors at mid-life. *American Journal of Epidemiology, 136,* 146–154.

Smith, T. W. (1992). Hostility and health: Current status of a psychosomatic hypothesis. *Health Psychology, 11,* 139–150.

Smith, T. W., & Frohm, K. D. (1985). What's so unhealthy about hostility? Construct validity and psychosocial correlates of the Cook and Medley HO scale. *Health Psychology, 4,* 503–520.

Smith, T. W., Pope, M. K., Sanders, J. D., Allred, K. D., & O'Keeffe, J. L. (1988). Cynical hostility at home and work: Psychosocial vulnerability across domains. *Journal of Research in Personality, 22,* 525–548.

Sussman, S., Dent, C. W., Flay, B. R., Hansen, W. B., & Johnson, C. A. (1987). Psychosocial predictors of cigarette smoking onset by White, Black, Hispanic, and Asian adolescents in Southern California. *Morbidity and Mortality Weekly Reports, 36,* 11–16.

Teichman, M., Barnea, Z., & Ravov, G. (1989). Personality and substance use among adolescents: A longitudinal study. *British Journal of Addiction, 84,* 181–190.

Terman, L. M. (1925). *Genetic studies of genius: I. Mental and physical traits of a thousand gifted children.* Stanford, CA: Stanford University Press.

Terman, L. M., & Oden, M. H. (1947). *Genetic studies of genius: IV. The gifted child grows up: Twenty-five years' follow-up.* Stanford, CA: Stanford University Press.

Tucker, J. S., Friedman, H. S., Tomlinson-Keasey, C., Schwartz, J. E., Wingard, D. L., Criqui, M. H., & Martin, L. R. (1995). Childhood psychosocial predictors of adulthood smoking, alcohol consumption, and physical activity. *Journal of Applied Social Psychology, 25,* 1884–1899.

Tucker, J. S., Friedman, H. S., Wingard, D. L., & Schwartz, J. E. (1996). Marital history at mid-life as a predictor of longevity: Alternative explanations to the protective effect of marriage. *Health Psychology, 15,* 1–8.

U.S. Department of Health and Human Services. (1989). *Reducing the health consequences of smoking: 25 years of progress.* Report of the Surgeon General. DHHS Pub. No (CDC) 89-8411. Rockville, MD: Public Health Service.

U.S. Department of Health and Human Services. (1990). *Seventh special report to the U.S. Congress on alcohol and health.* Rockville, MD: Public Health Service.

Webb, J. A., Baer, P. E., McLaughlin, R. J., McKelvey, R. S., & Caid, C. D. (1991). Risk factors and their relation to initiation of alcohol use among early adolescents. *Journal of the American Academy of Child and Adolescent Psychiatry, 30,* 563–568.

CHAPTER 18

Quality of Life and Affect in Later Life

M. Powell Lawton

Polisher Research Institute
Philadelphia Geriatric Center and
Temple University School of Medicine
Philadelphia, Pennsylvania

This chapter addresses the research literature on psychological well-being, quality of life (QOL), and affect as they apply to older people and suggest a new way of accounting for their interrelationships. The literature on affect experience will be examined in relation to Helson's (1964) adaptation level (AL) theory. QOL is asserted to represent a subjective processing of the overall duration and intensity of affect states over a self-chosen period of time (the hedonic integral) augmented by stable personality characteristics and cognitive affective schemata built up over variable periods of time. The person will tend to select the reference time period in such a way as to optimize the excess of positive over negative affect.

I. CONCEPTUALIZATIONS OF QUALITY OF LIFE AND PSYCHOLOGICAL WELL-BEING

Attempts to organize knowledge regarding the meaning of psychological well-being in gerontology may be found in Lawton (1991) and George and Bearon (1980). My definition of psychological well-being is the self-evaluated level of the person's competence and the self, weighted in terms of the person's hierarchy of goals. One conception of QOL was offered in which psychological well-being was one of four sectors, the others being behavioral competence, environment, and perceived QOL (Lawton, 1983; 1991). The larger QOL construct was defined as, "The multidimensional evaluation, by both intrapersonal and social-normative criteria, of the person-environment system of an individual in time past, present, and anticipated" (Lawton, 1991, p. 6). This conceptual definition simply suggested that all four sectors were aspects of QOL. Further reflection has suggested, however, the necessity for a revision that includes some casual hypotheses.

The revision was suggested by the research of Burt, Wiley, Minor, and Murray (1978), who used a measurement model to define the hypothesized latent variable of happiness. From several large national surveys, they tested a model that included positive affect (PA), negative affect (NA), domain-specific satisfactions (perceived QOL), and generalized life satisfaction. Domain-specific satisfactions represented perceived QOL in the areas studied by Andrews and Withey (1976) and Campbell, Converse, and Rodgers (1976), such as family life, work, marriage, and housing.

Burt et al.'s conception led to my revised conception. Behavioral competence and environment were viewed as exogenous variables contributing to psychological well-being both directly and indirectly, through perceived QOL. In my present view, QOL, in turn, is a subjective judgment whose components are PA, NA, temperament, and cognitive-affective schemata, linked to specific domains of life. QOL and its components can be understood only in terms of their dynamics over time. The next sections consider how affect is related to personality and how affect is cumulated into a subjective assessment of QOL.

A. Affect and Personality

Personality in its broadest conception encompasses aspects of behavior, cognition, and affect. Affect has had less attention than the other two, although Epstein (1983) demonstrated that the recurrence of affect states over time converged on personality traits, and Costa and McCrae (chap. 20, this volume) suggested that neuroticism is defined almost exclusively by a constellation of affect traits. Affect is usually construed in terms of short states or traits that are stable over time. In fact, the state–trait dichotomy is better seen as a continuum. The time-related continuum ranges from momentary affect states to periods of minutes, hours, days, and years over which affect is experienced. As the reference time increases, the recurrent pattern approaches the stability or predictability of a trait.

The most stable pattern deserves the name *temperament,* with its implications of a genetic basis and very stable manifestations. The clearest forms of temperament appear to be neuroticism and introversion–extroversion; as Costa and McCrae note (chap. 20, this volume), other members of the five-factor model may also have similar stability and heritability. Whether there are behavioral patterns, cognitive styles, and affect propensities that lie midway between temperament and states in their stability and ability to be influenced by ongoing context—midlevel traits—remains to be investigated. For the present purpose, the existence of affective experiences based on a variety of time spans are seen to be central to QOL.

B. A Hedonic Calculus

Quality of daily life is a dynamic, multidetermined process; its character is determined by a hedonic calculus in which the duration, intensity, and quality of subjective experience is the active ingredient. The origin of affect input is usually the domains that compose QOL in the conceptions of Burt et al. (1978) and Campbell et al. (1976). The integral of affect duration and intensity over a reference period of time is the dynamic component of QOL. Specifically, a single affect's onset and cessation represents the duration of that state. That affect and other affects may be experienced in multiple episodes over a reference time period. Whatever the reference time period, the impact of the immediate affect will be augmented by varying influences of temperament, contemporary cognitive appraisal of one's environmental context, cognitive schemata of past affect states, and cognitive appraisals of present affect states. The basic distinction between PA and NA, including their partial independence (Diener & Emmons, 1984), is an essential component of the hedonic calculus. Figure 1 represents in the abscissa the time interval (continuum from trait to state) over which QOL is estimated. The ordinate represents the proportions of QOL accounted for by temperament, cognitive–affective schemata, and the focal hedonic integral. Temperament's contribution is seen as relatively constant, whether the time frame is long (trait) or short (state). As the time frame becomes very short the hedonic integral constitutes the major influence on perceived QOL—intense emotion overwhelms all else in the person's world. With smaller inputs of affect, and with the time frame encompassing longer periods, cognitive–affective schemata in the form of memories of past affects, cog-

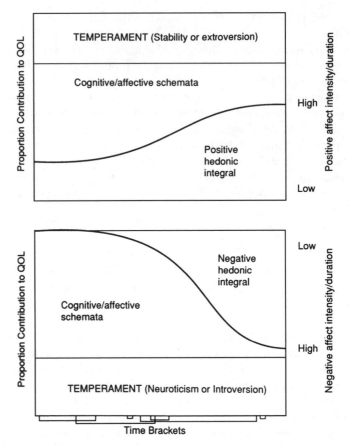

Figure 1 Schematic model of time-related contributions of temperament, cognitive-affective schemata, and hedonic integral of positive and negative affect states to quality of life.

nitive standards against which to compare contemporary affects, learned affect-regulating mechanisms, and expectations dominate judgments of QOL. Over very long periods of time, QOL merges into psychological well-being in such a way that the hedonic integral is dominated by temperament.

One difference between the PA and NA figure is that the percentage contribution for PA even in the absence of major affective state input is above zero (the neutral level), whereas that for NA can be zero. This represents hypotheses of Frijda (1988) and Taylor (1991) that resting state affect is mildly positive. It is consistent with evidence reviewed by Diener and Diener (1996) suggesting that across methods, statuses, and countries, mild PA is the usual state.

Another asymmetry between the positive and negative is the depiction in Figure 1 that the absolute magnitude of the PA contribution may be less than that of NA. Again Taylor (1991, pp. 68–73) reviews a large amount of research supporting the propensity of negative over positive events in influencing behavior, cognition, and affect. In the present instance, when the negative integral is very high, it dominates.

II. ADAPTATION LEVEL AND QUALITY OF LIFE

The dynamics proposed here and illustrated in Figure 1 may be elaborated with reference to Helson's (1964) AL theory. The experience of any phenomenon may be understood in terms of three features: the nature of the focal stimulus, past experience with that stimulus, and the field, or context, in which the focal stimulus appears. This psychophysical theory proposed AL as a moving standard through which qualitative judgments of properties such as brightness, loudness, or intensity were made. The threshold for the perception of magnitude and change in magnitude vary as a function not only of the physical intensity of the stimulus but also of the quality of the surrounds (for example, contrast effects) and the history and timing of previous experiences with similar stimuli (including adaptation over time). The following sections will discuss QOL from perspectives organized around each of these three realms with respect to emotion, making age-related predictions where possible, but usually, because of lack of data, taking an age-neutral position.

In order to apply AL theory, some stretching of the original psychophysical model is required. In AL theory, the focal stimulus had known physical qualities and the response was a subjective experience of that quality. In this QOL model, the focal stimulus is itself subjective (i.e., an experienced emotion), and the response is the judgment of QOL. Past experience brings in historical experiences with the emotion, along with stored traces of the cognition that developed in association with the original affects, the cognitive-affective schema. The environmental context includes both the specific elicitor and the broader context in which the affect is experienced.

A. *The Focal Stimulus*

The major components of the hedonic integral are the duration or frequency of affect, the intensity of the affect, and the valence of the affect over time.

1. FREQUENCY

Frequency of affect experience is the usual metric by which affects are studied. Frequency of affects by age is not definitively known at this time. If measured simply in terms of broad dimensions of positive and negative affect, cross-sectional comparisons on national samples have shown both NA and PA to be slightly lower in older samples, when measured with the "past few weeks" time anchor provided by the Affect Balance Scale (Bradburn, 1969; Campbell et al., 1976). Studies of more differentiated affects have generally not been performed on representative samples. Among the relatively privileged people across the adult age span studied by Lawton, Kleban, and Dean (1993), older people reported less frequent depression, anxiety, hostility, and shyness, more contentment, and did not differ in PA from younger people, when estimating frequencies over the past year. Depression is the most studied affect. In Newmann's (1989) analysis of 14 published surveys using representative community, state, or national samples, age trends varied with the measures and age ranges studied. Although the young-aged (through age 69) appeared to report less depression than younger adults, there was some suggestion that depression might increase at older ages. More recently Gatz, Johansson, Pedersen, Berg, and Reynolds (1993) presented data from two Swedish surveys, which also showed an increase in depression in old age.

The critical longitudinal and sequential data are not available to separate age change from other types of change. Costa and McCrae (chap. 20, this volume), however, in reporting a 2-year longitudinal study of depression, cite stability measures considerably lower than those for the five basic personality traits, together with a zero correlation between depression and age, suggesting that one must look beyond either age or temperament for additional factors to explain affect frequency.

2. INTENSITY

Intensity, however, is another matter. Larsen & Diener (1987) make a convincing case for the separateness of frequency and intensity. Their data indicated that psychological well-being was determined primarily by subjects' estimates of the frequency (which is duration, when aggregated over time) of various affect states. Intensity judgments represent a different dimension of experiencing affect; PA intensity and NA intensity ratings were positively correlated, but neither was related to well-being. Schulz (1982) also discussed duration and intensity as different facets of experiencing emotion. Reasoning from knowledge regarding the greater persistence and level of neurological activation once elicited, Schulz hypothesized that both duration and intensity would be higher among the aged.

3. TWO VALENCED INTENSITY FACTORS

If frequency and intensity are such different dimensions, it would be reasonable to expect that people would distinguish between them in the concepts they use in reporting their meta-experiences with emotion; that is, that they would form different factors. Lawton, Kleban, Rajagopal, and Dean (1992) embedded about half (randomly chosen) of the items of the Larsen (1985) Affect Intensity Measure (AIM) and, following Schulz (1982), constructed a number of items expressing the subjective experience of the duration, persistence, and intensity of both positive and negative affective states. These and other items describing ways of experiencing emotion were embedded in an instrument designed to assess a variety of aspects of the subjective experience of emotion. Ratings of a total of 71 items, responded to on three-point scales of "very true of me," "somewhat true of me," and "not at all true of me," were obtained for 828 participants in the Elderhostel program (ages 60–92), 251 children of some of the Elderhostels subjects (ages 31–59), and 207 grandchildren of Elderhostelers plus undergraduate students (18–30). Two-sample confirmatory factor analyses produced seven replicated factors representing dimensions of experiencing affect (one was not appropriate for the youngest group), all of which will be discussed in different sections of this chapter.

Among these dimensions, these subjects neither identified intensity as a nonvalenced construct nor distinguished intensity from duration. Instead, AIM items and intensity and duration appeared in two highly valenced factors along with other items from the pool. The factors represented, first, high-intensity PA (named Surgency) characterized by high-loading items such as, "When I'm happy I feel like bursting with joy" and "When I'm happy I feel very energetic." The second factor represented Stability, a more complex factor. On one end, items expressed both evenness of mood ("I feel the same every day, rarely changing from happy to unhappy"), long durations of positive states ("My good moods are short," reverse-coded), and short and infrequent intrusions of negative states ("My negative moods are pretty mild"). On the opposite end of the same factor, which might be characterized as moodiness, affect states are seen as highly subject to change, and often for the worse ("I'm a person of quick mood changes" or "If I feel elated I know I will turn to feeling depressed").

The mixing of duration, intensity, and, to some extent, the separation of positive from negative valence intensity suggest that people do, in fact, perform the hedonic calculus. They do not readily distinguish intensity from duration and find the integration of intensity and duration difficult to perform without also distinguishing the favorable from the unfavorable.

On the two factors related to intensity, duration, and valance, older people were significantly lower in Surgency but higher in Stability than middle-aged and younger-adult groups. In their treatment of the single dimension of intensity, Larsen and Diener (1987) studied individual differences in AIM responses. Among their several productive explorations of affect intensity, a cross-sectional comparison of 237 age-grouped members of 63 families on a 21-item AIM showed a systematic decline of affect intensity as age increased (Diener, Sandvik, & Larsen, 1985). Lawton (unpublished data from the Lawton et al., 1992, research on dimensions of affective experience cited earlier) used a 16-item version of the AIM. Systematic significant pairwise age differences were found between young adult, middle aged, and older adults.

Psychophysiological, particularly autonomic, changes appear to be markers of the perceived intensity of emotion in both psychological research and in literature and popular culture. Levinson, Carstensen, Friesen, and Ekman (1992) studied heart rate and finger temperature responses of younger and older subjects to two types of experimentally induced emotion: Directed facial action (tensing emotion-specific facial muscles at the instruction of the examiner without mention of any affect state) and imaginal-induced emotions based on the recall of personal emotion states that matched a prototype experience described by the experimenter (e.g., sadness after bereavement). Autonomic displacements in the predicted directions were much greater among young subjects than among old for all emotions (anger, fun, sadness, and disgust). Consistent findings from the subjective experiential perspective were found by Lawton et al. (1992). A factor clearly descriptive of perceived autonomic activation emerged among the dimensions of experienced emotion; both middle-aged and older subjects reported less frequent autonomic manifestations of emotion than did younger subjects.

These findings seem very clear in pointing to age-related decline in affect intensity. Some other evidence is inconsistent with age-related reduction in intensity however. In the Levinson et al. (1991) study, despite their notably lower autonomic responses, older and younger subjects did not differ in the self-rated intensity of their feelings. Malatesta and Kalnok (1984) factored a number of statements about the types and experiences of emotion. Like Lawton et al. (1992), they found that items relating to intensity split into NA and PA factors. No mean difference in these factors were noted between young, middle-aged, and older groups of 80 subjects each. In another study (Malatesta, Izard, Culver, & Nicolich, 1987) involving emotion induction in women of different ages, no age differences were observed in self-rated intensity, nor did decoders of facial expression intensity reveal any age differences. In a study of anger induction and the type A personality, Malatesta-Magai, Jonas, Shepard, and Culver (1992) found that older people reported *more* overt behavioral expression of anger than did younger people, and in judges' ratings of facial expression ratings of induced emotion, they were significantly more likely to express anger, sadness, fear, and interest under eliciting conditions that targeted each of these affects.

These conflicting findings indicate a need for considerably more research on the topic. It is clear, first, that intensity is difficult for people to characterize independently of frequency. The splitting of intensity measures between positive and negative instances in the research of both Lawton et al. (1992) and Malatesta and Kalnok (1984), as well as the fact that intensity and frequency ratings fell on the same factors, suggested that if these two parameters are to be understood separately, new study methods will be needed. It may be of note that contemporary induced subjective affect states measured on the spot also produced conflicting findings: No age difference in affect intensity was reported by Levinson et al. (1991), but significantly less anger and anxiety by the Malatesta-Magai et al. (1992) older subjects.

4. INTENSITY AND HEALTH

Although health was not investigated as such, Malatesta-Magai et al. (1992) posited that type A individuals who were more expressive of their feelings would be healthier than those who did not exhibit behavioral signs of anger in response to the subjective experience of anger. If this is true, the lesser link between type A and heart disease found in older subjects might be due to the survivorship into old age of the more affectively expressive type A personality. Their results showing more behavioral expression among the older subjects is consistent with this reasoning. Another of their findings raises other questions, however. Despite their greater behavioral indicators, older subjects reported less subjective trait anger and anxiety than younger subjects. It is worth considering further the hypothesis that less intense affect may be experienced subjectively at the same time as (or even because of) greater behavioral expression. This would be consistent with Buck's (1984) distinction between people who internalize and who externalize.

5. RECENCY

Recency of affect as an influence on QOL has not been tested with older people. Indirect evidence regarding the recency effect may be found in the research relating measures of QOL to time following major events. An example is provided by the negative event of spousal bereavement. Most research (see review by Murrell & Meeks, 1992) has shown significant depression following the death of a spouse. Research mapping depression against postbereavement time has shown a slow return to prebereavement levels (Lund, Caserta, & Dimond, 1989; Murrell & Himmelfarb, 1989; Mendes de Leon, Kasl, & Jacobs, 1994; Thompson, Gallagher-Thompson, Futterman, Gilewski, & Peterson, 1991). It should also be noted that a very different trajectory is shown in a more domain-specific indicator of QOL, that of mourning or feeling of loss, which may be much more persistent (Thompson et al., 1991). In another study, cross-sectional research noted a significant difference between depression frequency among those bereaved for 6–8 months and those with longer postbereavement intervals (Winter, Lawton, Casten, & Sando, 1996). This study tested an analogous hypothesis for PA, showing selective elevation of PA among elders married 6–8 months previously, as compared to married elders unselected for duration of marriage. These data also underlined the potency of the two-factor structure of affect, in showing no influence of bereavement on PA or of recent marriage on depression. Such suggestive findings underline the potential usefulness of mapping the course of multiple affect states across time in such a way as to study the lagged effects of single affect states upon subsequent hedonic integrals of varying durations. Another study among younger adults showed that "only recent events matter"; that is, subjective well-being was influenced only by events that occurred within the past 3 months (Suh, Diener, & Fujita, 1996).

6. Positive and Negative Affect

Positive and negative affect need always to be differentiated as they were in Figure 1. The dynamics of PA appear to differ from those of NA. Taylor (1991) reviewed evidence suggesting that physiological arousal is greater for NA than for PA, although there is a tendency for NA to decay more quickly and to a lower level than PA (the "mobilization–minimization hypothesis"). The possible age functions of such processes have not been studied, however.

7. The Timing of Hedonic Calculus

The time span over which one's estimate of QOL is assessed may vary infinitely. QOL may be construed to represent one's entire life so far, stages of life (a happy childhood), a historical period (the Depression), major life events (parent loss, marriage, retirement), minor events, or simple nonevent-related slices of time ("during the past week," "today so far," "right now"). Research data are not available on the mechanics by which people invoke differing time frames and integrate their super-imposed QOL schemata, particularly whether age differences in the de-gree of "chunking" of calendar time increase as the overall length of life-time lived so far increases. A hypothesis is advanced to account for the ability to enhance QOL even in the face of poor health, losses, and other stressors.

a. The Temporal Optimization Principle of Subjective QOL.   When a per-son conceptualizes her own QOL at a given time, the time span over which the hedonic calculus is performed is selected so as to bracket affect states within maximum PA and minimum NA. Thus responding to "How happy are you in general?" might involve excluding input from an earlier pe-riod of life when one was happier than one is now. One may also invoke a social comparison (Carp & Carp, 1981) standard where a more contem-porary time bracket allows the person to compare herself with others less fortunate. On a bad day, "How happy are you right now?" might be refer-enced back a day or two in time to encompass good days and lessen the influence of today's health symptoms or bad mood.

No argument is made here for the age-specificity of temporal opti-mization. Nonetheless, such an idea may help explain the findings of Williamson and Schulz (1995) and the less than expected intrusion of physical symptoms and pain into the daily lives of older people. A similar dynamism was suggested to apply to the maintenance of personal control among disabled elders who were confined to their homes, a single room, or a chair in a room (Lawton, 1985). Many of these people appeared to have established physical "control centers," a location, often a fixed posi-tion in a chair, from which stimulation, knowledge, and security could be maximized: A view of the street, the front porch, the front door; location in a high-resource living room; reachable surfaces for books, food, per-sonal objects, medicine; and communication with the world outside the home through telephone, television, and radio. This principle of "den-sity of control" represents a cognitive-ecological maximization of benefits despite their severely constricted behavioral space. The temporal opti-mization principle represents an analogous cognitive-affective maximiza-tion of benefits. In each instance the boundaries of one's life space were proactively altered in the direction of preserving the most desirable out-comes possible in the face of threats of physical and psychological stress.

Looking back at the use of AL theory to examine properties of the "focal stimulus," the analogy with the hedonic integral is only approxi-mate. In psychophysics one can measure physical amounts, whereas many attributes of affects are psychological. Thus stimulus and response are innately confounded in this application of AL theory to QOL. Nonetheless, looking at the structure of the experience of affect identifies a process whose relationship to the other two determinants of QOL can be examined.

B. Past Experience, Adaptation, and Affect Regulations

Of the three sources of influence on AL, past experience is the one where age effects might be most logically expected. As one ages one cumulates experience in every sense, including affect experience. Thus a longer lifetime may mean both more affect input and more learning how to make the most of one's affect. Two processes may be distinguished that differ in the role taken by the subject. Adaptation refers to reactive change from repeated exposure to affect-inducing situations, whereas self-regulation refers to more active processes of mastery of affect input and response. Not all change or perceived change over time in affect dynamics can be assigned definitively to adaptation or self-regulation.

1. ADAPTATION

The nervous system has limits beyond which attention cannot be maintained in the face of continuous stimulation. One adapts to ongoing stimulation and becomes more receptive to novel stimulation. However, novel or very complex stimuli may be threatening at first. They may become less threatening through repetition and ultimately become affectively nonactivating with continued exposure. As Schulz (1982) suggested, it might well be that simple repetition of either PA or NA states over a lifetime might result in raising the threshold for the experience of either affect valence, producing a restriction in range of intensity, frequency, duration, or quality ("dampening," Diener, Colvin, Pavot, & Allman, 1991). One could hypothesize that such cognitive strategies repeated over life could also moderate or augment affect experience. The data from Diener et al. (1985) on age and intensity would be consistent with dampening of both PA and NA.

a. Dampening the Negative.   In the Lawton et al. (1992) study, several items of the type "I have the same worries and bad moods that I always have had but they bother me less at this stage of life" were endorsed more frequently by older people. Such meta-experiential statements could also be consistent with more proactive self-management strategies. Other strategies are more clearly active and focused, as expressed in the item, "Part of maturity is being able to arrange your life so there are fewer highs and fewer lows." This factor, labeled Emotional Maturity Through Moderation, contained other more passive content, such as, "My feelings are likely to become more moderate as I grow older." Older subjects perceived such age-related maturity to a much greater degree than did middle-aged and younger subjects.

   b. Dampening the Positive.   Although the desirability of dampening NAs cannot be argued, if the same thing happens to PAs, QOL may suffer. In the Lawton et al. (1992) research on dimensions of experience, another factor emerged that was named Leveling of Positive Affect. This factor included three items referring to novelty or excitement, all of which, as well as the factor score as a whole, showed more leveling among older as compared to middle-aged subjects. Two other items failed to show an age difference; they referred to differences in elation and interest, compared to similar feelings "during my twenties." Thus one concludes that dampening may have occurred for the more extreme degrees of engagement with external objects but not with the capacity for moderate engagement and the positive feelings that go with it.

   Does the opponent-process hypothesized by Solomon (1980) put people at risk for an excessively intense negative rebound after a highly positive affective experience? Are people aware of this risk and do they exert active preventive effort? Although Sandvik, Diener, and Larsen (1989) found that adaptation to both positive and negative stimuli occurred, opposite-valence affect as hypothesized in opponent-process theory did not become greater as a function of the length of exposure to the original valence. Other evidence inconsistent with PA dampening was seen in the very low endorsement rate for the item, "If I feel exceptionally elated for a while, I know I will soon turn to feeling depressed"; and elders were significantly less likely to agree with this statement than were younger adults (Lawton et al., 1992).

   c. Health.   A special instance is health, symptoms, and pain. Surprisingly, the evidence as to whether the pain experience differs by age remains rather ambiguous, despite the clear increase in morbidity due to pain-producing illnesses such as arthritis. The prevalence of pain appears to vary little with age (Gibson, Katz, Corran, Farrell, & Helme, 1994). Little agreement is found regarding age differences in other qualities of pain or pain management strategies. Nonetheless, pain is a major correlate of negative QOL. Is there such a thing as adaptation to pain and other distressing physical symptoms? Where pain is reported it is related to depression (Parmelee, Katz, & Lawton, 1991; Williamson & Schulz, 1995). The latter authors review evidence suggesting that "similar levels of disease-related chronic pain seem to be tolerated better by older than by younger adults," perhaps because "they view such changes as a normal part of the aging process" (p. 370). Williamson and Schulz (1995) also suggested that the cognition that illness is "normal" for age is a control mechanism that leads to lowered emotional distress.

d. Control. Attempting to control one's feelings actively is a more directive process than adaptive dampening, whose purpose is to limit the impact rather than the onset of the affect. An eight-item factor named Emotional Control was much higher in the older adult group studied by Lawton et al. (1992). Illustrative items include, "I try to avoid reacting emotionally, whether the emotion is positive or negative" and "Detachment or cool judgment is my best way to meet most life situations." McConatha, Lightner, and Deaner (1994) used the Emotional Control Questionnaire (Roger & Najarian, 1989) to test differences between a young-adult and middle-aged group. They found the middle-aged group to endorse control mechanisms of Rehearsal and Emotion Inhibition more than the young.

e. Mood Repair. One other aspect of the effect of past experience and practice upon affect is the possibility of deliberately changing the valence of the affect. An example of such an attempt to change affect has been studied in the general psychological literature under the name "mood repair" and similar terms. The research of Thayer, Newman, and McClain (1994) suggested that people seek to optimize their activation levels by raising or lowering their energy expenditures to combat depression. Although age differences were tested, they tended to appear in relation to individual indicators of mood management rather than as a total stylistic pattern.

In summary, past experience is the source of the cognitive-affective schemata that compose varying proportions of the determinants of QOL for a given reference time period. The person actively constructs the schemata and in addition to their contribution to QOL (the person as object), the schemata are actually utilized to give meaning to contemporary experiences and to optimize QOL in a dynamic process. Past experience with affective stimuli tends to lead to adaptation, or habituation, but the cognitive and affective learning also gives the power to repair mood, control affect, and change the mix of contributors to QOL.

C. The Environmental Context of Quality of Life

In AL theory, the field in which the focal stimulus is embedded exerts a major influence on the character of the experience, analogous to contrast or assimilation effects of background hue on the judged color of a stimulus patch. As in the discussion of the focal stimulus, the analogy of context with the stimulus field in AL theory is only approximate. The material to be presented treats influences on QOL deriving from factors outside the individual, broadly classed as social contexts, external events, and the external environment. As in the discussion of past experience, contextual effects may occur in both reactive and proactive modes.

1. SOCIAL CONTEXTS

Frederickson and Carstensen (1990) provided experimental documentation of a mechanism by which cognitive and behavioral control of emotion was attained by older, middle-aged, and younger adults. The research was designed to test Carstensen's socioemotional selectivity theory. This theory suggests that as people age they conserve their personal resources by regulating the amount of contact they have with others and the degree to which they invest emotionally in social relationships. Using groups with ages across the full adult life span, they asked subjects to perform similarity sorts for 18 prototypic types of people, such as a close friend, a family member, a stranger your age, or a poet or artist you admire. Multidimensional scaling identified three dimensions underlying the judgments: Probability of high versus low future contact, anticipated positive or negative affect in interaction with the person, and high versus low information seeking. Elders organized their social partner choices most in terms of affect expected, rather than either future contact or information. In a second study, they asked subjects to choose between a familiar partner (family member) and two novel partners (new acquaintance or an author) to spend time with, first under no specified conditions, and second, under the condition of having a free evening before moving to a distant location (the social ending condition). Although younger subjects were much more likely to choose the novel social partner, when they were given the condition that included the social ending they made the affectively based choice of a family member. Frederickson and Carstensen concluded that older people were not less desirous of, or less emotionally involved in, social relationships, but were more selective and resource conserving about the conditions of such investment. Furthermore, the selective use of resources had more to do with the prospective social ending than with age itself. It thus seems that there is no affective disengagement from best friends or closest family members. The question remains to be investigated, however, as to whether the quality of the affect (e.g., intensity or valence) is influenced by age, health, or the social ending.

2. EXTERNAL EVENTS

The effects of major events have been previously noted and will not be discussed further. The full exploration of the effects of minor events on

QOL is still in process. Daily hassles and daily uplifts were shown to affect estimates of stress and well-being (Delongis, Coyne, Dakof, Folkman, & Lazarus, 1982). This research led to the discovery of a variety of relationships between affect states, health indicators, and daily events (Stone, 1981; Tennen, Suls, & Affleck, 1991). General congruence between event valence and affect was demonstrated among community-resident adults (Zautra & Reich, 1983) and older people in residential care (Lawton, Devoe, & Parmelee, 1995). Specialized methodologies are necessary for the study of such intrapersonal processes (Tennen et al., 1991; Zautra, Affleck, & Tennen, 1994).

Leisure-time activities are prototypic proactive event manipulations. They are usually self-initiated. In the Lawton et al. (1992) study, the item, "I choose activities carefully so as to give me just the right amount of emotional stimulation, neither too much nor too little" was endorsed more frequently by older people. Participation in such activities has usually been associated with PA (Lawton, 1994; Lawton et al., 1995).

Two important dimensions of events were singled out for study by Reich, Zautra, and their colleagues. Zautra and Reich (1983) distinguished between events that simply happen to a person ("pawn" events, de Charms, 1968) and those that occur as the result of active effort by the person ("origin" events). They also contrasted "desires" and "demands," activities engaged in because of the active wish to gratify personal wishes versus those performed through some obligatory or instrumental motive (Reich & Zautra, 1983). Origin events and desire behaviors tended to result in PA but influenced NA minimally. Pawn experiences and demands, even positive ones, showed a tendency to be associated with negative affective consequences. Further evidence for the affective consequences of proactivity are seen in Langston's (1994) demonstration that expressive, self-initiated actions in response to positive events further amplified the positive affective responses to the events themselves. Among older people, however, the clear relationships noted above were less regular (Reich, Zautra, & Hill, 1987). Active responding to events was associated with both positive and negative well-being, and even demand–event responding was associated with PA; responding to "desire" events was also associated with decreased negative well-being, in contrast to the lack of such cross-category relationships among younger subjects in their earlier study. Reich et al. speculated that these results are consistent with the idea that all types of events may hover around the challenge–stress boundary for older subjects and thus have broader affective outcomes. This is also consistent with the daily events study of Lawton et al. (1995), which showed both same valence and crossover effects of event valence on both PA and NA, rather than the affect specificity found in the study of bereaved and recently married people (Winter et al., 1996). It is possible that the "smallness" of events intrinsically has more diffused effects on affect states than do major events.

Reich & Zautra (1987) defined an event as "a change from usual everyday occurrences," as distinguished from ongoing daily activities. AL is reestablished in response to a change in input from any source, whether the focal stimulus, the relevance of past experience, or the character of the stimulus field. Thus novelty and routine are important features of the context. Sensation seeking (Zuckerman, 1978) is an expression of personal need and behavioral proactivity to search for novel experiences with a resulting increase in experienced intensity, whether sensory, cognitive, or affective. In the Lawton et al. (1992) study of dimensions of experiencing, items from the Reducer Index (Herzog, Williams, & Weintraub, 1985) were included in the factor analysis. All items formed a single cluster, but some items failed to load on the common factor because of near-zero endorsement rates by older people. Three items nonetheless formed a factor replicable across ages, expressing liking for excitement, variety, and noisy parties. Middle-aged and older people were much lower in this stimulus-seeking factor than younger adults. Reich and Zautra (1987) also examined "routinization" as an individual-difference trait expressing a cautious route to controlling everyday events. Extended discussion of novelty versus familiarity among older people may be found in Lawton (1989). Much research remains to be done to investigate which aspects of event proactivity and change management are related to age and which are more like individual differences irrespective of age.

3. ENVIRONMENT

Environmental proactivity describes the process where a person chooses or creates an environmental context, one of whose properties is that events will occur with differing probabilities (Lawton, 1985). These probabilities may be comprehended by the person and used to optimize the affect outcomes associated with that context. Long-term choices such as moving to planned housing (Carp, 1966) or making "amenity moves" (Wiseman & Roseman, 1977) to retirement areas of the country have been associated with affective-cognitive indicators of QOL such as housing satisfaction. In a detailed analysis of the mechanisms underlying the high housing satisfaction of older people, Campbell et al. (1976) suggested that both the internal affect-regulation mechanism of adaptation and liking through familiarity (Zajonc, 1968), as well as the objectively higher housing quality obtained over one's life by successive approximation to one's ideal housing, contributed to such age-specific QOL. Strong affective attachment to home (Rubinstein, 1989) is implied by the low wish of elders to relocate, even in the face of apparent objective "push" factors such as old housing or crime-ridden locations.

To conclude this section on context, daily events, ongoing daily life, and complex environments all represent influences of the environmental surrounds on affect outcomes. Thus they constitute a major aspect of QOL. In addition, sometimes change in context is at least as important an influence as the absolute character of the context. One dimension of environmental change, the agency of the person in producing the change and the desired affective outcome, has been shown to be important. Others need to be investigated.

IV. CONCLUSION

The connection between events and QOL is clearly mediated by affect and the hedonic integral of these states. Events may be protracted in time, as in the case where the event of residential location in turn creates, or allows the person to form, an ongoing set of new daily events. In contexts that are ongoing and relatively stable, the person's familiarity and sense of personal competence in living in that context contribute to the mild sense of PA that constitutes most people's baseline level of QOL. Intrusions of negative events are more likely as personal competence decreases and as contexts become imposed rather than chosen. Internally focused affect management processes such as adaptation and cognitive control come into play at that point. Thus the continuing motivation to remain proactive, together with the use of reactive affect management mechanisms, accounts for the surplus of PA over NA states.

QOL has been defined as the subjective judgment of the net valence of one's life as marked by time intervals from very brief to very long. Contributors to this experienced valence are relatively stable temperament, cognitive-affective schemata from past experiences, and the hedonic integral of the duration, intensity, and quality of the affects encompassed in the targeted time interval. People evaluate QOL utilizing a time interval that will optimize the net of PA and NA qualities. QOL in these terms contributes to overall psychological well-being and mental health, as do the environment and behavioral competence. QOL among older people appears positive by comparison with other age groups in some estimates of the frequencies of PA and NA, although research shows some conflicting findings. Older people appear to experience emotion in somewhat different ways than do younger people, the differences showing greater selectivity in responding and increased control. Adaptation-level theory provides a convenient structure in which to examine affect-management learning over the life span.

ACKNOWLEDGMENTS

Much of the research described in this chapter and support for its writing was provided by a MERIT award grant from the National Institute on Aging (Grant AG07001).

REFERENCES

Andrews, F. M., & Withey, S. B. (1976). *Social indicators of well-being.* New York: Plenum Press.

Bradburn, N. M. (1969). *The structure of psychological well-being.* Chicago: Aldine.

Buck, R. (1984). *The communication of emotion.* New York: Guilford Press.

Burt, R. S., Wiley, J. A., Minor, M. J., & Murray, J. R. (1978). Structure of well being. *Sociological Methods & Research, 6,* 365–407.

Campbell, A., Converse, P., & Rogers, W. (1976). *Quality of life in America.* New York: Russell Sage.

Carp, F. (1966). *A future for the aged.* Austin: University of Texas Press.

Carp, F., & Carp, A. (1981). It may not be the answer, it may be the question. *Research on Aging, 3,* 85–100.

de Charms, R. (1968). *Personal causation.* New York: Academic Press.

DeLongis, A., Coyne, C., Dakof, G. Folkman, S., & Lazarus, R. S. (1982). Relationship of daily hassles, uplifts, and major life events to health status. *Health Psychology, 1,* 119–136.

Diener, E., Colvin, C. R., Pavot, W. G., & Allman, A. (1991). The psychic costs of intense positive affect. *Journal of Personality and Social Psychology, 61,* 492–503.

Diener, E., & Diener, C. (1996). Most people are happy. *Psychological Science, 7,* 181–185.

Diener, E., & Emmons, R. (1984). The independence of positive and negative affect. *Journal of Personality and Social Psychology, 47,* 1105–1117.

Diener, E., Sandvik, E., & Larsen, R. J. (1985). Age and sex effects for emotional intensity. *Developmental Psychology, 21,* 542–546.

Epstein, S. (1983). Aggregation and beyond: Some basic issues on the prediction of behavior. *Journal of Personality, 51,* 360–392.

Frederickson, B. L., & Carstensen, L. L. (1990). Choosing a social partner: How old age and anticipated endings make people more selective. *Psychology and Aging, 5,* 335–347.

Frijda, N. H. (1988). The laws of emotion. *American Psychologist, 43,* 349–358.

Gatz, M., Johansson, B., Pederson, N., Berg, S., & Reynolds, C. (1993). A cross-national self-report measure of depressive symptomatology. *International Psychogeriatrics, 5,* 147–156.

George, L. K., & Bearon, L. B. (1980). *Quality of life in older persons. Meaning and measurement.* New York: Human Sciences Press.

Gibson, S. J., Katz, B., Corran, M., Farrell, M. J., & Helme, R. D. (1994). Pain in older persons. *Disability and Rehabilitation, 16,* 127–139.

Helson, H. (1964). *Adaptation-level theory.* New York: Harper and Row.

Herzog, T. R., Williams, D. M., & Weintraub, D. J. (1985). Meanwhile, back at personality ranch: The augmenters and reducers ride again. *Journal of Personality and Social Psychology, 48,* 1342–1352.

Langston, C. A. (1994). Capitalizing on and coping with daily life events: Expressive responses to positive events. *Journal of Personality and Social Psychology, 67,* 1112–1125.

Larsen, R. J. (1985). *The Affect Intensity Measure (AIM). Preliminary manual.* Psychology Department, Purdue University, Lafayette, IN.

Larsen, R. J., & Diener, E. (1987). Affect intensity as an individual difference characteristic. A review. *Journal of Research in Personality, 21,* 1–39.

Lawton, M. P. (1977). Morale: What are we measuring? In C. Nydegger (Ed.), *Measuring morale: A guide to effective assessment* (pp. 6–14). Washington, DC: Gerontological Society.

Lawton, M. P. (1983). Environment and other determinants of well-being in older people. *The Gerontologist, 23,* 349–357.

Lawton, M. P. (1985). The elderly in context: Perspectives from environmental psychology and gerontology. *Environment and Behavior, 17,* 501–519.

Lawton, M. P. (1989). Environmental proactivity and affect in older people. In S. Spacapan & S. Oskamp (Eds.), *Social psychology of aging* (pp. 135–164). Newbury Park, CA: Sage.

Lawton, M. P. (1991). A multidimensional view of quality of life. In J. E. Birren, J. E. Lubben, J. C. Rowe, & D. E. Deutchman (Eds.), *The concept and measurement of quality of life in the frail elderly* (pp. 3–27). San Diego: Academic Press.

Lawton, M. P. (1994). Personality and affective correlates of leisure activity participation by older people. *Journal of Leisure Research, 26,* 138–157.

Lawton, M. P., Devoe, M. R., & Parmelee, P. (1995). The relationship of events and affect in the daily lives of an elderly population. *Psychology and Aging, 19,* 469–477.

Lawton, M. P., Kleban, M. H., & Dean, J. (1993). Affect and age: Cross-sectional comparisons of structure and prevalence. *Psychology and Aging, 8,* 165–175.

Lawton, M. P., Kleban, M. H., Rajagopal, D., & Dean, J. (1992). The dimensions of affective experience in three age groups. *Psychology and Aging, 7,* 171–184.

Levinson, R. W., Carstensen, L. L., Friesen, W. V., & Ekman, P. (1991). Emotion, physiology, and expression in old age. *Psychology and Aging, 6,* 28–35.

Lund, D. A., Caserta, M. S., & Dimond, M. F. (1989). Impact of spousal bereavement on subjective well-being of older adults. In D. A. Lund (Ed.), *Older bereaved spouses* (pp. 3–15). New York: Hemisphere.

Malatesta, C. Z., Izard, C. E., Culver, C., & Nicholich, M. (1987). Emotion communication skills in young, middle-aged, and older women. *Psychology and Aging, 2,* 193–203.

Malatesta-Magai, C., Jonas, R., Shepard, B., & Culver, L. C. (1992). Type A behavior pattern and emotion expression in younger and older adults. *Psychology and Aging, 7,* 551–561.

Malatesta, C. Z., & Kalnok, M. (1984). Emotional experience in younger and older adults. *Journal of Gerontology, 39,* 301–308.

McConatha, J. T., Lightner, E., & Deaner, S. L. (1994). Culture, age and gender as variables in the expression of emotions. *Journal of Social Behavior and Personality, 9,* 481–488.

Mendes de Leon, C. F., Kasl, S. V., & Jacobs, S. (1994). A prospective study of widowhood and changes in symptoms of depression in a community sample of the elderly. *Psychological Medicine, 24,* 613–624.

Murrell, A., & Himmelfarb, S. (1989). Effects of attachment bereavement and pre-event conditions on subsequent depressive symptoms in older adults. *Psychology and Aging, 4,* 166–172.

Murrell, S. A., & Meeks, S. (1992). Depressive symptoms in older adults: Predispositions, resources and life experiences. In K. W. Schaie (Ed.), *Annual review of gerontology and geriatrics* (pp. 261–286). New York: Springer Publishing Company.

Newmann, J. P. (1989). Aging and depression. *Psychology and Aging, 4,* 150–165.

Parmelee, P. A., Katz, I. R., & Lawton, M. P. (1991). The relation of pain to depression among the institutionalized aged. *Journal of Gerontology: Psychological Sciences, 46,* 15–21.

Reich, J., & Zautra, A. (1983). Demands and desires in daily life: Some influences on well-being. *American Journal of Community Psychology, 11,* 41–58.

Reich, J. W., & Zautra, A. J. (1987, June). *An event-based approach to personality mediation of subjective well-being.* Paper presented at Conference on Subjective Well-Being, Bad Homberg, Germany.

Reich, J. W., Zautra, A. J., & Hill, J. (1987). Activity-event transactions and quality of life in older adults. *Psychology and Aging, 2,* 116–124.

Roger, D., & Najarian, B. (1989). The construction of a new scale for measuring emotion control. *Personality and Individual Differences, 10,* 845–853.

Rubinstein, R. (1989). The home environment of older people and description of the psycho-social process linking person to place. *Journal of Gerontology: Social Sciences, 44,* S45–S53.

Sandvik, E., Diener, E., & Larsen, R. J. (1985). The opponent process theory and affective reactions. *Motivation and Emotion, 9,* 407–418.

Schulz, R. (1982). Emotionality and aging: A theoretical and empirical analysis. *Journal of Gerontology, 37,* 42–51.

Solomon, R. L. (1980). The opponent-process theory of acquired motivation: The costs of pleasure and the benefits of pain. *American Psychologist, 35,* 691–712.

Stone, A. A. (1981). The association between perceptions of daily experiences and self and spouse rated mood. *Journal of Research in Personality, 15,* 510–522.

Suh, E., Diener, E., & Fujita, F. (1996). Events and subjective well-being: Only recent events matter. *Journal of Personality and Social Psychology, 70,* 1091–1102.

Taylor, S. E. (1991). Asymmetrical effects of positive and negative events: The mobilization-minimization hypothesis. *Psychological Bulletin, 110,* 67–85.

Tennen, H., Suls, J., & Affleck, G. (Eds.). (1991). Personality and daily experience. *Journal of Personality* (Whole No. 3), *59.*

Thayer, R. E., Newman, J. R., & McClain, T. M. (1994). *Journal of Personality and Social Psychology, 67,* 910–925.

Thompson, L. W., Gallagher-Thompson, D., Futterman, A., Gilewski, M. J., & Peterson, J. (1991). The effects of late-life spousal bereavement over a 30-month interval. *Psychology and Aging, 6,* 434–441.

Williamson, G. M., & Schulz, R. (1995). Activity restriction mediates the association between pain and depressed affect: A study of younger and older cancer patients. *Psychology and Aging, 10,* 369–378.

Winter, L., Lawton, M. P., Casten, R. J., & Sando, R. (1996). *The relationship between external events and affect states of moderate temporal span in older people.* Unpublished manuscript.

Wiseman, R. F., & Roseman, C. C. (1977). A typology of elderly migration based on the decision-making process. *Economic Geography, 55,* 324–337.

Zajonc, R. B. (1968). Attitudinal effects of mere exposure. *Journal of Personality and Social Psychology Monographs, 9,* (Part 2), 1–28.

Zautra, A. J., Affleck, G., & Tennen, H. (1994). Assessing life events among older adults. In M. P. Lawton & J. A. Teresi (Eds.), *Annual review of gerontology and geriatrics* (vol. 14, pp. 324–352). New York: Springer Publishing Company.

Zautra, A. J., & Reich, J. W. (1983). Life events and perceptions of life quality; Developments in a two-factor approach. *Journal of Community Psychology, 11,* 121–132.

Zautra, A. J., Reich, J. W., & Guarnaccia, C. A. (1990). Some everyday life consequences of disability and bereavement for older adults. *Journal of Personality and Social Psychology, 59,* 550–561.

Zuckerman, M. (1978). *Sensation-seeking: Beyond the optimal level of arousal.* Hillsdale, NJ: Lawrence Erlbaum.

CHAPTER 19

Religion,

Emotions,

and Health

Susan H. McFadden *and* Jeffrey S. Levin
Department of Psychology   *Department of Family and Community*
University of Wisconsin—Oshkosh   *Medicine*
Oshkosh, Wisconsin   *Eastern Virginia Medical School*
                      Norfolk, Virginia

I. INTRODUCTION

One of the pervading effects of religion's role in societies and in individual lives is the selection and orchestration of emotions through public ritual observances and private meditative acts. Religions also shape beliefs about "holy" and "unholy" emotions (Pruyser, 1968). Given the renewed vigor of the psychological study of emotion, as well as recent methodological and theoretical advances in the psychology of religion, the time seems right for an explicit consideration of (a) how religion shapes and modulates emotion and (b) the outcomes of religious influences on emotion. One of these outcomes—health—is suggested in accumulating evidence about the impact of psychosocial variables on physical well-being and the mediating role of emotion (Leventhal & Patrick-Miller, 1993).

Because other chapters in this volume review research on health and emotion, this chapter focuses on epidemiologic studies of religion and health. It begins with a review of key issues in gerontological research on religion followed by a discussion of recent findings about the epidemiology of religion. Possible etiologic mechanisms for salutary religious effects are described and then examined in detail to elaborate on their emotional components. John Bowlby's attachment theory applied to adult life (see Berman & Sperling, 1994; Weiss, 1982) provides an organizing framework for this discussion. Although some of the studies cited include young and middle-aged adults, the majority focus on older persons. Because gerontologists investigating the parameters of well-being in later life have increasingly noted the contribution of religious variables (McFadden, 1996), the literature on aging has produced the largest and most coherent body of evidence about the effects of religion on health.

II. GERONTOLOGICAL RESEARCH ON RELIGION

Among the factors influencing the growth of research on religion and aging is the high degree of religiosity among the current cohort of older adults. Religious beliefs, behaviors, and experiences along with a more general sense of spirituality have been shown to contribute to the variance in measured well-being in the older population. High-quality quantitative and qualitative research on religion and spirituality has begun to appear in the gerontological literature, and many have interpreted this trend as reflecting efforts to find alternatives to biomedical views of aging and old age that focus on physical decline. Recent social gerontological research has begun to focus on (a) multidimensional measures, (b) patterns, (c) predictors, and (d) psychosocial and health-related outcomes of religious involvement in older adults and across the life course.

The *measurement* of religiosity is an important but often neglected issue for researchers who are nonspecialists in the study of religion. Much epidemiologic research on religiosity has emphasized simple constructs such as religious denomination or attendance (see Levin & Vanderpool, 1987), and thus has focused on only a narrow portion of religious life. Recent gerontological work, on the other hand, has utilized validated scales and multidimensional measures, thus capturing a fuller range of religious involvement. Here, the construct of religiosity has been taken to encompass those behaviors that reflect organizational (i.e., public, institutional, formal) or nonorganizational (i.e., private, noninstitutional, informal) religious involvement, as well as subjective religious feelings or attitudes. This multidimensional approach is the prevailing conceptual model of religiosity used in aging research.

Although the ways religiosity is expressed are common across age cohorts, particular *patterns* of involvement are more or less predominant depending upon one's age and functional status (Levin & Vanderpool, 1987). For example, as older adults age and, on average, experience declining functional health, a concomitant decline in organizational religious participation may be offset by nonorganizational expression of religiosity (Witter, Stock, Okun, & Haring, 1985). Notwithstanding these health-related declines in organizational participation among the oldest cohorts, findings from the 1990 General Social Survey (GSS) reveal that at least weekly religious attendance is more common with successively older age cohorts and among those aged 65 years and older, it is over 46% (Levin, 1995), a rise of nearly 10% over 1978 data (Markides, 1987). Furthermore, among respondents aged 75 years and older in 1990, nearly three-fourths pray at least daily (Levin, 1995), almost twice as many as in the youngest cohort. Because these data are cross-sectional, it is not possible to conclude whether they indicate increased religiosity with age or greater religiosity among older cohorts. However, the comparison with earlier data raises the possibility that both cohort *and* aging effects may be present (see Moberg, 1990).

Research on *predictors* of religious involvement has been hampered by a lack of studies drawing on large, national probability surveys. A notable exception is the work of Taylor and associates using data from the National Survey of Black Americans. Both over the life course (Taylor, 1988) and among older adults (Taylor, 1986), several sociodemographic characteristics significantly predict religious attendance, nonorganizational involvement, and subjective religiosity in African Americans, including age, education, and marriage, as well as being female and living in rural areas in the South. Data on older adults from four national surveys document clear and consistent gender and racial differences in nearly every religious indicator examined (Levin, Taylor, & Chatters, 1994). African Americans and women are more religious than Whites and men, respectively, even after controlling for the effects of age, education, marital status, family income, region, urbanicity, and subjective health.

Finally, researchers have identified statistically significant, salutary religious effects on many psychosocial and health-related *outcomes* in older adults. These include subjective health, functional disability, mortality, symptomatology, hypertension prevalence, cancer prevalence, smoking and drinking behavior, coping, self-esteem and mastery, and dimensions of mental health and well-being, such as life satisfaction, depressive symptoms, chronic anxiety, loneliness, happiness, and emotional adjustment (see Levin, 1994a, for a review).

III. THE EPIDEMIOLOGY OF RELIGION

Over the past century, the impact of religious involvement on physical health and illness has been a popular, though not publicized, topic of empirical research in epidemiology and medicine. More than 200 published studies have identified religious differences in a broad range of health outcomes and have investigated the effects of religious involvement, variously defined, on many health status measures and rates of morbidity and mortality (Levin & Vanderpool, 1989). Until recently, however, this literature was not widely known, perhaps because few of these studies were designed to focus specifically on the effects of religion on health. Rather, in typical epidemiologic fashion, investigators charged with directing large-scale studies of heart disease, cancer, life expectancy, or other outcomes, and wishing to ensure the collection of data on as many psychosocial and biological variables as possible, likely permitted a few religion variables to slip seredipitously into their studies. As a result, statistical findings bearing on these variables are often buried in tables and not even discussed in the papers in which they appear.

Results of these studies are remarkably consistent. Although there are exceptions, findings mostly point to a salutary effect of religious involvement on health status. It is especially noteworthy that findings suggestive of a protective effect for religiosity have been found across populations regardless of gender, race, or ethnicity (e.g., Caucasians, African Americans, Hispanics), age (from adolescents to the old-old), national origin (U.S., Europe, Africa, Asia), study design (prospective, retrospective, cohort, case-control, cross-sectional), religious affiliation (e.g., Protestants, Catholics, Jews, Parsis, Buddhists, Hindus, Muslims), the religious measures employed (e.g., denomination, religious attendance, belief in God, religious experience, frequency of prayer), and, most importantly, the outcomes under study. These encompass self-limiting acute conditions, fatal chronic diseases, and illnesses with lengthy, brief, or absent latency periods between exposure and diagnosis and mortality (Levin, 1994b), including outcomes related to atherosclerosis, myocardial infarction, most cancer sites, hypertension and stroke, colitis and enteritis, and various cause-specific and overall morbidity and mortality rates.

The preponderance and consistency of findings linking religion and health suggests that something of considerable clinical and basic scientific significance may be revealed through further exploration of this relationship. The most pressing issue for biomedical and behavioral researchers is to identify those characteristics, functions, expressions, or manifestations of being religious or practicing religion that are health-related. Alternative explanations for this association have been proposed, each one representing a possible etiologic mechanism based on respective social, behavioral, psychological, or biological factors already believed to influence health and illness (see Levin & Vanderpool, 1989).

First, religious commitment is associated, on average, with lower rates of smoking, drinking, drug use, and other deleterious *health behaviors* that are known through numerous studies to increase disease risk (Hamburg, Elliott, & Parron, 1982; Jarvis & Northcott, 1987). Second, religious participation and fellowship can lead to integration into *social support* networks and to positive social relationships (Ellison & George, 1994; Tobin, 1991) that exert protective effects on health (House, Landis, & Umberson, 1988). Third, religious worship and prayer can engender a wide range of positive *emotional experiences* such as relaxation, hope, forgiveness, empowerment, catharsis, and love. Research has begun to demonstrate psychoneuroimmunological, neuroendocrine, and psychophysiological pathways through which emotions influence health (Ader, Felten, & Cohen, 1991). Fourth, particular religious beliefs or worldviews are conceptually consonant with certain *health beliefs* and, in many cases, represent the origins of such beliefs (Spector, 1991). Many studies, in turn, show such health-related cognitions to be significantly associated with rates of health and illness (see Jenkins, 1985). Fifth, religious faith may, by itself, lead to optimism or positive expectations regarding health or healing. Research suggests that these positive mental *attitudes* may, through something akin to the placebo effect, promote physical and emotional well-being (Taylor, 1989).

A sixth possibility is that a *multifactorial combination* of the above mechanisms is required to explain the observed effects of religious measures on health outcomes. The joint influence of the various risk factors for the diseases most prevalent in the developed world are often characterized as a "web of causation" (McMahon, Pugh, & Ipsen, 1960)—a multifactorial confluence of multiple etiologic agents. For example, findings linking religious involvement to lower rates of hypertension and cardiovascular diseases (Levin & Vanderpool, 1989) may best be understood by accounting for each of the above mechanisms: religiously committed people are less likely to smoke and consume alcohol, are more likely through regular religious fellowship to receive social support that helps them cope with the stresses of life, are more likely through worship to experience positive emotions that engender a relaxation response and vasodilation, may be less likely to possess or value personality styles or belief patterns that are thought to increase cardiovascular risk, and may benefit from religious beliefs that promote the expectation that their faith will protect them from harm. This latter mechanism may be especially salient among faith communities in which fellow congregants, as a whole, appear to be blessed with good health (e.g., as in the especially low rates of blood pressure and cardiovascular-related morbidity and mortality among Seventh-day Adventists and Mormons).

Each of these etiologic mechanisms can be understood as involving emotion in some way. Even religious proscriptions and prescriptions regarding health behaviors, which seem more rule-focused than emotion-focused, contain an emotional element because those who adopt them do so out of strong conviction, a type of attitude involving emotional commitment (Abelson, 1988). If indeed "emotional processes are the key factors linking psychosocial factors to disease" (Leventhal & Patrick-Miller, 1993, p. 375), then the evidence accumulated in the literature on the epidemiology of religion invites theoretical integration through investigation of the emotional parameters of religion. One promising pathway to this integration is provided by attachment theory.

In the sections that follow, we apply attachment theory to religious behaviors and experiences that have been identified as related to health outcomes. In doing so, we consider the ways these expressions of religiosity engender positive emotions that may have salutary effects (Malatesta, 1989). We recognize that our suggestions are highly speculative, although we find support in research showing the salience of emotion in later life (Carstensen & Turk-Charles, 1994), the significance of religion for many older persons (McFadden, 1996), and the modulation of autonomic and hormonal processes by psychological variables (Maier, Watkins, & Fleshner, 1994). By no means do we wish to imply simple relationships among these complex variables; we acknowledge the high degree of heterogeneity among older persons, the variability among religions, and the redundancy in the neuroendocrinological and immune systems.

IV. ATTACHMENT THEORY AND RELIGION

Theistic religions are essentially relational. For this reason, Bowlby's (1969, 1973, 1980) attachment theory has recently been suggested as a way of organizing and interpreting a wide range of religious behaviors including prayer and meditation, public worship, conversion, and religious coping (Kirkpatrick, 1992). Kirkpatrick (1992, 1995) proposed that religion can be conceptualized as an attachment process wherein religious beliefs and behaviors function as an extension of the attachment system in humans. This biobehavioral system shapes the interpersonal relationship between infants and caregivers; it enables infants to feel safe in the presence of the attachment figure and also secure enough to explore their environments. Based upon early attachment experiences, the child develops cognitive-emotional schemas about interpersonal relationships that later may be associated with a supernatural attachment figure. Kirkpatrick suggested that the God image may function either as a compensation for early failures to develop secure attachment or as a continuation of early parental relationships (either secure or insecure). He wrote,

> *The religious person proceeds with faith that God (or another figure) will be*
> *available to protect and comfort him or her when danger threatens; at other*
> *times, the mere knowledge of God's presence and accessibility allows him or her to*
> *approach the problems and difficulties of daily life with confidence. (Kirkpatrick,*
> *1992, p. 6)*

Researchers now need to test Kirkpatrick's compensation and correspondence hypotheses and to evaluate the effects of individual differences in religious attachment on emotion regulation, religiosity across the life span, and the contribution of religion to health and well-being. The origins and outcomes of hostility, apathy, and indifference to religion also merit further investigation.

To support his contention that religion functions as an attachment process, Kirkpatrick (1992) noted that under conditions of threat, many humans seek a haven of safety in their attachment relation to God. Research on religious coping has demonstrated that both public and private religious behaviors are employed by many individuals when faced with stressful situations (Pargament, in press). Older adults, in particular, spontaneously mention religious coping strategies significantly more often than nonreligious approaches to coping with the major stressors in their lives (Koenig, George, & Siegler, 1988), with prayer being the type most often mentioned (Manfredi & Pickett, 1987). Maton (1989) found that under conditions of high life stress (parents mourning the death of a child), a sense of a relationship with God was inversely related to depression and positively related to self-esteem. For these parents and for many older persons facing situations over which they have no control, religious coping appears to have a positive effect on well-being by offering the emotional comfort of a safe haven and by ordering a structure of meaning for the interpretation of stressful events.

A belief in a just and loving God (presumably indicative of a secure attachment relationship), a perceived supportive relationship with God, participation in religious rituals, and the search itself for support from religion have been found to be significantly associated with positive outcomes to stressful situations (Pargament et al., 1990). These religious coping strategies not only reflect efforts to seek protective haven with an attachment figure; they also reflect confidence in the availability of the attachment figure. This assurance that support and assistance are readily available represents what Bowlby depicted as the secure base.

Considerable theoretical and empirical work is needed to elaborate on the differential origins and outcomes of religious attachment processes. One such possible outcome is health. Epidemiological findings have identified (a) support from membership in religious organizations, (b) public religious participation, and (c) private religious observance as significant protective factors against morbidity and mortality. Each of these types of religious involvement can be interpreted as expressions of attachment processes that have the potential to produce positive emotions and buffer against stress.

A. Social Support in Religious Communities

As many authors have noted, social support is a complex construct encompassing many different kinds of interactive behaviors (Leventhal & Patrick-Miller, 1993) that may function protectively against life stressors, especially when there is some form of attachment relationship with the person or persons providing support (Reite & Boccia, 1994). Given the long-term, reliable, and close relationships that develop in many religious communities, it is not surprising that social support contributes to the stress-buffering effects of religious participation (Friedlander, Kark, & Stein, 1986; Krause & Tran, 1989). Although the actual physiological mechanisms mediating the effect of interpersonal relationships on immune function are not well understood (Kiecolt-Glaser & Glaser, 1989), and the protective effects of social support may not apply to all stress-induced illnesses (Leventhal & Patrick-Miller, 1993), nevertheless there are enough suggestions of a protective function of religious participation to warrant scrutiny of their emotional dynamics.

Religious congregations often refer to themselves as families and indeed, for many older persons, the religious institution is the most trusted social institution besides the family (Payne, 1988). Like families, religious communities can confer a sense of identity and belonging. People grow up and grow older in religious communities, much like they do in families. Religious organizations provide a context for a sense of continuity over the life span, an important characteristic of close social relationships (Antonucci, 1994). Many religious groups reinforce the familial sense through the use of kinship language and imagery, referring to fellow congregants as "brother" and "sister" and thus encouraging the kind of helping behavior often reserved for close family members (Batson, 1983). For some elders, the religious community may even be more important than the family in providing a sense of social integration and support. One study found that older persons' social involvement in a religious organization was significantly more likely to reduce feelings of loneliness than their involvement in family and friendship relations (Johnson & Mullins, 1989).

Actual social interaction may not even be as important for maintaining positive affect as the anticipation that support will be available if needed (Murrell, Chipley, & Norris, 1992). Confidence that clergy and laypersons can be called upon if necessary may be yet another reason why older persons value the social support offered in their religious communities. This support is not only emotional, but may also be instrumental when short-term financial support, goods and services, or assistance during illness are offered. This is particularly true of the kind of support African-American elders receive from their religious communities (Taylor & Chatters, 1986).

A recent study of the relation between religious involvement and social ties found that persons who attend religious services frequently report larger social networks and a greater perceived quality in social interactions. Compared to less frequent attenders and nonattenders, frequent religious attenders were "especially likely to report feeling cared for and valued, and feeling that they are a part of ongoing networks of communication and mutual obligation" (Ellison & George, 1994, p. 57).

For many persons, this sense of interpersonal caring is more significant than the actual content of religious belief. An interview study of 300 Lutherans found great reluctance to discuss basic Christian beliefs. What seemed most central to their religious commitment was the bond these persons felt with co-religionists (Johnson, cited in Wulff, 1991). A similar finding is reported by Ozorak (1996), who interviewed Protestant, Catholic, and Jewish women about their ability to tolerate inhospitable patriarchal beliefs and practices in their religious communities. Such inequalities, while recognized, were deemed less significant than the opportunities to care and be cared for in their religious congregations. In terms of attachment theory, the religious community appears to provide some persons a context for relationships that reinforce a sense of emotional security.

B. Public Religious Participation

Older persons, including the very frail, are active in managing their close emotional relationships; they behave proactively to optimize these relationships in order to maintain a sense of social integration (Lang & Carstensen, 1994). This may be one way of explaining the high level of religious participation among older persons: they strategically determine that investment of time and energy in attending religious services maintains important social ties and contributes to emotion self-regulation.

In addition to fostering social ties by eliciting feelings of interpersonal trust, mutuality, and intimacy (Ellison & George, 1994), religious rituals structure encounters with the divine. Thus, they activate attachment processes that connect individuals not only to other persons and but also to God. Rituals occur within environments designated as sacred.

Many religions call these sacred spaces "sanctuaries," a word that recalls Bowlby's (1973) description of the "safe haven" and "secure base" of attachment relationships. It is possible that if salutogenic emotions have predominated in these spaces, the spaces themselves may become conditioned stimuli eliciting feelings of calm, peace, and joy. Anticipation of these positive feelings as well as the social support of fellow congregants may have motivated the 98 severely disabled older women studied by Idler (1987) who managed to attend religious services at least once a week. These women needed assistance in feeding themselves, toileting, and walking, but they nevertheless made the effort to engage in public worship.

Some tangential support for a connection between well-being and the strong emotional responses elicited in public religious observance comes from studies of African-American churches, many of which encourage the expression of emotion through testimony, glossolalia, dancing, singing, and spirit possession. Participants report leaving such services feeling infused with hope and joy as well as a sense of closeness to fellow congregants (Gilkes, 1980; Griffith, Young, & Smith, 1984).

Measures of the types and intensities of emotions associated with religious observances need to be developed and tested. This type of research in conjunction with continued study of psychoneuroimmunology is needed to advance understanding about the impact of religious observance on health. In addition, the effect of age on participation in the more intensely emotional and physically active aspects of some public religious observances should be studied.

C. Private Religious Observance

Older adults' participation in nonorganizational, private religious activities is high (Levin, 1995; McFadden, 1996). Behaviors such as prayer, Bible study, and daily devotions may increase with age and functional disability as organizational involvement declines. The impact of these activities on older persons' ability to cope with physical difficulties (Koenig, George, & Siegler, 1988) is better understood than their possible direct effects on neuroendocrine and immune system functioning. Data from research on the psychophysiological correlates of various meditative practices suggest that certain forms of private religious observance may have salutary effects (see Wulff, 1991, pp. 172–182, for a review). Unfortunately, much of this research suffers from a lack of control groups, confounded independent variables, and poorly defined dependent measures. To date, no one has shown that observations of Zen masters, Hindu yogis, and American practitioners of transcendental meditation apply also to older adults who pray before meals, read Bible verses every morning, and engage in nightly devotions and meditation.

Much more needs to be learned about whether private religious behaviors can actually synchronize or entrain biorhythms (Hofer, 1984) or whether this synchronization affects health. If, as Hofer (1984) suggested, internal object representations can serve as biologic regulators, then daily prayer and other forms of contact with the "exalted attachment figure" (Kirkpatrick, 1992, p. 13) that generate positive emotions may indeed have salutary effects.

V. SUGGESTIONS FOR FUTURE RESEARCH

The ideas about religion and emotion offered in this chapter suggest new possibilities for psychological and medical research on the biopsychosocial dynamics undergirding human life. Further research on religion, emotions, and health will benefit from increased methodological sophistication, notably (a) the use of longitudinal and multiwave panel designs, (b) the use of midrange theoretical perspectives to frame and specify testable models, (c) attention to gender as a source of variation in both patterns and outcomes of religious involvement, (d) a focus on intraethnic differences and of racial- and ethnic-comparative approaches, and (e) cross-denominational and cross-national investigations.

Evidence of both cohort and aging effects in religious involvement and the much discussed possible confounding of behavioral measures of religiosity and functional or somatic measures of health or well-being in older adults, underscore the value of *longitudinal research* for this area. Prospective epidemiologic cohort studies, multiwave panel analyses, time series, aging-period-cohort designs, and other longitudinal research all have much to offer. Lifelong continuities in religious outlook as well as discontinuities engendered by conversion or shattered faith need to be examined for their effects on the management of emotion. Longitudinal studies of religious attachment processes also promise to reveal important information about the development and outcomes of religious beliefs and coping strategies.

Within research on religion, aging, and well-being over the past 25 years, half a dozen *midrange theoretical perspectives* have been identified (Levin, 1989), although they are often more implicit than explicit in the justification for particular analyses. Also, as noted, gerontologists in this area recently have begun to more explicitly evaluate alternative theoretical perspectives (Krause & Tran, 1989); test well-specified multifactorial structural models (Krause & Tran, 1989; Levin, Chatters, & Taylor, 1995), and develop comprehensive, integrated theoretical frameworks for understanding religious effects on particular well-being outcomes such as depression (Ellison, 1994). This chapter has suggested that attachment theory offers testable hypotheses about individual differences in religiosity in older adults, changes in religiosity over the life course, and the nature of religion's impact on health and well-being over time.

As recently noted (Levin, Taylor, & Chatters, 1994), considerable work within the psychology and sociology of religion indicates that *gender* is the strongest, most consistent sociodemographic correlate of religious involvement, such that women tend to be more religious than men, regardless of the type of religious involvement. Furthermore, reviews have emphasized the accumulation of significant, if inconsistent, findings linking gender and well-being (Chatters, 1988; Diener, 1984; Larson, 1978) and gender and emotion (Brody & Hall, 1993). Religious involvement, aging, gender, and emotion appear to be related in a complex, multifactorial fashion that merits further investigation.

Considerable developmental research has shown the effects of socialization on emotional elicitors, emotional expression, and emotional experience (Saarni, 1993). Participation in religious organizations may be an important—though, to date, unexamined—source of learning about emotion, particularly among *racial and ethnic minority groups* for whom religion has functioned as a particularly salient haven of safety (Maldonado, 1995). Studies of patterns and outcomes of religious involvement among older African Americans (e.g., Brown, Ndubuishi, & Gary, 1990; Levin, Chatters, & Taylor, 1995) and older Mexican Americans (e.g., Markides & Cole, 1984; Markides, Levin, & Ray, 1987) indicate the importance of religion for these groups. Examination of religious attachment processes as well as the influence of religion on emotion self-regulation among these individuals is warranted.

Researchers interested in the ways emotion mediates the relation between religion and health need to begin to attend to differences in degrees of social cohesiveness in faith communities, emotion expression in worship, and emphasis on private religious practice and experience. *Cross-denominational and cross-national research* is essential. Existing studies have focused almost entirely on U.S. citizens and have tended to eschew analyses of religious effects stratified by affiliation. Where religious denomination has been used in particular analyses, which is rarely, it is typically for purposes of zero-order comparisons of an outcome variable between widely heterogeneous groups, such as Christians and Jews, without attention to more substantive religious issues. In addition to considering differences between and within major world religions, researchers might also choose to examine the patterns, predictors, and outcomes of participation in groups embracing New Age spiritualities, especially because many also advocate alternative approaches to health and medicine.

VII. CONCLUSION

Given the complexity of the issues under discussion here, great caution must be exercised in drawing conclusions. Many potential confounds exist—for example, between social class and religious expression; functional health and religious participation; and personality variables like shyness or hostility and receipt of social support from religious communities. Simplistic impressions drawn from correlational studies that employ unidimensional measures of religiosity and health may delight newspaper feature writers but they are clearly inadequate for advancing understanding of the mechanisms through which differential emotions associated with various religious beliefs and behaviors affect physiological systems. Nevertheless, evidence is accumulating from many quarters that suggests abundant challenges and possibilities for further study of these intriguing expressions of biopsychosocial holism.

In this chapter, we have reviewed research evidence of salutary effects of religiosity, particularly among older persons. We have suggested that attachment theory offers a promising way of integrating data on the etiologic mechanisms that may explain the observed effects of religion on health. The implication has been that religion can evoke positive, salutogenic emotions given a secure religious attachment and positive cognitive-emotional schemas of the self and others born out of secure familial attachment. However, we do not have data about the health and well-being of those who experience fearful, preoccupied, or dismissing religious attachments nor do we not know the outcomes for individuals who grow up in households permeated with religious anger or fear. Do such religious environments produce toxic effects? Emerging research on the relation between hostile right-wing authoritarianism and fundamentalist religions (Altemeyer & Hunsberger, 1992) ought to catch the attention of psychologists seeking to understand the effects of early emotional climate on personality development and health and well-being in adulthood.

We do not mean to imply that religious faith is *only* a reflection of early attachment relations nor do we believe that religion can be reduced to the neuroendocrinology of emotion. Rather, we suggest that the scientific study of religion—an enduring and multifaceted aspect of human experience—can contribute in many ways to ongoing efforts to understand the relation between emotion and health.

REFERENCES

Abelson, R. P. (1988). Conviction. *American Psychologist, 43,* 267–275.

Ader, R., Felten, D. L., & Cohen, N. (Eds.). (1991). *Psychoneuroimmunology* (2nd ed.). San Diego: Academic Press, Inc.

Altemeyer, B., & Hunsberger, B. (1992). Authoritarianism, religious fundamentalism, quest, and prejudice. *International Journal for the Psychology of Religion, 2,* 113–133.

Antonucci, T. (1994). Attachment in adulthood and aging. In M. B. Sperling & W. H. Berman (Eds.), *Attachment in adults: Clinical and developmental perspectives* (pp. 256–272). New York: Guilford.

Batson, C. D. (1983). Sociobiology and the role of religion in promoting prosocial behavior: An alternative view. *Journal of Personality and Social Psychology, 45,* 1380-1385.

Berman, W. H., & Sperling, M. B. (1994). The structure and function of adult attachment. In M. B. Sperling & W. H. Berman (Eds.), *Attachment in adults: Clinical and developmental perspectives* (pp. 3–28). New York: Guilford.

Bowlby, J. (1969). *Attachment and loss: Vol. 1. Attachment.* New York: Basic.

Bowlby, J. (1973). *Attachment and loss: Vol. 2. Separation: Anxiety and anger.* New York: Basic.

Bowlby, J. (1980). *Attachment and loss: Vol. 3. Loss.* New York: Basic.

Brody, L. R., & Hall, J. A. (1993). Gender and emotion. In M. Lewis & J. M. Haviland (Eds.), *Handbook of emotions* (pp. 447–460). New York: Guilford.

Brown, D. R., Ndubuishi, S. C., & Gary, L. E. (1990). Religiosity and psychological distress among Blacks. *Journal of Religion and Health, 29,* 55–68.

Carstensen, L. L., & Turk-Charles, S. (1994). The salience of emotion across the adult life span. *Psychology and Aging, 9,* 259–274.

Chatters, L. M. (1988). Subjective well-being among older Black adults: Past trends and current perspectives. In J. S. Jackson (Ed.), *The Black American elderly: Research on physical and psychosocial health* (pp. 237–258). New York: Springer Publishing Company.

Diener, E. (1984). Subjective well-being. *Psychological Bulletin, 95,* 542–575.

Ellison, C. G. (1994). Religion, the life stress paradigm, and the study of depression. In J. S. Levin (Ed.), *Religion in aging and health: Theoretical foundations and methodological frontiers* (pp. 78–121). Thousand Oaks, CA: Sage Publications.

Ellison, C. G., & George, L. K. (1994). Religious involvement, social ties, and social support in a Southeastern community. *Journal for the Scientific Study of Religion, 33,* 46–61.

Friedlander, Y., Kark, J. D., & Stein, Y. (1986). Religious orthodoxy and myocardial infarction in Jerusalem: A case control study. *International Journal of Cardiology, 10,* 33–41.

Gilkes, C. T. (1980). The black church as a therapeutic community: Suggested areas for research into the black religious experience. *Journal of the Interdenominational Theological Center, 8,* 29–44.

Griffith, E. E. H., Young, J. L., & Smith, D. L. (1984). An analysis of the therapeutic elements in a black church service. *Hospital and Community Psychiatry, 35,* 464–469.

Hamburg, D. A., Elliott, G. R., & Parron, D. L. (Eds.). (1982). *Health and behavior: Frontiers of research in the biobehavioral sciences.* Washington, DC: National Academy Press.

Hofer, M. A. (1984). Relationships as regulators: A psychobiologic perspective on bereavement. *Psychosomatic Medicine, 46,* 183–197.

House, J. S., Landis, K. R., & Umberson, D. (1988). Social relationships and health. *Science, 241,* 540–545.

Idler, E. L. (1987). Religious involvement and the health of the elderly: Some hypotheses and an initial test. *Social Forces, 66,* 226–228.

Jarvis, G. K., & Northcott, H. C. (1987). Religion and differences in morbidity and mortality. *Social Science and Medicine, 25,* 813–824.

Jenkins, C. D. (1985). New horizons for psychosomatic medicine. *Psychosomatic Medicine, 47,* 3–25.

Johnson, D. P., & Mullins, L. C. (1989). Subjective and social dimensions of religiosity and loneliness among the well elderly. *Review of Religious Research, 31,* 3–15.

Kiecolt-Glaser, J. K., & Glaser, R. (1989). Interpersonal relationships and immune function. In L. L. Carstensen & J. M. Neale (Eds.), *Mechanisms of psychological influence on physical health with special attention to the elderly* (pp. 43–59). New York: Plenum.

Kirkpatrick, L. A. (1992). An attachment-theory approach to the psychology of religion. *International Journal for the Psychology of Religion, 2,* 3-28.

Kirkpatrick, L. A. (1995). Attachment theory and religious experience. In R. W. Hood (Ed.), *Handbook of religious experience* (pp. 446–475). Birmingham, AL: Religious Education Press.

Koenig, H. G., George, L., & Siegler, I. C. (1988). The use of religion and other emotion-regulating coping strategies among older adults. *The Gerontologist, 28,* 303–310.

Krause, N., & Tran, T. V. (1989). Stress and religious involvement among older blacks. *Journal of Gerontology: Social Sciences, 44,* S4–S13.

Lang, F. R., & Carstensen, L. L. (1994). Close emotional relationships in late life: Further support for proactive aging in the social domain. *Psychology and Aging, 9,* 315–324.

Larson, R. (1978). Thirty years of research on the subjective well-being of older Americans. *Journal of Gerontology, 33,* 109–125.

Leventhal, H., & Patrick-Miller, L. (1993). Emotion and illness: The mind is in the body. In M. Lewis & J. M. Haviland (Eds.), *Handbook of emotions* (pp. 365–379). New York: Guilford.

Levin, J. S. (1989). Religious factors in aging, adjustment, and health: A theoretical overview. In W. M. Clements (Ed.), *Religion, aging and health: A global perspective* (pp. 133–146). Compiled by the World Health Organization. New York: Haworth.

Levin, J. S. (Ed.). (1994a). *Religion in aging and health: Theoretical foundations and methodological frontiers.* Thousand Oaks, CA: Sage Publications.

Levin, J. S. (1994b). Religion and health: Is there an association, is it valid, and is it causal? *Social Science and Medicine, 38,* 1475–1482.

Levin, J. S. (1995). Religion. In G. L. Maddox (Ed.), *The encyclopedia of aging* (2d ed.) (pp. 799–802). New York: Springer Publishing Company.

Levin, J. S., Chatters, L. M., & Taylor, R. J. (1995). Religious effects on health status and life satisfaction among Black Americans. *Journal of Gerontology: Social Sciences, 50B,* S154–S163.

Levin, J. S., Taylor, R. J., & Chatters, L. M. (1994). Race and gender differences in religiosity among older adults: Findings from four national surveys. *Journal of Gerontology: Social Sciences, 49,* S137–S145.

Levin, J. S., & Vanderpool, H. Y. (1987). Is frequent religious attendance *really* conducive to better health?: Toward an epidemiology of religion. *Social Science and Medicine, 24,* 589–600.

Levin, J. S., & Vanderpool, H. Y. (1989). Is religion therapeutically significant for hypertension? *Social Science and Medicine, 29,* 69–78.

Maier, S. F., Watkins, L. R., & Fleshner, M. (1994). Psychoneuroimmunology. *American Psychologist, 49,* 1004–1017.

Malatesta, C. Z. (1989). Differential emotions model for the study of health and illness processes in aging. In L. L. Carstensen & J. M. Neale (Eds.), *Mechanisms of psychological influence in physical health with special attention to the elderly* (pp. 105–127). New York: Plenum.

Maldonado, D. (1995). Religion and persons of color. In M. Kimble, S. McFadden, J. Ellor, & J. Seeber (Eds.), *Aging, spirituality, and religion: A handbook* (pp. 119–128). Minneapolis: Fortress.

Manfredi, C., & Pickett, M. (1987). Perceived stressful situations and coping strategies utilized by the elderly. *Journal of Community Health Nursing, 4,* 99–110.

Markides, K. S. (1987). Religion. In G. L. Maddox (Ed.), *The encyclopedia of aging* (pp. 559–561). New York: Springer.

Markides, K. S., & Cole, T. (1984). Change and continuity in Mexican American religious behavior: A three-generation study. *Social Science Quarterly, 65,* 618–625.

Markides, K. S., Levin, J. S., & Ray, L. A. (1987). Religion, aging, and life satisfaction: An eight-year, three-wave longitudinal study. *The Gerontologist, 27,* 660–665.

Maton, K. I. (1989). The stress-buffering role of spiritual support: Cross-sectional and prospective investigations. *Journal for the Scientific Study of Religion, 28,* 310–323.

McFadden, S. H. (1996). Religion, spirituality, and aging. In J. E. Birren & K. W. Schaie (Eds.), *Handbook of the psychology of aging* (4th ed.) (pp. 162–177). San Diego: Academic Press.

McMahon, B., Pugh, T. F., & Ipsen, J. (1960). *Epidemiologic methods.* Boston: Little, Brown & Co.

Moberg, D. O. (1990). Religion and aging. In K. F. Ferraro (Ed.), *Gerontology: Perspectives and issues* (pp. 179–205). New York: Springer Publishing Company.

Murrell, S. A., Chipley, Q. T., & Norris, F. H. (1992). Functional versus structural social support, desirable events, and positive affect in older adults. *Psychology and Aging, 7,* 562–570.

Ozorak, E. W. (1996). The power, but not the glory: How women empower themselves through religion. *Journal for the Scientific Study of Religion, 35,* 17–29.

Pargament, K. I. (in press). *Religion and coping: The sacred and the search for significance in stressful times.* New York: Guilford.

Pargament, K. I., Ensing, D. S., Falgout, K., Olsen, H., Reilly, B., Van Haitsma, K., & Warren, R. (1990). God help me: 1. Religious coping efforts as predictors of the outcomes of significant negative life events. *American Journal of Community Psychology, 18,* 793–824.

Payne, B. (1988). Religious patterns and participation of older adults: A sociological perspective. *Educational Gerontology, 14,* 255–267.

Pruyser, P. W. (1968). *A dynamic psychology of religion.* New York: Harper & Row.

Reite, M., & Boccia, M. L. (1994). Physiological aspects of adult attachment. In M. B. Sperling & W. H. Berman (Eds.), *Attachment in adults: Clinical and developmental perspectives* (pp. 155–178). New York: Guilford.

Saarni, C. (1993). Socialization of emotion. In M. Lewis & J. M. Haviland (Eds.), *Handbook of emotions* (pp. 435–446). New York: Guilford.

Spector, R. E. (1991). *Cultural diversity in health and illness* (3rd ed.). Norwalk, CT: Appleton & Lange.

Taylor, R. J. (1986). Religious participation among elderly Blacks. *The Gerontologist, 26,* 630–636.

Taylor, R. J. (1988). Structural determinants of religious participation among Black Americans. *Review of Religious Research, 29,* 114–125.

Taylor, R. J., & Chatters, L. M. (1986). Church-based informal support among elderly Blacks. *The Gerontologist, 26,* 637–642.

Taylor, S. E. (1989). *Positive illusions: Creative self-deception and the healthy mind.* New York: Basic Books.

Tobin, S. S. (1991). Preserving the self through religion. In S. S. Tobin, *Personhood in advanced old age: Implications for practice* (pp. 119–133). New York: Springer Publishing Company.

Weiss, R. S. (1982). Attachment in adult life. In D. M. Parkes & J. Stevenson-Hinde (Eds.), *The place of attachment in human behavior* (pp. 171–184). New York: Basic Books.

Witter, R. A., Stock, W. A., Okun, M. A., & Haring, M. J. (1985). Religion and subjective well-being in adulthood: A quantitative synthesis. *Review of Religious Research, 26,* 332–342.

Wulff, D. M. (1991). *Psychology of religion: Classic and contemporary views.* New York: John Wiley & Sons.

PART V

Continuity and Change
in Emotion Patterns
and Personality

CHAPTER 20

Mood and

Personality

in Adulthood

Paul T. Costa, Jr. *and* Robert R. McCrae
Gerontology Research Center
National Institute on Aging
National Institutes of Health
Baltimore, Maryland

I. THE LONG-TERM PREDICTION OF TRANSIENT MOODS

How will you feel two months and three days after your 78th birthday? After some thought, this odd question is likely to elicit one of two answers. The first is that you will feel "old," meaning tired, apathetic, irritable, and lonely. The second is that the answer depends on a host of factors that cannot be foreseen—your health and your spouse's, your financial situation, recent life events, daily hassles and uplifts (Kanner, Coyne, Schaefer, & Lazarus, 1981); there is thus no meaningful way to make such a prediction.

Both of these answers are wrong. Gerontologists, if not laypersons, have long been aware that stereotypes depicting the elderly as chronically depressed and withdrawn are incorrect both in neglecting the wide range of individual differences in mood that are found at every age and in suggesting that, on average, older individuals have lower hedonic levels than younger individuals (Lawton, Kleban, & Dean, 1993; Walker, 1952). Gerontologists and psychologists are perhaps less aware that affect is predictable years in advance, not from foreknowledge of the situations that induce affective responses, but from an understanding of the enduring dispositional basis of affect: personality traits (Costa, McCrae, & Zonderman, 1987).

That point can be illustrated with some new data on depression. Major depression (American Psychiatric Association, 1994) is a debilitating disorder that poses a major challenge for public health. Subclinical depression—feelings of sadness, loneliness, grief, discouragement, despair—is far more prevalent, and though it may not impede social functioning, it robs the individual of the full enjoyment of life.

If we ask why people are sometimes so unhappy, the commonsense answer is that they have encountered adversities: loss of a friend or job, sickness or disability, or limited prospects for the future. Because older individuals are disproportionately burdened by bereavement and disease and have little time left to live, it would seem that old age ought to be a depressing period of life, and it is so viewed by many young people.

But in fact older individuals as a group are not markedly depressed, either at clinical or subclinical levels (Costa & McCrae, 1993), and that fact makes a reconsideration of common sense necessary. Clinical psychologists are accustomed to the idea that there is a subset of individuals who are constitutionally prone to depressive disorders (Moldin, Reich, & Rice, 1991); from there it is a small extrapolation to hypothesize that normal variations in depressive mood are also related to enduring features of the individual, namely, personality traits. A test of that hypothesis is offered by data from the Baltimore Longitudinal Study of Aging (BLSA; Shock et al., 1984).

Since 1990 the Center for Epidemiologic Studies Depression scale (CES-D; Radloff, 1977) has been administered to participants in the BLSA at each 2-year visit to the Gerontology Research Center. The CES-D includes 20 items covering such symptoms of depression as poor appetite, difficulty in concentrating, and feelings of depression, fear, and social isolation. Scores of 16 and above on this widely used measure are regarded as evidence of possible clinical depression.

BLSA participants are generally healthy, well-educated, community-dwelling volunteers, so it is not surprising that about 90% of them score within the normal range. Yet most respondents showed some degree of depressive affect, and a few participants scored as high as 50. Depressive symptoms are by no means confined to psychiatric patients.

In completing the CES-D, participants are asked to describe how they have felt "in the past week"; consequently, responses ought to be sensitive to relatively transient influences on mood. Some evidence that they are is provided by the 2-year retest correlation of .51, $N = 1{,}032$, $p < .001$. This fairly modest value stands in clear contrast to retest correlations as high as .85 over intervals of up to 30 years in measures of personality traits (Costa & McCrae, 1992b).

A subset of participants had completed personality measures several years earlier. Within this group, CES-D scores showed slight associations with female gender, $r = .14$, $N = 323$, $p < .01$, and years of education, $r = -.12$, $N = 307$, $p < .05$, but no correlation at all, $r = .00$, with age across the range from 35 to 95 ($M = 65.4$ years).

In striking contrast to these weak associations is the correlation of CES-D with the personality dimension of Neuroticism (N), measured by a scale from the NEO Personality Inventory (NEO-PI; Costa & McCrae, 1988). Neuroticism is a basic factor of personality defined primarily by stable tendencies to experience negative affects such as fear, anger, and shame. The correlation between NEO-PI N measured in 1980 and CES-D assessed after an interval of at least 10 and as much as 15 years was .42, $N = 266$, $p < .001$. This association was replicated in men ($r = .46$) and women ($r = .32$). N scores from 1980 differentiated those who would and would not exceed the clinical cutoff for the CES-D 10 or more years later, $t(264) = 6.52$, $p < .001$; they also predicted CES-D scores within the restricted group of individuals in the normal range, $r = .26$, $N = 239$, $p < .001$.

The NEO-PI N scale includes six subscales, or facets, one of which measures trait Depression. That facet was indeed related to subsequent CES-D scores, $r = .38$; but so were facets measuring Anxiety, Hostility, Self-Consciousness, Impulsiveness, and Vulnerability, $rs = .20$ to $.37$. Finally, these predictive associations cannot be attributed solely to shared method, such as a persistent response-style bias, because self-reports of depressive symptoms were also predicted by spouse ratings of N collected on a subset of participants in 1980, $r = .25$, $N = 121$, $p < .01$.

These are not isolated findings; they can be replicated over longer intervals and with different measures. Women first joined the BLSA in 1978, but personality data on men had been gathered since 1959. The major instrument used (in the years before the development of the NEO-PI) was the Guilford-Zimmerman Temperament Survey (GZTS; Guilford, Zimmerman, & Guilford, 1976), one scale of which, Emotional Stability, assesses the low pole of the N dimension. This scale was completed by 194 men between 1959 and 1978; its correlation with CES-D scores gathered after 1990 was $-.40$, $p < .001$. That dramatic prediction of a mood score from a personality measure obtained an average of 26.5 years earlier is testimony to the enduring influence of personality traits on human emotions. How you will feel at age 78 is to a considerable extent predictable from your personality traits today.

II. TRAIT BASICS: CONTEMPORARY VIEWS OF ADULT PERSONALITY

The dominant paradigm in current personality psychology is a reinvigorated version of one of the oldest approaches, trait psychology. As the basis for a systematic analysis of personality and mood, it is useful to review what is known about personality traits—much of it learned from longitudinal studies over the past 20 years (Costa & McCrae, 1992a). Personality traits are "dimensions of individual differences in tendencies to show consistent patterns of thoughts, feelings, and actions" (McCrae & Costa, 1990, p. 23), and both laypersons and psychologists have identified a host of traits. *Trait structure* refers to the pattern of covariation among individual traits, usually expressed as dimensions of personality identified in factor analyses. For decades the field of personality psychology was characterized by competing systems of trait structure; more recently a consensus has developed that most traits can be understood in terms of the dimensions of the Five-Factor Model (Digman, 1990; McCrae, 1992).

We have already described one of these factors, Neuroticism (N). Its companion in Eysenck's (Eysenck & Eysenck, 1964) system, Extraversion (E), is defined chiefly by sociability, but also includes assertiveness, energy level, and—most relevant to this chapter—the tendency to experience positive emotions such as joy and mirth. Indeed, the dimension is sometimes labeled *Positive Emotionality* (Watson & Clark, in press). Less familiar as a global dimension is Openness to Experience (O; McCrae, 1993–1994), which combines aesthetic sensitivity, intellectual curiosity, and liberal attitudes. Agreeableness (A) is another interpersonal dimension that contrasts trust, cooperation, and sympathy with suspicion, antagonism, and tough-mindedness. Finally, Conscientiousness (C) includes both inhibitive traits, such as orderliness and punctuality, and proactive traits, such as achievement striving and industriousness.

One or more of these five factors recur in various guises in almost all personality trait measures. For example, needs for Achievement, Cognitive Structure, Endurance, and Order in the Personality Research Form (Jackson, 1984) all measure aspects of C; the Intuition scale of the Myers-Briggs Type Indicator (Myers & McCaulley, 1985) can be construed as a measure of O (McCrae, 1993–1994). The five factors can thus be measured with a variety of self-report instruments; perhaps more important, they can also be assessed with observer ratings, which show substantial agreement with self-reports that cannot be attributed solely to shared method variance (McCrae, 1994).

There is increasing evidence that all five factors are substantially heritable (Loehlin, 1992), and that they are closely related to measures of temperament (Angleitner & Ostendorf, 1994). Because temperament in turn is closely related to the experience and expression of emotion, these lines of research reinforce conclusions about the close links between mood and personality.

The developmental course of the five factors in adults is fairly clear. Between age 20 and age 30, there is consistent cross-sectional and longitudinal evidence that both men and women become somewhat lower on N and E, and somewhat higher on A and C—as they age they become less emotionally volatile and more completely socialized (Costa & McCrae, 1994b). Thereafter, with a few exceptions (Helson & Wink, 1992), people show little change, either in mean levels or in rank order. The 40-year-old who is cheerful, enthusiastic, and fun-loving is likely to become a cheerful, enthusiastic, and fun-loving 80-year-old (Costa & McCrae, 1994a). It is precisely this stability that accounts for the long-term prediction of mood from personality scores.

III. EMPIRICAL LINKS BETWEEN PERSONALITY AND MOOD

A. Parallel Structures in Traits and Moods

The consensus on personality trait structure is not paralleled by consensus on the structure of affects. Indeed, it is far from clear what kinds of states ought to be subsumed by the term *affect,* or whether and in what ways affects differ from moods, emotions, or feelings (Batson, Shaw, & Oleson, 1992). Mehrabian (1995) has proposed a three-dimensional model, defined by Pleasure, Arousal, and Dominance factors in which it is possible to classify such state-descriptive terms as *mighty, fascinated, unperturbed, docile, insolent, aghast, uncaring,* and *bored.* More common are two-dimensional systems with axes of Pleasure and Arousal (Russell, 1980) or Positive and Negative Affect (Watson & Tellegen, 1985). These two schemes have been interpreted as rotational variants: Positive Affect is midway between Pleasure and Arousal, whereas Negative Affect lies between Arousal and low Pleasure.

One argument in favor of adopting the Positive and Negative Affect rotation is that these two poles correspond respectively to the personality factors of E and N (Costa & McCrae, 1980; Warr, Barter, & Brownbridge, 1983). Extraverts experience more positive emotions, although they are not necessarily spared negative feelings. Individuals high in N are prone to distressing emotions such as fear, resentment, and gloom, although they are not necessarily deprived of positive feelings. Individuals who combine high N with high E are subject to the most intense emotions, and may occasionally merit a diagnosis of histrionic personality disorder. In contrast, those who are low in both N and E have flattened affect, and in extreme cases might be regarded as having a schizoid personality disorder (Widiger, Trull, Clarkin, Sanderson, & Costa, 1994).

The other combinations—low N with high E and high N with low E—describe temperamentally happy and unhappy people, respectively, who differ markedly on various measures of psychological well-being, from morale to affect balance to life satisfaction (Costa & McCrae, 1984). E and N together appear jointly to define an affective plane at the temperament level that corresponds to the circular ordering or circumplex structure of mood noted by Watson and Tellegen (1985).

However, the neat alignment of two dimensions of personality with two axes of affect does not exhaust the associations between traits and affective states. The two dimensions of A and C also appear to make independent contributions to the prediction of happiness: Loving and hardworking people enjoy life more (McCrae & Costa, 1991). Although O is unrelated to global measures of happiness, it, too, is relevant to affect. Highly open people have deep, subtle, and sometimes ambivalent emotional responses; it is because they are sensitive to negative as well as positive moods that they are on balance no happier than closed people.

There is a great deal more to emotions than merely feeling good or bad, even if those two dimensions characterize most affects at a broad level. Many researchers prefer to work on a more specific level, differentiating such affects as anger, disgust, and contempt (Dougherty, Abe, & Izard, chap. 2, this volume; Izard, 1972; Malatesta, 1990). Watson and Clark (1992) linked measures of these more specific emotions to the dimensions of the Five-Factor Model and noted several associations beyond the usual pairing of E and N with positive and negative affects. Specifically, A was negatively related to hostility and positively related to joviality, and C was strongly related to attentiveness, a state marked by the terms *alert, attentive, concentrating,* and *determined.* Wild, Kuiken, and Schopflocher (1995) argued that states described by such terms as *awe, fascination,* and *flow* (Csikszentmihalyi, 1975) are likely to be related to O. With a sufficiently broad specification of the universe of affects, we might discover that five dimensions, rather than two, are needed to define the full structure of affect.

B. The Generalizability of Findings

It is sometimes suggested that personality plays an important role in determining levels of happiness only for the fortunate few to whom economic and social resources have given the luxury of a truly subjective perspective on well-being (Thomae, 1992). Because participants in the BLSA are predominantly white, healthy, well-educated, community-dwelling volunteers, findings on personality and well-being in that sample (Costa & McCrae, 1984) might not be generalizable to less elite populations. In fact, however, they are (Diener, Sandvik, Pavot, & Fujita, 1992).

Consider the relation between E and CES-D. Although depression is chiefly related to N, there is consistent evidence that it also has a small negative association with E, reflecting the lack of positive feelings in depressed individuals (Watson & Clark, 1992). In the 10-year predictive study in the BLSA described in Section I, the correlation of NEO-PI E with CES-D was $-.18$ in men, $N = 191$, $p < .05$, and $-.24$ in women, $N = 75$, $p < .05$. For comparison, data are also available from the National Health and Nutrition Examination I—Epidemiologic Follow-up Survey (NHANES; Cornoni-Huntley, et al., 1983). In that large national probability sample, the CES-D was included along with a brief, eight-item version of the NEO-PI E scale.

Table 1 shows correlations between the two scales in the total group and in demographically defined subsamples. With few exceptions, the correlations support the inverse association between E and depression, even in individuals with limited education and income and only fair to poor self-rated health. The small group of individuals who were institutionalized at the time of the follow-up showed the same association seen in the community-dwelling BLSA. E influenced depression in black as well as white, widowed as well as married respondents.

The importance of enduring personality dispositions for determining levels of happiness is particularly striking when contrasted with the relatively weak influences of objective life circumstances. In one analysis, concurrent age, race, sex, income, education, and marital status combined accounted for only 6% of the variance in measures of well-being (Costa et al., 1987; cf. Campbell, Converse, & Rodgers, 1976). By contrast, E and N together account for 19% of the variance in CES-D scores 10 to 15 years later in the BLSA study. The relative lack of effect of life circumstances on well-being is attributable to the operation of processes

Table 1

Correlation between CES-Depression and a Short E Scale in Demographic Subgroups of a National Sample

Group	N^a	r
Total	9,371	−.17***
Race		
White	8,090	−.16***
Black	1,185	−.20***
Other	96	−.12
Years of education		
12 or more	5,849	−.14***
Less than 12	3,473	−.18***
Family income		
Over $10,000	6,249	−.15***
Under $10,000	2,456	−.17***
Self-rated health		
Good to excellent	7,329	−.12***
Fair to poor	2,038	−.18***
Housing		
Private home, apartment	9,226	−.17***
Nursing home, institution	94	−.21*
Marital status		
Married	6,437	−.16***
Widowed	1,443	−.18***
Divorced	778	−.21***
Separated	253	−.18***
Never married	455	−.06
Age group		
32 to 64	6,549	−.16***
65 to 88	2,820	−.17***

[a]Subgroups do not sum to total because of missing data.
*$p < .05$; ***$p < .001$.

of adaptation, which quickly accustom the individual to his or her situation (Costa & McCrae, 1980). It is adaptation, in part, which explains why old age, which may seem so terrible to young people, is cheerfully tolerated by most old people (Andrews & Withey, 1976).

IV. INTERPRETING THE ASSOCIATIONS BETWEEN TRAITS AND MOODS

In section II, personality traits were defined in terms of "patterns of thoughts, feelings, and actions." That definition is controversial; some theorists argue that traits proper comprise only patterns of overt behavior (Pervin, 1994). In a careful analysis of these issues, Malatesta (1990) argued that affective responsiveness can show trait-like qualities, and proposed the term *emotional biases* to indicate the tendency of individuals to perceive and respond to the world with certain kinds of affect.

Many traits are manifested in a constellation of attributes including wishes, activities, preferences, needs, and habits. But some personality traits—particularly those related to N—are almost purely affective dispositions: They are defined and assessed in terms of the frequency or intensity with which specific affects are experienced. Items in a trait measure of anxiety may be indistinguishable from the items in a state measure of anxiety, except that they are used to describe chronic rather than acute affects. This fact has suggested to some writers (e.g., Lawton, 1983) that the prediction of mood from personality is tautological, because affective traits are nothing more than the running average of mood states.

If the only data supporting a link between personality and mood were concurrent correlations between trait and state measures of the same affect, that view would be tenable. But traits, although inferred from patterns of behavior, have surplus meaning that endows them with explanatory power (McCrae & Costa, 1995). Affective traits demonstrate substantial heritability (Tellegen, et al., 1988), which could hardly be explained unless there is something in the genetic makeup of the individual that predisposes him or her to experience specific emotions. The fact that trait measures predict state measures decades in advance also shows that enduring characteristics of the individual—affective traits—influence transient moods.

By what mechanisms do traits affect moods? To the extent that moods are purely spontaneous, they may be direct reflections of temperament. A cheerful person may wake up singing with no provocation at all. More commonly, perhaps, mood is in response to circumstance—but not all people are equally responsive. Larsen and Ketelaar (1989) showed experimentally that people high in E were more susceptible to positive mood inductions, whereas those high in N were more susceptible to negative mood inductions.

There are also indirect ways in which personality influences mood, through instrumental behaviors (McCrae & Costa, 1991). People who are high in A score higher on measures of psychological well-being, presumably because their trusting and affectionate interpersonal behaviors bring more interpersonal rewards. Similarly, the organization and diligence of highly Conscientious people lead to pride in achievement. These instrumental routes to well-being are sometimes frustrated in old age, when the loss of spouse and friends can make the expression of love difficult, and when disease and disability limit productive work. Interventions that provide a way to express affection (such as companion animal visitation programs in nursing homes) and sustain feelings of usefulness may promote morale.

Many of the chapters in this volume detail the centrality of interpersonal relationships in determining affect, and relationships are shaped at least in part by personality traits. For example, Shaver and Brennan (1992) showed that attachment styles were related to N, E, and A. Through their effects on interpersonal behaviors and relationships and the selection of social roles, enduring dispositions shape affective experience.

Again, stress and coping processes are often identified as important determinants of affect. But perceptions of stress, ways of coping, and adaptational outcomes are all profoundly affected by personality traits (Costa, Somerfield, & McCrae, 1996). Indeed, Bolger (1990) has claimed that "coping is personality in action under stress" (p. 525). People high in N use wishful thinking and escapist fantasy to deal with their problems, whereas those high in C take resolute action. Is it any wonder that in the long run perceived stress is higher among the former than the latter?

V. UNDERSTANDING EMOTIONS IN OLDER MEN AND WOMEN

We have stressed the links between personality and mood because a good deal is already known about personality and aging that may provide clues to understanding emotions in old age. The central fact in adult personality development, replicated by a host of longitudinal studies, is that personality shows little change after age 30 and until the advent of dementing disorders (Costa & McCrae, 1994a). To the extent that affect is a reflection or result of the operation of personality traits, we would expect few age differences in affect, and that is in fact a recurrent finding (Malatesta & Kalnok, 1984; Pasupathi, 1995). In this respect, as in many others, older adults are simply adults who happen to be older.

In other respects, of course, age is of central importance for understanding emotions. Older men and women face a different set of losses, threats, and challenges. Death of a spouse, for example, is an emotionally charged experience that is rare for young persons but normative for older women. Emotions have a physiological as well as a psychological aspect, and age-related changes in physiology may significantly alter the manifestation of emotion. There is some evidence that the reduced mobility of facial muscles in older adults can lead to impairments in the communication of feelings (Bromley, 1978; Malatesta & Izard, 1984). Personality and its stability are a necessary but not sufficient basis for understanding emotion in aging adults.

In moving from generalizations about older individuals as a group to implications for individuals, the stability of rank ordering is the most salient fact. The personality traits that characterize the middle-aged man or woman are still likely to be present decades later. Those whose chronic affects are anxiety, depression, or anger ought not to suppose that they will "mellow" with time; instead, they should perhaps consider psychotherapeutic intervention. Conversely, those whose current emotional life can be described in such terms as *calm, cheerful, fascinated, affectionate,* and *determined* need not fear the loss of these feelings in old age. Whatever the vicissitudes of life, people's emotional responses remain an expression of their enduring dispositions.

ACKNOWLEDGMENTS

The NHANES I Epidemiologic Follow-up Study was jointly initiated by the National Institute on Aging and the National Center for Health Statistics, and has been developed and funded by the National Institute on Aging, National Center for Health Statistics, National Cancer Institute, National Heart, Lung, and Blood Institute, National Institute of Arthritis, Diabetes, and Digestive and Kidney Diseases, National Institute of Mental Health, National Institute of Alcohol Abuse and Alcoholism, National Institute of Allergy and Infectious Diseases, and the National Institute of Neurological and Communicative Disorders and Stroke.

REFERENCES

American Psychiatric Association. (1994). *Diagnostic and statistical manual of mental disorders* (4th ed.). Washington, DC: Author.

Andrews, F. M., & Withey, S. B. (1976). *Social indicators of well-being: Americans' perceptions of life quality.* New York: Plenum.

Angleitner, A., & Ostendorf, F. (1994). Temperament and the Big Five factors of personality. In C. F. Halverson, G. A. Kohnstamm, & R. P. Martin (Eds.), *The developing structure of temperament and personality from infancy to adulthood* (pp. 69–90). Hillsdale, NJ: Lawrence Erlbaum Associates.

Batson, C. D., Shaw, L. L., & Oleson, K. C. (1992). Differentiating affect, mood, and emotion: Toward functionally based conceptual distinctions. In M. S. Clark (Eds.), *Emotion, Review of personality and social psychology* (pp. 294–326). Newbury Park, CA: Sage.

Bolger, N. (1990). Coping as a personality process: A prospective study. *Journal of Personality and Social Psychology, 59,* 525–537.

Bromley, D. B. (1978). Approaches to the study of personality changes in adult life and old age. In A. D. Issacs & F. Post (Eds.), *Studies in geriatric psychiatry* (pp. 17–40). New York: Wiley.

Campbell, A., Converse, P. E., & Rodgers, W. L. (1976). *The quality of American life: Perceptions, evaluations, and satisfactions.* New York: Russell Sage Foundation.

Cornoni-Huntley, J., Barbano, H. E., Brody, J. A., Cohen, B., Feldman, J. J., Kleinman, J. C., & Madans, J. (1983). National Health and Nutrition Examination I—Epidemiologic Followup Survey. *Public Health Reports, 98,* 245–251.

Costa, P. T., Jr., & McCrae, R. R. (1980). Influence of extraversion and neuroticism on subjective well-being: Happy and unhappy people. *Journal of Personality and Social Psychology, 38,* 668–678.

Costa, P. T., Jr., & McCrae, R. R. (1984). Personality as a lifelong determinant of well-being. In C. Malatesta & C. Izard (Eds.), *Affective processes in adult development and aging* (pp. 141–157). Beverly Hills, CA: Sage.

Costa, P. T., Jr., & McCrae, R. R. (1988). Personality in adulthood: A six-year longitudinal study of self-reports and spouse ratings on the NEO Personality Inventory. *Journal of Personality and Social Psychology, 54,* 853–863.

Costa, P. T., Jr., & McCrae, R. R. (1992a). Multiple uses for longitudinal personality data. *European Journal of Personality, 6,* 85–102.

Costa, P. T., Jr., & McCrae, R. R. (1992b). Trait psychology comes of age. In T. B. Sonderegger (Ed.), *Nebraska Symposium on Motivation: Psychology and aging* (pp. 169–204). Lincoln, NE: University of Nebraska Press.

Costa, P. T., Jr., & McCrae, R. R. (1993). Depression as an enduring disposition. In L. S. Schneider, C. F. Reynolds III, B. D. Lebowitz, & A. J. Friedhoff (Eds.), *Diagnosis and treatment of depression in late life: Results of the NIH consensus development conference* (pp. 173–187). Washington, DC: American Psychiatric Press.

Costa, P. T., Jr., & McCrae, R. R. (1994a). "Set like plaster"? Evidence for the stability of adult personality. In T. Heatherton & J. Weinberger (Eds.), *Can personality change?* (pp. 21–40). Washington, DC: American Psychological Association.

Costa, P. T., Jr., & McCrae, R. R. (1994b). Stability and change in personality from adolescence through adulthood. In C. F. Halverson, G. A. Kohnstamm, & R. P. Martin (Eds.), *The developing structure of temperament and personality from infancy to adulthood* (pp. 139–150). Hillsdale, NJ: Lawrence Erlbaum Associates.

Costa, P. T., Jr., McCrae, R. R., & Zonderman, A. B. (1987). Environmental and dispositional influences on well-being: Longitudinal followup of an American national sample. *British Journal of Psychology, 78,* 299–306.

Costa, P. T., Jr., Somerfield, M. R., & McCrae, R. R. (1996). Personality and coping: A reconceptualization. In M. Zeidner & N. M. Endler (Eds.), *Handbook of coping* (pp. 44–61). New York: Wiley.

Csikszentmihalyi, M. (1975). *Beyond boredom and anxiety: The experience of play in work and games.* San Francisco: Jossey-Bass.

Diener, E., Sandvik, E., Pavot, W., & Fujita, F. (1992). Extraversion and subjective well-being in a U.S. national probability sample. *Journal of Research in Personality, 26,* 205–215.

Digman, J. M. (1990). Personality structure: Emergence of the five-factor model. *Annual Review of Psychology, 41,* 417–440.

Eysenck, H. J., & Eysenck, S. B. G. (1964). *Manual of the Eysenck Personality Inventory.* London: University Press.

Guilford, J. S., Zimmerman, W. S., & Guilford, J. P. (1976). *The Guilford-Zimmerman Temperament Survey Handbook: Twenty-five years of research and application.* San Diego, CA: EdITS Publishers.

Helson, R., & Wink, P. (1992). Personality change in women from the early 40s to the early 50s. *Psychology and Aging, 7,* 46–55.

Izard, C. (1972). *Patterns of emotions: A new analysis of anxiety and depression.* New York: Academic Press.

Jackson, D. N. (1984). *Personality Research Form manual (3rd. ed.).* Port Huron, MI: Research Psychologists Press.

Kanner, A. D., Coyne, J. C., Schaefer, C., & Lazarus, R. S. (1981). Comparison of two modes of stress measurement: Daily hassles and uplifts versus major life events. *Journal of Behavioral Medicine, 4,* 1–39.

Larsen, R. J., & Ketelaar, T. (1989). Extraversion, neuroticism, and susceptibility to positive and negative mood induction procedures. *Personality and Individual Differences, 10,* 1221–1228.

Lawton, M. P. (1983). The varieties of well-being. *Experimental Aging Research, 9,* 65–72.

Lawton, M. P., Kleban, M. H., & Dean, J. (1993). Affect and age: Cross-sectional comparisons of structure and prevalence. *Psychology and Aging, 8,* 165–175.

Loehlin, J. C. (1992). *Genes and environment in personality development.* Newbury Park, CA: Sage.

Malatesta, C. Z. (1990). The role of emotions in the development and organization of personality. In R. A. Thompson (Eds.), *Socioemotional development: Nebraska Symposium on Motivation, 1988* (pp. 1–56). Lincoln, NE: University of Nebraska Press.

Malatesta, C. Z., & Kalnok, M. (1984). Emotional experience in younger and older adults. *Journal of Gerontology, 39,* 301–308.

Malatesta, C. Z., & Izard, C. E. (1984). The facial expression of emotion: Young, middle-aged, and older adult expressions. In C. Z. Malatesta & C. E. Izard (Eds.), *Emotion in adult development* (pp. 253–273). Beverly Hills: Sage.

McCrae, R. R. (1992). The Five-Factor Model: Issues and applications [Special issue]. *Journal of Personality, 60*(2).

McCrae, R. R. (1993–1994). Openness to experience as a basic dimension of personality. *Imagination, Cognition and Personality, 13,* 39–55.

McCrae, R. R. (1994). The counterpoint of personality assessment: Self-reports and observer ratings. *Assessment, 1,* 159–172.

McCrae, R. R., & Costa, P. T., Jr. (1990). *Personality in adulthood.* New York: Guilford.

McCrae, R. R., & Costa, P. T., Jr. (1991). Adding *Liebe und Arbeit:* The full five-factor model and well-being. *Personality and Social Psychology Bulletin, 17,* 227–232.

McCrae, R. R., & Costa, P. T., Jr. (1995). Trait explanations in personality psychology. *European Journal of Personality, 9,* 231–252.

Mehrabian, A. (1995). Framework for a comprehensive description and measurement of emotional states. *Genetic, Social, and General Psychology Monographs, 121,* 341–361.

Moldin, S. O., Reich, T., & Rice, J. P. (1991). Current perspectives on the genetics of unipolar depression. *Behavior Genetics, 21,* 211–242.

Myers, I. B., & McCaulley, M. H. (1985). *Manual: A guide to the development and use of the Myers-Briggs Type Indicator.* Palo Alto: Consulting Psychologists Press.

Pasupathi, M. (1995, June). *Adult age differences in emotion experience and expression.* Paper presented at the 103rd Annual Convention of the American Psychological Society, New York.

Pervin, L. A. (1994). A critical analysis of current trait theory. *Psychological Inquiry, 5,* 103–113.

Radloff, L. S. (1977). The CES-D Scale: A self-report depression scale for research in the general population. *Applied Psychological Measurement, 1,* 385–401.

Russell, J. A. (1980). A circumplex model of affect. *Journal of Personality and Social Psychology, 39,* 1161–1178.

Shaver, P. R., & Brennan, K. A. (1992). Attachment styles and the "Big Five" personality traits: Their connection with each other and with romantic relationship outcomes. *Personality and Social Psychology Bulletin, 18,* 536–545.

Shock, N. W., Greulich, R. C., Andres, R., Arenberg, D., Costa, P. T., Jr., Lakatta, E. G., & Tobin, J. D. (1984). *Normal human aging: The Baltimore Longitudinal Study of Aging* (NIH Publication No. 84-2450). Bethesda, MD: National Institutes of Health.

Tellegen, A., Lykken, D. T., Bouchard, T. J., Jr., Wilcox, K. J., Segal, N. L., & Rich, S. (1988). Personality similarity in twins reared apart and together. *Journal of Personality and Social Psychology, 54,* 1031–1039.

Thomae, H. (1992). Personality and its attributes. In J. C. Brocklehurts, R. C. Tallis, & H. M. Fillit (Eds.), *Textbook of geriatric medicine and gerontology* (pp. 110–121). New York: Churchill Livingstone.

Walker, K. (1952). *Commentary on age.* London: Jonathan Cape.

Warr, P., Barter, J., & Brownbridge, G. (1983). On the independence of positive and negative affect. *Journal of Personality and Social Psychology, 44,* 644–651.

Watson, D., & Clark, L. A. (1992). On traits and temperament: General and specific factors of emotional experience and their relation to the five-factor model. *Journal of Personality, 60,* 441–476.

Watson, D., & Clark, L. A. (in press). Extraversion and its positive emotional core. In R. Hogan, J. A. Johnson, & S. R. Briggs (Eds.), *Handbook of personality psychology.* San Diego: Academic Press.

Watson, D., & Tellegen, A. (1985). Toward a consensual structure of mood. *Psychological Bulletin, 98,* 219–235.

Widiger, T. A., Trull, T. J., Clarkin, J. F., Sanderson, C., & Costa, P. T., Jr. (1994). A description of the DSM-III-R and DSM-IV personality disorders with the five-factor model of personality. In P. T. Costa, Jr., & T. A. Widiger (Eds.),

Personality disorders and the five-factor model of personality (pp. 41–56). Washington, DC: American Psychological Association.

Wild, T. C., Kuiken, D., & Schopflocher, D. (1995). The role of absorption in experiential involvement. *Journal of Personality and Social Psychology, 69,* 569–579.

CHAPTER 21

Facial Expressions of Emotion and Personality

Dacher Keltner
Department of Psychology
University of Wisconsin—Madison
Madison, Wisconsin

I. INTRODUCTION

Emotion is central to the structure and processes of personality and the conflicts and crises that accompany personality development (Malatesta, 1990; Pervin, 1993). Establishing the links between emotion and personality offers great promise for the studies of personality and emotion: Such research points to the social and biological mechanisms underlying the structure and continuity of personality, and presents a framework for thinking about the elaboration, stability, and social consequences of specific emotion tendencies.

This chapter reviews the evidence relating facial expressions of emotion to personality. It begins with a presentation of the discrete emotions perspective, which specifies how specific emotion tendencies observed early in life elaborate into personality traits. The chapter then outlines how facial expressions of emotion mediate the interaction between personality and the social environment. Following a review of the empirical relations between facial expressions of emotion and personality, the concluding section discusses the role personality-related facial expressions may play in the social lives of people across the life course.

II. DISCRETE EMOTIONS AND PERSONALITY TRAITS

"A trait is a generalized and focalized neuropsychic system . . . with the capacity to render many stimuli functionally equivalent, and to initiate and guide consistent (equivalent) forms of adaptive and expressive behavior" (Allport, 1937, p. 295).

"Emotions evolved for their adaptive value in dealing with fundamental life tasks . . . can be identified not only in expression but in . . . appraisal, probable behavioral response, physiology, etc." (Ekman, 1992, p. 171).

It is more than coincidence that emotion and personality-trait researchers find themselves on similar quests, seeking to parse human nature in terms of a limited number of universal traits and emotions (Costa & McCrae, 1992a; Ekman, 1992; Izard, 1977; John, 1990). Both emotions and personality traits are multicompetent constructs with biological substrates, serve adaptive, organizational functions, and are expressed in distinct, observable behaviors that evoke responses in others (Allport, 1937; Ekman, 1984; Eysenck, 1990; Izard & Malatesta, 1987).

There is convergent evidence that personality is defined by specific tendencies to experience and express certain emotions. Analyses of the trait lexicon reveal numerous words that refer to specific emotion tendencies (e.g., "irritable" "melancholy"), suggesting that the links between personality and emotion have long been encoded in language (John, 1990). Emotion researchers have speculated that emotional traits such as hostility and melancholy are the product of labile, tonic, or "flooded" emotions (Ekman, 1984; Izard, 1972; James, 1884; Tomkins, 1963). Temperament and adult personality traits have been redefined as the tendencies to experience and express specific emotions (Goldsmith, 1993; Tellegen, 1985; Watson & Clark, 1992). Underlying these converging lines of inquiry is the question that is the focus of this chapter: how are emotions and personality related?

Although several answers to this question have been offered (for review, see Malatesta, 1990), this chapter will focus on the account offered by discrete emotions theory (Izard & Malatesta, 1987; Magai & McFadden, 1995; Malatesta, 1990). According to discrete emotions theory, emotions are evolutionary-based adaptations to fundamental life tasks, such as fleeing danger, negotiating social dominance, or forming social bonds (Ekman, 1992; Izard, 1977). To fulfill these functions, the emotions have evolved into coherent, differentiated motivational systems that organize perception, physiology, communication, and action. For example, fear motivates a perceptual vigilance for threat cues (Mineka & Sutton, 1992), produces a physiological response well suited to escape behavior (Levenson, Ekman, & Friesen, 1990), is associated with flight or freeze action tendencies and actions (Frijda, 1986), and is marked by a facial expression that communicates the potential threat to others accurately and quickly (Ekman, 1984). The other discrete emotions, such as anger, disgust, or embarrassment, are also associated with unique and distinct facial expressions (Ekman, 1992; Izard, 1977; Keltner, 1995), autonomic and central nervous physiology (Davidson, Ekman, Saron, Sennulis, & Friesen, 1990; Levenson et al., 1990), and phenomenology (Lazarus, 1991) that facilitate adaptive responses to the challenges that are specific to each emotion.

The discrete emotions are present early in development (Izard & Malatesta, 1987), as are individual differences in emotion (Barrett & Campos, 1987; Izard & Malatesta, 1987). According to discrete emotions theory, individual differences in emotion, which appear to be stable over time, are elaborated into more complex personality traits in the course of development. For example, some young children are fearful early in life and develop into inhibited, shy young adults (Kagan & Snidman, 1991). How do specific emotion tendencies, in the previous example fear, develop into complex personalities? Discrete emotions theory points to three relevant processes.

First, discrete emotions direct attention to the potential causes of the emotion and adaptive responses (Schwarz, 1990), and therefore exert specific effects upon perception and judgment (Keltner, Ellsworth, & Edwards, 1993). For example, angry people attend to insults, injustice, and the causal salience of others' actions, whereas sad people attend to situational causes and hopelessness (Keltner et al., 1993). Specific emotion tendencies are likely to be associated with habitual beliefs and percepts that are part of personality. For example, fear proneness is likely to be associated with the acute awareness of threat and uncertainty, anger proneness with the awareness of insult and injustice, and shame proneness with humiliation.

Second, emotions prepare individuals for actions, such as flight, aggression, submission, or affection, that redress the causes of the emotion (Frijda, 1986). These action tendencies are supported by specific autonomic responses (Levenson et al., 1990) that retain their distinctness over the life course (Levenson, Carstensen, Friesen, & Ekman, 1991). These action tendencies, according to discrete emotions theory, characterize the habitual response tendencies of personality. Fearful individuals are likely to "freeze" up or engage in escape behavior, whereas hostile individuals are prone to aggression and elevated sympathetic nervous system activity.

Third, emotions are communicated to others in distinct patterns of facial, postural, vocal, and verbal behavior (Ekman, 1992; Izard, 1977). The pattern of communication associated with each emotion is likely to be part of the "expressive style" of personality (Magai & McFadden, 1995; Malatesta, 1990). Facial expressions of emotion mediate the influence of an individual's personality upon the social environment, it will be argued, through their informative and evocative functions.

As a product of emotion-related cognition, action, and expressive communication, individuals develop cognitive-affective structures and interaction styles that define their personalities. An illustration of this view is found in the findings related to the anger-prone personality. Certain infants appear to be irritable and prone to anger (Field, 1990). Angry, hostile children perceive hostility in others' ambiguous actions (Dodge, Price, Bachorowski, & Newman, 1990) and engage in more hostile, conflictual interactions with peers (Lemerise & Dodge, 1993). Later in life children prone to angry outbursts tend to fail academically, professionally, and in romantic relations (Caspi, Elder, & Bem, 1987).

III. FACIAL EXPRESSION, PERSONALITY, AND THE SOCIAL ENVIRONMENT

Expressive behavior, the social manifestation of personality traits, shapes social contexts, interactions, and relations in at least two ways. First, observers rely upon others' expressive behavior to make accurate judgments of others' personalities (Funder, 1993). Second, expressive behavior is an evocative process, defined as "actions, strategies, upsets, conflicts, coercions, and reputations that are unintentionally elicited by individuals displaying certain characteristics" (Buss, 1992, p. 479), that creates social conditions that promote the consistent expression of personality (Caspi & Bem, 1990; Scarr & McCartney, 1983). For example, competitive individuals' unremitting competitiveness elicits competition in others, which further enhances their competitiveness (Kelley & Stahelski, 1973).

Early studies of expressive behavior suggested that personality could be judged from the eyes, the shapes of people's heads, and profiles (Allport, 1937), but ignored the relation between facial expressions of emotion and personality. This oversight is especially surprising in light of the role facial expressions of emotion play in the establishment and maintenance of social relationships (Barrett & Campos, 1987), ranging from parent–child attachment (Bowlby, 1982) to negotiations between romantic partners (Levenson & Gottman, 1983). Facial expressions are proposed to mediate the influence of personality upon the social environment by communicating social significant information and by evoking emotional responses in others.

A. The Informative Functions of Facial Expression

Within the course of social interaction, facial expressions of emotion signal several kinds of information, which, given the spontaneous, involuntary nature of facial expression, tend to be judged as truthful and sincere (Ekman, 1992). Facial expressions of emotion are a quick, reliable, and seemingly universal signal to others of an individual's emotion (Ekman, 1992; Izard, 1977), which is an important source of information within social interactions. For example, parents may express anger when a child engages in a disapproved of behavior, discouraging the child from engaging in the disapproved of act. When low-status individuals tease high-status peers, disrupting the social hierarchy, high-status peers frequently express anger and contempt to disapprove of the action, whereas low-status individuals display embarrassment as an apology (Keltner & Heerey, 1995).

Beyond signaling momentary emotional states, facial expressions of emotion serve as cues in observers' inferences about the actor's personality and social role. For example, observers infer dominance from nonverbal behaviors such as the frown (Ellyson & Dovidio, 1985), and other personality traits from facial expressions of emotion. Observers infer how likable, outgoing, sociable, and extroverted people are from their Duchenne smiles[1] (Frank, Ekman, & Friesen, 1993) and how shy, nervous, and self-conscious people are from displays of embarrassment (Keltner, 1995). In the ongoing stream of social behavior, facial expressions provide rich information about others' emotions and personalities.

B. The Evocative Functions of Facial Expression

Facial expressions of emotion also evoke emotions in others, a process that may itself be universal (Darwin, 1872). The emotions that facial expressions of emotion evoke in others contribute to the bonds between

---

[1]Duchenne smiles are smiles that are accompanied by the movement of the *orbicularis oculi* (FACS Action Unit 6), which moves the cheeks upward, and are related to feelings of enjoyment, whereas non-Duchenne smiles are not. Duchenne laughter is defined as a Duchenne smile accompanied by an open mouth and head tilted back.

parents and children, romantic partners, and groups members (Barrett & Campos, 1987; Bowlby, 1982; Levenson & Gottman, 1983; Keltner, & Heerey, 1995). Two processes link one individual's facial expressions to another individual's emotion.

First, facial expressions of emotion evoke emotions in others through emotional contagion, which is defined as the transmission of one individual's emotion to another individual (Hatfield, Cacioppo, & Rapson, 1992). One individual's embarrassment produces embarrassment in observers (Miller, 1987); one person's distress elicits distress in others (Eisenberg et al., 1989). Negative emotional contagion predicts marital dissatisfaction (Levenson & Gottman, 1983), "burn out" in jobs that require people to cope with others' distress (Hatfield et al., 1992), and the reduced likelihood of helping others (Eisenberg et al., 1989). Whereas negative emotional contagion seems to relate to negative social consequences, positive emotional contagion is likely to predict enhanced interpersonal functioning.

Second, facial expressions of emotion evoke emotions in others that facilitate the adaptive response to the emotion-producing event (Darwin, 1872; Malatesta, 1990). For example, facial displays of embarrassment increase amusement, liking, and sympathy in observers, reducing observers' aggressive and punitive tendencies (Keltner, Young, & Buswell, in press). People's displays of distress and sadness elicit sympathy in others, increasing offers of succorance that reestablish social bonds (Eisenberg et al., 1989; Malatesta, 1990). Displays of anger produce fear in the target of the display (Dimberg & Ohman, 1983), which would deter the target of the anger display from carrying out anger-provoking actions. Nonhuman primates display threatening glares to the mothers of misbehaving infants to discourage disruptive behavior (Cheney & Seyfarth, 1980). Human parents may display anger when scolding a child to elicit fear and deter the child from engaging in inappropriate actions.

C. Implications for Personality

Facial expressions of emotion appear to be markers of more than just evanescent emotional states; rather, they signal information about the individual's likely action, social role and personality, and they evoke emotions in others that shape social interactions. If personality is manifest in tendencies to display specific emotions, the implications are several. First, the inferences people make about an individual's personality, beginning early in life, are likely to be strongly influenced by that individual's predispositions to express certain emotions. Second, an individual prone to express certain emotions should tend to consistently evoke certain emotions and actions in others, which would contribute to the character of the person's social relations. The predisposition to express positive emotion would evoke positive emotion in others and establish friendly interactions and relationships, whereas the consistent expression of anger and contempt would produce negative emotions in others, and establish conflictual and avoidant interactions and relationships. In sum, consistently displayed facial expressions are likely to define how the individual is perceived by others and the character of the individual's interactions and relations.

IV. EVIDENCE LINKING FACIAL EXPRESSIONS OF EMOTION TO PERSONALITY

A. *Facial Expressions of Emotion and the Five-Factor Model of Personality*

The Five Factor Model (FFM) of personality is a set of five traits derived from factor-analytic studies of people's descriptions of their own and others' personalities (see John, 1990, for review). The FFM is comprised of five traits; Extroversion, defined as active, enthusiastic, outgoing, and sociable; Neuroticism, defined as emotionally unstable, anxious, self-pitying, and worrying; Agreeableness, defined as kind, sympathetic, friendly, and warm; Conscientiousness, defined as dependable, reliable, thorough, and careful; and Openness to Experience, defined as artistic, creative, imaginative, and cultured. Although there are several criticisms of the FFM (Block, 1995), the FFM captures people's representation of their own and others' personalities across cultures (John, 1990), and the traits demonstrate impressive heritability and stability (Costa & McCrae, 1992b).

Motivated by the hypothesis that Extroversion and Neuroticism are defined by core emotional tendencies (Tellegen, 1985), several studies, beginning with Costa and McCrae's seminal study (1980), have yielded consistent correlations between the FFM and *self-reports* of emotion. Extroversion has consistently predicted self-reports of increased positive emotion, as has Openness to Experience, Agreeableness, and Conscientiousness. With similar consistency, Neuroticism has predicted self-reports of increased negative emotion (Costa & McCrae, 1980; Larsen & Ketelaar, 1991; Watson & Clark, 1992).

Research linking the FFM to facial expressions of emotion has several benefits: such research remedies the semantic overlap problem of self-report measures of personality and emotion (Watson & Clark, 1992), offers convergent validity to previous studies, and pertains to the long-standing concern with identifying the social expression and consequences of personality traits (e.g., Allport, 1937; Buss, 1992). Motivated by these concerns, several studies have now examined the relations between the FFM and facial expressions of emotion.

Studies of the relations between the FFM and facial expressions of emotion have examined different age groups in different contexts using different measures of the FFM. A first study (Keltner, Bonanno, Caspi, Krueger, & Stouthamer-Loeber, 1995) examined the correlations between black and white adolescent males' facial expressions of emotion observed during a 2.5-min portion of an IQ test and the mother's ratings of their adolescent's personality. A second study examined the correlations between adults' facial expressions shown during a 6-min portion of bereavement interview regarding their deceased spouse and their self-rated personality on Costa and McCrae's NEO inventory (Keltner et al., 1995). The study of adults is important because as people age they acquire increased knowledge of emotion display rules (Gordon, 1989) and control over facial muscles (Ekman, Roper, & Hager, 1980), and as a consequence may inhibit certain emotions, such as anger or contempt, that may be related to personality. A final study examined the emotional behavior of college students in response to two events: first, as they watched another person struggle to perform a task, an elicitor of sympathy and distress; and second, after being singled out and praised for their verbal skills in front of strangers (Buswell & Keltner, 1995). In all studies participants' facial expressions were reliably coded with the Facial Action Coding System (FACS; Ekman & Friesen, 1978), which is an anatomically based system that allows researchers to code the intensity of discrete facial expressions of emotion. The measures of facial expression were composite measures combining measures of the number, intensity, and duration of facial expressions of each emotion. Were individuals' facial expressions observed in these brief interactions systematically related to the FFM?

1. Extroversion and Facial Expressions of Social Approach

Several findings support the claim that Extroversion is defined by positive emotionality (Tellegen, 1985). Extroverted adolescents showed increased Duchenne smiles of enjoyment while taking the IQ test. Extroverted adults showed increased Duchenne smiles of enjoyment *and* amusement during the bereavement interview, demonstrating that Extroversion predicts positive emotions in highly distressing contexts.

In both the IQ and bereavement studies, however, Extroversion was also positively correlated with facial expressions of sadness, which contradicts documented negative correlations between Extroversion and self-reports of negative emotion (Watson & Clark, 1992), and challenges the view that Extroversion is best defined as positive emotionality. If, however, one views sadness as a facial expression that evokes social approach in others (Malatesta, 1990), this apparent contradiction is resolved. Extroverted people may show increased facial expressions of sadness to stimulate social approach and engagement, which is consistent with the social approach tendencies of Extroversion. Consistent with this interpretation, bereaved adults' facial expressions of sadness were positively correlated with the size of participants' social networks, indicating that displays of sadness relate to increased social contacts. In sum, whereas Extroversion consistently predicts only the experience of positive emotion, it predicts facial expressions of both positive *and* negative emotion that encourage positive social contact.

2. Neuroticism and Negative Emotion, Empathic Distress, and Decreased Positive Emotion

Neuroticism has been linked to three tendencies to display emotion in the face that point to the potential social problems associated with this trait. First, consistent with the definition of Neuroticism as negative emotionality (Tellegen, 1985), Neuroticism has consistently correlated with increased facial expressions of negative emotion. In the IQ study, neurotic adolescents showed increased facial expressions of anger, contempt, and fear. In the adult bereavement study, neurotic adults showed increased facial expressions of anger.

A second finding suggests that neuroticism may be associated with avoidant responses to others' distress (Buswell & Keltner, 1995). Individuals watched another individual awkwardly struggle to make an embarrassing face, and responded with a variety of emotions, including sympathy, amusement, embarrassment, and distress. Neuroticism was correlated with increased facial expressions of distress, which predict avoidance of the distressed individual (Eisenberg et al., 1989). This tendency may undermine the neurotic individual's opportunities for social closeness and increase the negativity of distressing experiences.

Finally, a recent study has linked Neuroticism to the conspicuous *absence* of positive emotion (Buswell & Keltner, 1995). College students were praised for the verbal skills following the completion of a word-association task. Most college students displayed intense, enduring Duchenne smiles when praised. Neuroticism, however, was negatively correlated with Duchenne smiles. The sum of these findings suggest that Neuroticism is defined by a general negative emotionality and reduced positive emotionality in positive contexts.

3. Agreeableness and Amusement, Sympathy, and Inhibited Negative Emotion

Across studies, Agreeableness was positively correlated with facial expressions of emotion that would encourage cooperative, friendly social interactions, consistent with the defining attributes of this trait. In both the IQ and bereavement studies, Agreeableness was positively correlated with Duchenne laughter, which reduces social tension and increases social approach (Ruch, 1993). In the bereavement interview, Agreeableness was also negatively correlated with facial expressions of anger and disgust. Finally, in the study in which college students watched another student struggle to make a ridiculous face, Agreeableness was positively correlated with displays of sympathy, identified by the oblique eyebrows of sadness and a head movement forward (Eisenberg et al., 1989). These findings are consistent with defining attributes of Agreeableness, which include kindness, sympathy, and warmth, and quite suggestive of the enduring, positive social bonds that agreeable people are likely to form.

4. Conscientiousness and Amusement, Embarrassment, and Inhibited Negative Emotion

Studies have documented correlations between Conscientiousness and facial expressions of emotion that are consistent with the tendency to inhibit impulses that is characteristic of this trait. In the bereavement study, Conscientiousness, like Agreeableness, was negatively correlated with general measures of facial expressions of negative emotion, anger, and disgust. In the bereavement study Conscientiousness was correlated with Duchenne laughter (amusement) but not with self-reports of positive emotion, suggesting that Conscientious people laugh for reasons other than pleasure, such as the interest in having pleasant social interactions.

In the study in which participants were praised for their verbal skills, Conscientiousness was positively correlated with displays of embarrassment, which involve a controlled smile, gaze aversion, head movements down, and face touching (Keltner, 1995). This finding is sensible when one considers the conceptual similarities between Conscientiousness and embarrassment: both are defined by adherence to social norms, conventional behavior, and the inhibition of impulses (John, 1990; Keltner, 1995). More fine-grained analyses showed that Conscientiousness most strongly predicted the facial muscle actions that inhibited the smile, consistent with the role of impulse control in Conscientiousness (Watson & Clark, 1992).

5. OPENNESS TO EXPERIENCE AND AMUSEMENT

Openness to Experience was positively correlated with adolescents' Duchenne laughter while taking the IQ test. Perhaps more intellectually inclined adolescents, which defines Openness to Experience, found the test questions or their responses to the questions amusing.

B. Summary of Findings Linking Facial Expression to Personality Traits

The established links between facial expressions of emotion and personality traits reveal, like the self-report literature, that Extroversion predicts facial expressions related to social approach and Neuroticism predicts facial expressions of negative emotion. New relations between the FFM and emotion have been documented: Agreeableness predicts sympathy and Conscientiousness predicts embarrassment. Finally, certain traits were related to the absence or inhibition of emotion: Neuroticism was related to reduced positive emotion, and Agreeableness and Consciousness were related to reduced negative emotion. Theories attempting to account for the expressive behavior of personality must also account for occasions in which traits predict the absence of socially significant behavior.

These findings raise several questions regarding the study of personality and expressive behavior. First, are there unique emotional markers of different traits? Remaining within one system of personality, such as the FFM, may yield unique facial markers of traits: enjoyment marks Extroversion, anger marks Neuroticism, and perhaps embarrassment is the marker of Conscientiousness. Certain facial expressions of emotion were related to different traits depending on the context: Amusement was positively correlated with Openness to Experience in the IQ study and with Extroversion and Conscientiousness in the bereavement study.

The context specificity of certain facial expression–personality trait links raises the question of when personality traits will predict facial expressions of emotion. One possibility, following conceptions of "strong" and "weak" situations (Snyder & Ickes, 1985), is that each emotional context is a "strong" situation for certain typical, common emotions, and a "weak" situation for atypical, uncommon emotions. Common emotional responses to situations—sadness at the death of a loved one or joy at the birth of a child—are related to potent, universal characteristics of the event that should elicit fairly similar responses across individuals, except in instances in which people, because of their personalities, do *not* experience or express those emotions. Uncommon emotional responses that are not driven by the characteristics of the situation are more likely to reflect the individual's interpretive and responsive idiosyncracies and will be more highly correlated with personality traits.

Certain patterns in the findings presented in this chapter support these claims. In the IQ study, Neuroticism predicted anger, contempt, and fear, which were relatively uncommon (for example fear was observed in only 9% of the boys), but did not predict the most common negative emotion, disgust, observed in 43% of the boys. Other findings support the contention that personality traits predict the relative absence of common, typical emotions within a situation. Neuroticism was negatively related to Duchenne smiles, the dominant response to the overpraise induction. Agreeableness and Conscientiousness were negatively related to anger during the bereavement interview, which again was a common emotion in that context. These speculations need to be addressed in appropriately designed studies.

V. FACIAL EXPRESSION AND PERSONALITY ACROSS THE LIFE COURSE

Facial expressions of emotion are vital to social functioning and they relate systematically to personality traits. Over the life course, people increasingly base their social interactions and friendships on emotion (Carstensen, 1993), suggesting that the informative and evocative functions of facial expressions are more likely to shape people's social lives with age. This might account for the stability the traits of the FFM show over the life course, and the tendency for the stability of those traits to increase with age (Costa & McCrae, 1992b).

Yet there is a paradox: as people age, certain aspects of their emotionality, including their autonomic responsivity, levels of emotional traits such as Extroversion and Neuroticism, and facial expressions of emotion, become less intense (Costa & McCrae, 1992b; Levenson et al., 1991; Malatesta, Izard, Culver, & Nicolich, 1987). Facial expressions of emotion of elderly adults (65 to 80) compared with those of middle-aged (45 to 65) and young adults (30 to 45) are (a) marked by fewer components of the facial expression, (b) masked by smiles, and (c) blends of several emotions (Malatesta & Izard, 1984; Malatesta et al., 1987), and when presented to observers are judged (d) as less discrete (Levenson et al., 1991) and (d) less accurately (Malatesta et al., 1987). If facial expressions of emotion contribute to the stability of personality, how does one reconcile the findings that with age facial expressions of emotion become less intense but the stability of personality increases somewhat (Costa & McCrae, 1992b)? I offer these speculations to stimulate subsequent research.

First, the stability of personality in elderly adults may be based less on personality-related emotion and more on other factors than that of younger adults. The stability of elderly adults' personality may be more influenced by the increasing stability of their relationships, friendships, group membership, and living circumstances than that of younger adults, whose life circumstances are in more flux. In contrast, the stability of younger adults' personalities may be more based on their emotional tendencies, which provide continuity to their changing lives.

A second possibility contradicts this first speculation. Emotion actually figures *more* prominently in the interactions of elderly compared to younger adults (Carstensen, 1993). The reduced intensity of elderly adults' facial expressions of emotion may point to an explanation of this phenomenon. Elderly adults may evoke less emotion in others, but strategically rely on other means, including the choice of friends, interaction settings, conversational topics, and levels of disclosure, to continue to experience the emotions so central to social life.

A third possibility is that although elderly adults express less intense discrete facial expressions across the spectrum of emotions, they continue to consistently and clearly express certain emotions—specifically, those related to their personality—that influence the inferences and emotions of others. One study lends credence to this possibility (Malatesta, Fiore, & Messina, 1987). Elderly adults filled out self-report measures of their tendencies to express 10 different emotions, and afterwards were photographed while posing four emotions and a neutral face. Decoders did a poor job of ascertaining what expressions were being posed; the encoders' emotional dispositions leaked through and overrode posed expressions. Anger-prone elderly adults were perceived to be expressing anger, sad-prone adults sadness, contempt-prone adults contempt, and guilt-prone adults guilt. This would suggest that certain emotions, beginning early in development, increasingly suffuse the individuals' expressive and interactional style over the life course.

VI. CONCLUSIONS AND FUTURE PROSPECTS

In this chapter I have discussed how the informative and evocative functions of facial expressions of emotion contribute to how personality shapes social interactions and relations. Evidence shows that basic personality traits, such as Extroversion, Neuroticism, Agreeableness, and Conscientiousness, are marked by specific facial expressions of emotion that are likely to have distinct social consequences. The challenge is to now connect these personality–facial expression correlations to the hypothesized social functions of facial expression. In doing so, there is great promise in discovering *how* personality through facial expressions of emotion shapes the lives of people across the life course. The keys to such discovery lie in part in looking closely at the face, long believed to be the vessel of character and personality.

ACKNOWLEDGMENTS

The author expresses his gratitude to Avshalom Caspi for his thoughtful reading and insightful discussions pertaining to this chapter. This research was supported by the BSTART program of NIMH (Grant 144-FE-81 to Dacher Keltner).

REFERENCES

Allport, G. W. (1937). *Personality: A psychological interpretation.* New York: Holt.

Barrett, K. C., & Campos, J. J. (1987). Perspectives on emotional development II: A functionalist approach to emotions. In J. D. Osofsky (Ed.), *Handbook of infant development* (2nd ed., pp. 555–578). New York: Wiley-Interscience.

Block, J. (1995). A contrarian view of the Five-Factor approach to personality description. *Psychological Bulletin, 117,* 187–216.

Bowlby, J. (1982). *Attachment and loss* (2nd ed.). New York: Basic Books.

Buss, D. M. (1992). Manipulation in close relationships: Five personality factors in interactional context. *Journal of Personality, 60,* 477–500.

Buswell, B. N., & Keltner, D. (1995). *The themes and variants of embarrassment: A study of social facial expression across three embarrassing situations.* Unpublished manuscript.

Carstensen, L. L. (1993). Motivation for social contact across the life span: A theory of socioemotional selectivity. In J. E. Jacobs (Ed.), *Nebraska Symposium on Motivation* (pp. 209–254). Lincoln: University of Nebraska Press.

Caspi, A., & Bem, D. J. (1990). Personality continuity and change across the life course. In L. A. Pervin (Ed.), *Handbook of personality: Theory and research* (pp. 549–575). New York: Guilford Press.

Caspi, A., Elder, G. H., Jr., & Bem, D. J. (1987). Moving against the world: Life-course patterns of explosive children. *Developmental Psychology, 23,* 308–313.

Cheney, D. L., & Seyfarth, R. M. (1980). Vocal recognition in free-ranging vervet monkeys. *Animal Behaviour, 28,* 362–367.

Costa, P. T., & McCrae, R. R. (1980). Influence of extraversion and neuroticism on subjective well-being: Happy and unhappy people. *Journal of Personality and Social Psychology, 38,* 668–678.

Costa, P. T., & McCrae, R. R. (1992a). Four ways five factors are basic. *Personality and Individual Differences, 13,* 653–665.

Costa, P. T., & McCrae, R. R. (1992b). Trait psychology comes of age. In T. B. Sonderegger (Ed.), *Nebraska Symposium on Motivation* (pp. 169–204). Lincoln: University of Nebraska Press.

Darwin, C. (1872). *The expression of the emotions in man and animals.* New York: Philosophical Library.

Davidson, R. J., Ekman, P., Saron, C., Senulis, J., & Friesen, W. J. (1990). Emotional expression and brain physiology. I: Approach/Withdrawal and cerebral asymmetry. *Journal of Personality and Social Psychology, 58,* 330–341.

Dimberg, U. & Öhman, A. (1983). The effects of directional facial cues on electrodermal conditioning to facial stimuli. *Psychophysiology, 20,* 160–167.

Dodge, K. A., Price, J. M., Bachorowski, J., & Newman, J. P. (1990). Hostile attributional biases in severely aggressive adolescents. *Journal of Abnormal Psychology, 99,* 385–392.

Eisenberg, N., Fabes, R. A., Miller, P. A., Fultz, J., Shell, R., Mathy, R. M., & Reno, R. R. (1989). Relation of sympathy and personal distress to prosocial behavior: A multimethod study. *Journal of Personality and Social Psychology, 57,* 55–66.

Ekman, P. (1984). Expression and the nature of emotion. In K. Scherer & P. Ekman, (Eds.), *Approaches to emotion* (pp. 319–344). Hillsdale, NJ: Lawrence Erlbaum.

Ekman, P. (1992). An argument for basic emotions. *Cognition and Emotion, 6,* 169–200.

Ekman, P., & Friesen, W. V. (1978). *Facial action coding system: A technique for the measurement of facial movement.* Palo Alto, CA: Consulting Psychologists Press.

Ekman, P., Roper, G., & Hager, J. C. (1980). Deliberate facial movement. *Child Development, 51,* 886–891.

Ellyson, S. L., & Dovidio, J. F. (1985). *Power, dominance, and nonverbal behavior.* New York: Springer-Verlag.

Eysenck, H. J. (1990). Biological dimensions of personality. In L. Pervin (Ed.), *Handbook of personality theory and research* (pp. 244–276). New York: Guilford.

Field, T. (1990). *Infancy.* Cambridge, MA: Harvard University Press.

Frank, M., Ekman, P., & Friesen, W. V. (1993). Behavioral markers and recognizability of the smile of enjoyment. *Journal of Personality and Social Psychology, 64(1),* 83–93.

Frijda, N. (1986). *The emotions.* Cambridge, UK: Cambridge University Press.

Funder, D. C. (1993). Judgments of personality and personality itself. In K. H. Craik (Ed.), *Fifty years of personality psychology* (pp. 207–214). New York: Plenum Press.

Goldsmith, H. H. (1993). Temperament: Variability in developing emotion systems. In M. Lewis & J. Haviland (Eds.), *The handbook of emotions* (pp. 353–364). New York: Guilford.

Gordon, S. (1989). The socialization of children's emotions: Toward a unified constructionist theory. In C. Saarni & P. L. Harris (Eds.), *Children's understanding of emotion* (pp. 319–349). New York: Cambridge University Press.

Hatfield, E., Cacioppo, J. T., & Rapson, R. (1992). Primitive emotional contagion. *Review of Personality and Social Psychology,* Vol. 14, *Emotion and Social Behavior.* Newbury Park, CA: Sage.

Izard, C. E. (1972). *Patterns of emotions: A new analysis of anxiety and depression.* New York: Academic Press.

Izard, C. E. (1977). *Human emotions.* New York: Plenum Press.

Izard, C. E., & Malatesta, C. Z. (1987). Perspectives on emotional development: I. Differential emotions theory of early emotional development. In J. D. Osofsky (Ed.), *Handbook of infant development* (2nd ed.) (pp. 494–554). New York: John Wiley.

James, W. (1884). What is an emotion? *Mind, 9,* 188–205.

John, O. P. (1990). The "Big Five" factor taxonomy: Dimensions of personality in the natural language and in questionnaires. In L. Pervin (Ed.), *Handbook of personality theory and research,* (pp. 66–100). New York: Guilford.

Kagan, J., & Snidman, N. (1991). Temperamental factors in human development. *American Psychologist, 46,* 856–862.

Kelley, H. H., & Stahelski, A. J. (1973). Social interaction basis of cooperators' and competitors' beliefs about others. *Journal of Personality and Social Psychology, 33,* 66–91.

Keltner, D., Ellsworth, P. C., & Edwards, K. (1993). Beyond simple pessimism: Effects of sadness and anger on social perception. *Journal of Personality and Social Psychology, 64,* 740–752.

Keltner, D. (1995). The signs of appeasement: Evidence for the distinct displays of embarrassment, amusement, and shame. *Journal of Personality and Social Psychology, 68,* 441–454.

Keltner, D., Young, R., & Buswell, B. N. (in press). Social-emotional processes in human appeasement. *Journal of Aggressive Behaviour.*

Keltner, D., Bonanno, G. A., Caspi, A., Krueger, R. F., & Stouthamer-Loeber, M. (1995). *Personality and facial expressions of emotion.* Unpublished manuscript.

Keltner, D. & Heerey, E. A. (1995). *The social and moral functions of teasing.* Unpublished manuscript.

Larsen, R. J., & Ketelaar, R. (1991). Personality and susceptibility to positive and negative emotional states. *Journal of Personality and Social Psychology, 61,* 132–140.

Lazarus, R. S. (1991). *Emotion and adaptation.* New York: Oxford University Press.

Lemerise, E. A., & Dodge, K. A. (1993). The development of anger and hostile interactions. In M. Lewis & J. M. Haviland (Eds.), *Handbook of emotions* (pp. 537–546). New York: Guilford Press.

Levenson, R. W., & Gottman, J. M. (1983). Marital interaction: Physiological linkage and affective exchange. *Journal of Personality and Social Psychology, 45,* 587–597.

Levenson, R. W., Ekman, P., & Friesen, W. V. (1990). Voluntary facial activity generates emotion-specific autonomic nervous system activity. *Psychophysiology, 27,* 363–384.

Levenson, R. W., Carstensen, L. L., Friesen, W. V., & Ekman, P. (1991). Emotion, physiology, and expression in old age. *Psychology and Aging, 6,* 28–35.

Magai, C., & McFadden, S. (1995). *The role of emotion in social and personality research: History, theory, and research.* New York: Plenum Press.

Malatesta, C. Z. (1990). The role of emotions in the development and organization of personality. In R. A. Thompson (Ed.), *Nebraska Symposium on Motivation: Vol. 36, Socioemotional development* (pp. 1–56). Lincoln: University of Nebraska Press.

Malatesta, C. Z., Fiore, M. J., & Messina, J. J. (1987). Affect, personality, and facial expressive characteristics of older people. *Psychology and Aging, 2,* 64–69.

Malatesta, C. Z., & Izard, C. E., (1984). The ontogenesis of human social signals: From biological imperative to symbol utilization. In N. Fox & R. Davidson (Eds.), *The psychobiology of affective development* (pp. 161–206). Hillsdale, NJ: Erlbaum.

Malatesta, C. Z., Izard, C. E., Culver, C., & Nicholich, M. (1987). Emotion communication skills in young, middle-aged, and older women. *Psychology and Aging, 2,* 193–203.

Malatesta, C. Z., & Wilson, A. (1988). Emotion/cognition interaction in personality development: A discrete emotions, functionalist analysis. *British Journal of Social Psychology, 27,* 91–112.

Miller, R. S. (1987). Empathic embarrassment: Situational and personal determinants of reactions to the embarrassment of another. *Journal of Personality and Social Psychology, 53,* 1061–1069.

Mineka, S., & Sutton, S. K. (1992). Cognitive biases and the emotional disorders. *Psychological Science, 3,* 65–69.

Pervin, L. (1993). Affect and personality. In M. Lewis & J. Haviland (Eds.), *The handbook of emotions* (pp. 301–312). New York: Guilford.

Ruch, W. (1993). Exhilaration and humor. In M. Lewis & J. M. Haviland (Eds.), *The handbook of emotion* (pp. 605–616). New York: Guilford Publications.

Scarr, S., & McCartney, K. (1983). How people make their own environments: A theory of genotype-environment correlations. *Child Development, 54,* 424–435.

Schwarz, N. (1990). Feelings as information: Informational and motivational functions of affective states. In E. T. Higgins & R. M. Sorrentino (Eds.), *Handbook of motivation and cognition* (Vol. 2, pp. 527–561). New York: Guilford Press.

Snyder, M., & Ickes, W. (1985). Personality and social behavior. In G. Lindzey & E. Aronson (Eds.), *Handbook of social psychology* (3rd ed.) (Vol. 2, pp. 883–948). New York: Random House.

Tellegen, A. (1985). Structures of mood and personality and their relevance to assessing anxiety, with an emphasis on self-report. In A. H. Tuma & J. Mason (Eds.), *Anxiety and the anxiety disorders* (pp. 681–707). Hillsdale, NJ: Erlbaum.

Tomkins, S. S. (1963). *Affect, imagery, consciousness, Volume 2. The negative affects.* New York: Springer.

Watson, D., & Clark, L. A. (1992). On traits and temperament: General and specific factors of emotional experience and their relation to the five factor model. *Journal of Personality, 60,* 441–476.

CHAPTER 22

Personality Change
in Adulthood

Dynamic Systems, Emotions,
and the Transformed Self

Carol Magai *and* Barbara Nusbaum
Department of Psychology
Long Island University
Brooklyn, New York

I. INTRODUCTION

Poets and philosophers have long argued about the malleability of human personality and the desirability of change. W. H. Auden was of the opinion that "we would rather be ruined than changed." Henri Bergson, on the other hand, thought that for a conscious being, existence implied change, which implied movement towards maturity; moreover, to mature was to go on creating the self endlessly.

Psychologists are also of two minds about the potential for personality transformation. As recently as 1994, when asked to reflect on the question of whether personality can change (Heatherton & Weinberger, 1994), leading figures in the field advanced quite different positions, marshalling different kinds of evidence. Indeed, it appears that as much of an argument can be made for stability as for change, depending on one's focus and interpretation, and depending on the level at which one examines personality (McAdams, 1994). Our own opinion is that stability

Handbook of Emotion, Adult Development, and Aging

is patently a marked feature of personality, but that a distinct potential for change is also present. As Fogel and Thelen (1987) remarked, stability and change are both fundamental characteristics of biological systems.

It is now time to move the "debate" about stability and change to a new level. Like Pervin (1994), we believe that one of the more challenging questions confronting personality psychologists today is that of determining the processes underlying change—a topic that we address in this chapter. More specifically, we focus on the role of emotion in the process of change, pursuing a line of thought introduced in an earlier work (Magai & McFadden, 1995). Although several theorists have come to the realization that emotions may play a critical role in the modification of personality (e.g., Miller & C'deBaca, 1994), it is far more common to attribute change to cognitive processes (e.g., Baumeister, 1994; Diclemente, 1994). However, although one cannot deny the significance of mental processes, cognitive efforts alone cannot account for the kinds of substantial personality change that have been documented in several recent studies. In fact, these studies can be readily interpreted from an affect theoretical perspective, as we hope to illustrate.

In this chapter we explicitly consider the place of emotions and emotional processes as agents of personality change from a discrete emotions, functionalist perspective (Magai & McFadden, 1995; Malatesta, 1990). We then examine several sources of data from contemporary research to see how well the data conform to the theory. We also enlarge upon the issue by couching the discussion within the framework of dynamic systems theory, viewing both the emotion system and the personality system as dynamic systems.

II. DYNAMIC SYSTEMS AND CHANGE

Dynamic systems theory, which originally evolved within the mathematical and physical sciences and has been applied more recently to the biological sciences, attempts to account for the organized behavior of complex systems—systems whose component parts are capable of interacting in a nearly infinite number of actions or states. Though the component parts of complex systems tend to gravitate toward certain preferred patterns, it is also the case that they can develop independently of one another and that new forms of behavior can arise from small changes in any one of the system's components. As such, seemingly minor changes or perturbations can precipitate systemwide changes and the emergence of new behavior.

The emotion system would appear to comprise one of those complex organizations governed by dynamic systems principles. In fact, within the field of emotions research, there is growing awareness that emotion is a chaotic, unbounded system that can not be fully understood within the framework of the linear systems perspective that dominates so much contemporary research (Fogel & Thelen, 1987; Haviland & Walker-Andrews, 1992; Lewis, in press). The component features of the emotion system include (a) structural aspects (motor assemblies, neural command circuits), (b) stimulation from the social and physical environment, (c) innate temperament, and (d) certain kinds of mental activity and knowledge including metacognition (Haviland & Walker-Andrews, 1992). In development, the emotion system appears to change in nonlinear ways, as qualitatively different forms of behavior emerge. Examples include the shift from the endogenous smile of the neonatal period to social smiling at around 2 months and the rather sudden emergence of stranger anxiety at about 8 months. These examples illustrate the fact that the emotion system in development can change in saltatory, discontinuous ways. In the above examples we see a change in control parameters during these phase shifts—a shift from internal physical stimulation to that of the social world in the case of smiling, and from perceptual gestalts to cognitive schemas in the case of stranger anxiety.

In the present chapter we suggest that the emotion of "surprise"— a little studied and largely misunderstood affect, is typically present at phase shifts in human behavior—both in normative development as noted above and at junctures leading to personality change, as discussed later in the chapter. In the two cases above, small changes in cognitive maturation appear to shift emotional behavior in qualitatively different and novel ways. In both cases, the child manages to put together percepts and concepts in ways that produce a kind of primitive insight, or an "a-ha" reaction. In the past, these infant insights have been interpreted from within a strictly cognitive developmental perspective and have been linked to the constructs of recognitory assimilation and discrepancy hypothesis. In our view, these infant insights are not purely cognitive, but are developmentally continuous with what adults identify as the sensation of surprise, one of the fundamental human emotions.

Personality can also be conceived of as a dynamic system, and surprise appears to be present at the phase shifts in personality development as well as in the phase shifts in emotion development. Moreover, surprise may be functionally significant and not just epiphenomenol to personality change. This point applies to both gradual personality change of the kind noted in longitudinal research and psychotherapy process studies, as well as personality change of the more precipitous and dramatic kind described by various authors who have begun to study radical change.

We pause here to consider the phenomenology of surprise. Izard (1991), one of the few emotions researchers to address the properties of this emotion at any length (Izard, 1991), notes that it has some interesting and unique properties. In the first place, surprise tends to be activated by a sharp increase in external stimulation—as in the sudden appearance of a friend or in the crash of thunder during a storm. Second, the mind seems to be blank at the moment of surprise as if ordinary thought processes had come to a stop. Third, there is little thought content associated with the emotion—"it is a little like receiving mild electric shock" (p. 177). Fourth, despite the foregoing, most people associate surprise with a positive experience. Experientially, surprise has the quality of a sudden expansion of awareness or jolt of consciousness.

In terms of its functional significance, Tomkins's (1962) saw surprise as a "channel-clearing" affect. Surprise brings about a temporary interruption in thought processes; it clears the sensory channels for the reception of new information. The capacity to receive new information is maximized, which at the same time maximizes the potential to profit from fresh perspectives. In some cases, the expansion of consciousness is sustained, such that the individual examines his perceptions, motivations, and ongoing life choices in a new light.

The emotion of surprise has a sharp rise time. It makes its appearance in a singularly unbidden and abrupt fashion. At the neural level, at least theoretically, it shares features with other emotions. In terms of its rise time and the "density of neural firing" (Tomkins, 1962, 1981), surprise lies in the middle ground between interest at one end of the continuum, and fear or terror, at the other. Mild surprise creates a perturbation that momentarily opens the window of awareness, often with a quick return to baseline; under the higher density of traumatic shock, there may be a more violent disruption of prevailing ways of seeing and relating to the world, self, and others.

It is our thesis that any one of these sudden emotional experiences has the capacity to lay the groundwork for a phase shift in the system that comprises personality, such that emergent forms of behavior are potentiated. Thus, both terror and surprise are assumed to be active precipitants of personality change, although they may not in and of themselves be sufficient for enduring personality change, which we will discuss in more detail later.

As noted above, Izard (1991) associated the evocation of surprise with a sudden increase in external stimulation; however, we suggest that sudden internal sensations can also give rise to surprise. That is, a sudden internal percept—as in the sudden awareness of a connection between previously unlinked events or concepts. It is what we experience when we have a "flash of insight." We turn now to the larger context of the role of emotional process in personality change.

III. DISCRETE EMOTIONS AND THE FUNCTIONALIST PERSPECTIVE

In our earlier treatment of the processes underlying personality change (Magai & McFadden, 1995), we stressed that the antecedent to personality change is frequently a groundswell of negative emotion. Indeed, one of the most well-worked constructs in life span developmental psychology germane to the issue of personality change is the notion of life crises. As originally described by Jung, personal crises are junctures at which intense emotion is activated and released for either productive personality work or for constriction and conservation of pattern (Caspi & Moffit, 1993). In Jungian theory, as well as in the empirical work of Levinson, Darrow, Klein, and McKee (1978) and Gould (1980), crises are seen as turning points in the process of individuation.

However, negative emotion is neither the necessary nor sufficient agent of change. Strong positive emotion should have the capacity to set change into motion as readily as negative emotion, if it is the magnitude of effect that is crucial. In popular literature and theoretical works as well, positive emotion is quite often cited as a mutative agent (Magai & McFadden, 1995), as, for example, in romantic love (cf. Henry Murray, in Anderson, 1988) and in ecstatic religious conversion (James, 1902/1961).

With respect to the issue of sufficiency, highly charged affect cannot alone account for change. Indeed, in many cases strong affect results in strengthening old patterns (Caspi & Moffit, 1993). In order for personality change to endure, the emotional experiences that are galvanized during meaningful junctures in life must be followed by a period of sustained cognitive and emotional work. Perturbation in the working system that is personality creates conditions in which established feedback loops are temporarily disrupted, setting into motion novel positive and negative feedback interactions (Lewis, in press). There must also be support for changes, and these are largely interpersonal in nature (Magai & McFadden, 1995; Magai, in preparation).

It is thus our theory that for personality change to occur in any given individual, and for the change to consolidate, four essential ingredients are required: (a) highly charged emotional experience of either a positive or negative kind, (b) suspension of old patterns of thought and feeling, signalled by and perhaps mediated by a class of affects subsumed under the rubric of surprise, startle, or shock, (c) a period during which alternative ways of viewing the world and self are retained in consciousness for working through or trying out, and (d) an interpersonal component that supports change. Highly charged emotions provide an activation level sufficient to personality restructuring; surprise or shock acts as the fulcrum for a phase shift bringing new concepts and percepts into working consciousness; cognitive/emotional work over time functions to disable and replace old habits and patterns of defense; and the interpersonal component supports the externalization, elaboration, and enactment of tentative new ideas. The latter two processes—emotional/cognitive work and interpersonal support—are important elements that serve to stabilize the new views and emotional patterns until they become identified with the self and owned as an intrinsic part of the self.

Let us now turn to the relatively limited empirical work on personality change to assess the viability of this framework. We examine literature both on sudden, saltatory change as well as slow, gradual change.

IV. TYPES OF PERSONALITY CHANGE

A. *Sudden, Precipitous Change*

Massive or radical personality change of the kind found in posttraumatic stress disorder (Aldwin, Levenson, & Spiro, 1994) or in religious conversion (Ullman, 1989) has been described as quantum change by Miller and C'deBaca (1994)—that is, change that is sudden, transformational, and discontinuous. Several authors have begun to use micronarrative techniques—autobiographical descriptions that focus on specific events—to isolate the critical features of the change process. To this end we examine the work of Miller and C'deBaca (1994) and Baumeister (1994) on radical change.

Miller and C'deBaca (1994) studied individuals who had experienced a major change in core values, feelings, attitudes, or actions. The narrative accounts indicated that these persons were not expecting, nor were they prepared, for the changes that they experienced. One woman reported suddenly realizing, after an anger management workshop, that she had been living all her life with great shame and anger. After this epiphany, much emotion surfaced, she felt a great weight lifted from her, and her approach and experience of life radically and permanently improved. Although the specific antecedents to change varied widely among subjects' narratives, ranging from mundane activities such as cleaning the toilet, driving or being at work, to more profound activities such as praying or traveling in a foreign land, the majority of subjects reported an increase in emotional distress or upset prior to their change experience. They also made frequent reference to the experience of surprise and shock, which marked their excursions into change. So striking was the onset of change that the participants could identify the date and usually even the time of the change experience. Thus, emotional distress and surprise are common themes in these stories of change.

The changers also appear to have had a certain preexisting personality disposition conducive to openness to change, namely a self-reflective capacity. Scores on the Myers-Briggs Type Indicator scale, showed the quantum changers to be overrepresented as Intuitive Feeling types and especially Introverted, Intuitive Feeling types—at twice the adjusted population base rate. These Jungian personality types are especially inclined towards a focus on the inner life. Moreover, a majority of the subjects described themselves as spiritual or religious. Clearly these individuals were of a reflective disposition to begin with and took advantage of the opportunity to reorganize their personal identities and motives in productive, life-changing ways. Finally, there is some indication that interpersonal process may have been instrumental as well; it is noteworthy that one-fifth of the respondents had been in therapy and a number of narratives were striking for their depiction of the respondent's involvement with some kind of communal group such as a workshop or retreat where affiliative relationships were experienced.

Baumeister (1994), who has also studied profound or precipitous change, examined one particular step in the subjective process of change, namely the "crystallization of discontent." This process is well described in accounts of individuals who have left relationships or defected from religious groups. Although leaving a marriage or other committed relationship can be seen as a life change, as opposed to a change in personality, Baumeister argued that changes in behavior and lifestyle are often accompanied by alterations in fundamental, core values and priorities.

The people studied by Baumeister typically reported having "suddenly" perceived life in a radically new way, which then provoked a marked shift in how they interpreted life, with concomitant alteration in the values the individual attached to roles, relationships, and commitments. The process can be described as follows. A seemingly minor event (a "small change") is assimilated to a whole pattern, with a sudden insight; this then provokes an upsurge of negative emotion. Associative links are formed among many unpleasant, unsatisfactory, negative features of a situation. Although all these features may have been present prior to the crystallization of discontent, the person previously experienced them as unconnected. The crystallization gathers these negative features into a critical mass. Suddenly, they take on a new meaning that undermines and changes the nature of a role or relationship, as well as changes the commitment one has made to them. Baumeister makes it clear that focal events are not the source of change, but triggers that bring into focus dissatisfactions that previously had only been subliminal.

In summary, Baumeister's account of change in committed contexts highlights one particular element in the process of change—the sudden insight that profoundly transfigures the individuals' way of perceiving the relationship. At the heart of change then, according to Baumeister, is insight and emotional flooding. Although Baumeister has identified elements of cognition and emotion that are important in the change process, a systems perspective is missing.

Here it is important to appreciate that the phenomenological aspect of emotion is but a component of the larger emotion system, whose constituent parts include metacognitive aspects. In the instance of life change that involves leaving a committed relationship, the important metacognitions include views of the self and the self in relation. A person who has lived within a committed relationship of some duration and who has adapted to life with this person has also undergone alteration in the concept of the self—from a single individual to one in which the self is defined as a part of a pair. Discontent in the relationship then also threatens personal identity. When emotions are experienced as too powerful and threatening to the relationship, and, by association to the integrity of the self, defenses, such as repression, denial, minimization, reaction formation and splitting, are activated to keep volatile thoughts and emotions segregated from one another and out of consciousness. When this artificial segregation breaks down—through the intrusion of intense affect, and/or when information-processing channels are cleared in the midst of sudden insight—what appears to be a small incident becomes focal.

The above suggests that the emotion of surprise may be pivotal in the change process, precipitating the breakdown of defense, the ungating of negative emotion, and the kind of surge of energy that appears essential to change. Within dynamic systems, this kind of seemingly minor perturbation is all that is necessary to bring about systemwide changes. The operation of positive and negative feedback within the system as cognitions and emotions interact in new ways cause small effects to grow and large effects to recede (Lewis, in press). Personality has begun to change.

For personality change to be sustained, however, we contend that active self-reflection and interpersonal support may be necessary. These aspects are alluded to in the narratives of the studies cited above, but not given particular emphasis by Baumeister or Miller and C'deBaca. In our discussion of gradual personality change, these components came into more obvious play.

B. Gradual Change

Gradual change has been best documented in the context of longitudinal research and in psychotherapy process research. The first literature documents normative or developmental change; the second planful or deliberate change.

1. LONGITUDINAL RESEARCH

A good deal of longitudinal research has focused on the aspects of personality that appear to be relatively stable, as in the Baltimore Longitudinal Study (Costa & McCrae, chap. 20, this volume). Our own research (Magai, in preparation), and that of the Mills Longitudinal Study, has focused on change and the processes involved in change. In the Mills Longitudinal Study of Aging, Helson and colleagues (Helson & Moane, 1987; Helson & Roberts, 1994; Helson & Wink, 1992) identify aspects of personality that undergo change and attempt to draw profiles of those individuals most likely to show change, using concepts of ego status and ego development; this work highlights the role of self-reflective process in change. In our own research we have examined different facets of personality and focus on the role of the interpersonal in fostering and maintaining change.

  a. Developmental Change and Ego Processes.   The Mills study followed a cohort of women for nearly four decades. The women were first interviewed in their senior year at a private women's college in 1958 and 1960, with follow-ups in early, middle, and later adulthood. As reported by Helson and colleagues (Helson & Moane, 1987; Helson & Moane, 1994; Helson & Wink, 1992), the women depicted the period of their early 30s as tumultuous (Helson & Moane, 1987); they reported feeling disorganized, constricted, weak, lonely, and unrewarded for their efforts, particularly in the workforce where they had achieved only limited status. Of interest in this chapter is the differential response within this sample to these negative emotional experiences. Some women were able to make satisfying and productive changes in their lives in response to this negative period, whereas others were not. We interpret the Mills findings to indicate that the capacity to access and reflect upon internal emotions distinguished between those who successfully changed from those who did not. Equipped with the capacity for emotional reflection, women were able to make the kind of accommodative efforts that are necessary for progressive life change. In contrast, those without this capacity, when faced with negative emotional experiences, seemed to settle into a niche or even to retrogress (Helson & Roberts, 1994).

Although Helson and colleagues did not directly measure the women's ability to reflect upon and effectively use emotions, this capacity can be inferred from several of the constructs and measures that were employed, including ego-identity status, levels of ego development, and psychological mindedness. Women with the healthier ego identity statuses of achieved and moratorium were able to make adaptive change in their life, specifically in their chosen "social clock projects," whereas the foreclosed and diffuse women did not make such changes (Helson & McCabe, 1994).

Social clock projects are the major life tasks, like work and family, which, according to the norms of the society, women are expected to focus on at particular times in their lives. These life tasks are also the medium through which women develop their identities. Although the type of tasks and developmental periods are dictated by society, the degree of success with which the task is carried out varies (Helson, Mitchell, & Moane, 1984). By our reading, it was the reflective ability that distinguished the achieved and moratorium women from the foreclosed and diffuse. This crucial capacity appears to empower individuals to make positive changes; its absence makes such change unlikely.

Women high on the achieved prototype tended to be less defensive; as such they were open and able to integrate new information. They possessed insight into themselves as well. Insight makes it possible for individuals to dwell upon and utilize internal emotional experiences as important data for change. The moratorium group, like the achieved group, was introspective as well as verbally fluent; they possessed the motivation as well as the cognitive and verbal tools that fostered active self-reflection.

What is striking about the women high on the foreclosed and diffuse prototypes, in contrast to the first two statuses, is their closed-off nature. The coping style of women in the foreclosed group was defensive and characterized by a rigid repression of the experience of emotion and conflict. The diffuse group experienced much emotional conflict, but, like the foreclosed group, their ego defensive system was brittle. Thus, rather than being able to use their emotions productively, the foreclosed and diffuse women could only fall back on repression and withdrawal when faced with life's challenges and opportunities for growth.

Women with higher ego development levels (levels go from self-aware, to conscientious, to individuated, to autonomous, and finally integrated) were also better able to make positive change in their lives than were those with lower developmental levels (Helson & Roberts, 1994). The higher levels clearly reflect a more sophisticated and developed ability to deal with emotions. Increased levels of ego development mean an increased interest and understanding of the inner, emotional life of the self and of others. In addition, there is greater awareness and capacity to tolerate inner conflict and the ability to work through, rather than around, emotional issues. Thus, as our theory proposes, Helson and her co-workers found that those who were more able to reflect and work with their own emotions and the emotions of others, were also better able to effect positive change in their lives.

Finally, our hypothesis that emotional reflectivity is critical to personality change is well supported by Helson and Roberts's finding that psychological-mindedness in late adolescence predicted higher ego development in adulthood. The women who were psychologically minded as adolescents showed an early and keen interest in thinking about *why* people act as they do rather than in thinking about *what* they do. They were also good judges of how people feel and think about things. It can be argued that such a fundamental ability and interest in "differentiating and reflecting on the operations of the psyche" (Helson & Roberts, 1994, p. 918) is important in forging personality and life changes.

b. Interpersonal Process and Change.   In a recently completed longitudinal study based in New York, we examined the stability of personality at the level of basic tendencies or dispositions (Costa & McCrae, 1994)—in this instance trait emotions, as well as at the level of strivings and identity structures (McAdams, 1994)—in this case views of the self.

The study participants completed a battery of personality measures including a measure of Type A Behavior Pattern and the emotion traits of anxiety, interest, depression, anger-in, anger-out, and aggression, at two points in time—1986 (T1) and 1994 (T2); these served as our measures of basic dispositions. Our index of identity structure, administered at T2, was a self-report questionnaire that asked participants to reflect on whether their personal identities had changed over the past 8 years with respect to goals, perspectives, feelings, ways of relating to others, and personality. Prior to the administration of the personality tests at T2 we had participants complete a life graph depicting the most emotionally positive and negative events in their lives and asked them to describe these events. The events from the life graphs were subsequently coded into four categories that circumscribed both positive and negative interpersonal and noninterpersonal categories.

We predicted that dispositional aspects of personality would remain fairly stable, and that identity structures would show change. Moreover, we predicted that both positive and negative events would be associated with change, but that these changes would apply only in the domain of interpersonal events. Each of these hypotheses was confirmed. That is, stability coefficients for the emotion traits ranged from .47 to .75; matched pair *t*-tests indicated significant change in only one dimension—that of anger-out, which is a stylistic parameter of anger management. On the other hand, on the average, respondents reported "moderate" change in two of the dimensions of identity structure and mild-to-moderate change in three other dimensions. An aggregate measure of identity change was formed to test the relation between magnitude of identity change and the occurrence of negative and positive interpersonal and noninterpersonal life events during the 8-year interval between T1 and T2. As predicted, those life events that were relatively "noninterpersonal" (e.g., positive events involving personal achievements or negative events involving personal failures or dislocations in residence) were uncorrelated with identity change. In contrast, positive interpersonal events (falling in love, joining a religious group) and negative interpersonal events (the breakup of a relationship, getting divorced) were both significantly correlated with identity change.

The findings support our notion that personality change is more likely within interpersonal versus noninterpersonal contexts; however, we gain little sense of the actual processes involved. One place we should be able to observe more of the moment-to-moment processes is in the context of psychotherapy, a literature to which we now turn.

2. THERAPY

Psychotherapy presents individuals with an opportunity for elective personality change, and the growing body of literature on psychotherapy process presents personality theorists with opportunities to study the process of change more microscopically. Though our treatment of this literature is perforce limited due to constraints of space, we wish to make the point that the same elements that are involved in sudden, radical change appear to be at play, in modified form, during the more gradual changes of psychotherapy, namely the importance of intense emotion, the emotion of surprise (contained within the experience of insight), reflective work, and interpersonal process.

It should be obvious that psychotherapy capitalizes on reflective work and the interpersonal process, at least within most contemporary psychodynamic therapies, so we will not belabor these points. Insight has also been singled out as one of the more important agents of change, though it is not typically thought of or treated as an emotional experience. Curiously, it is the role of emotion, in an expanded sense of the term, that has been most neglected.

There are a few exceptions to this generalization. A number of writers have indicated that a high level of felt distress is associated with a positive therapeutic outcome and personality change (Luborsky & Spence 1971; Weiner, 1975). According to Weiner (1975), distress motivates a patient to work towards change because he wants and needs relief from painful affect. Greenberg and colleagues (Greenberg, 1993; Greenberg & Safran, 1984) have gone even further in their attention to the explicit use of emotion in psychotherapeutic work. Greenberg's premise is that effective and lasting personality change occurs only when patients meaningfully engage their emotions, thereby increasing awareness and knowledge of the role they play in the dynamic aspects of their lives. Emotions provide "orienting information" (Greenberg, 1993); they help the patient and therapist to become aware of and responsive to the behaviors that are prompted by particular feelings. In addition, they make a person's schemas accessible, and evoke underlying cognitive-affective structures. Emotions also give personal meaning to events, thereby helping to direct the therapist and patient to important content, moments, interactions, beliefs, and motivations. By examining emotional "triggers," the patient and therapist can gain clarity and insight concerning the relations among emotions, cognitions, and behavior. By examining emotional "reactions," they can determine if a reactive system in the personality is responding dysfunctionally or functionally to situations.

In Greenberg's experience, when emotions become the explicit focus of therapeutic work, connections can more readily be made between sectors of the personality that we know as feelings, thoughts, and behavior; when such connections are made, the patient typically experiences insight—one of the same elements that appear to figure so prominently in the analyses of radical change and as inferred in the developmental change described earlier. Similarly so for the other elements of personality change. In psychotherapy, as in quantum change and developmental change, emotions are brought into the foreground of consciousness. Moreover, there seems to be a constant movement back and forth among the elements of negative emotion, insight, and reflective work. And of course, the interpersonal process itself is intrinsic to the process and handmaiden to change, although the process itself could stand more scrutiny as discussed later.

The gradual change of psychotherapy process thus resembles the more precipitous and sudden change described earlier in this chapter. What differentiates them may be the intensity of affect and the suddenness of the "channel-clearing" process. In precipitous change there is a sudden and intense wave of insight, either secondary to or in advance of strong emotion. In the case of more gradual change, insights are also intrinsic to change, but they may be of a milder, less dramatic nature. According to Weiner (1975), in psychodynamic psychotherapy an interpretation is effective for a patient when it "identifies features of behavior that he has not been fully aware of" (Weiner, 1975, p. 115). Weiner instructed that a therapist effectively interprets "when the patient is verging (on awareness) . . . and is just one step away from full awareness" (p. 132). Thus, a moderate rather than precipitous jolt of channel-clearing insight seems called for. If it is too abrupt and intense, due, for example, to a poorly timed interpretation or one aimed at material too difficult, change is blocked rather than facilitated.

In summary, we can discern certain common elements cutting across precipitous and gradual change, elective and fortuitous change. Intense emotion provides the energic force necessary to propel movement and change. Small changes in the relation of thought to emotion signaled by the emotion of surprise and often indexed by the sensation of sudden insight also appear to be necessary; these seemingly "minor" changes in one component in the system, set into motion systemwide changes that can grow over time. The intense emotion can occur prior to the dawn of the new emotion–cognition linkage, or after, as in the cascade of negative emotion that is freed when discontent crystallizes or when defensive processes are lowered. For the change to grow, there needs to be cognitive-emotional work over time; there also needs to be interpersonal support during the consolidation of the new identity in order for the change to stabilize. We turn now to consider the implications of this theory for further research on stability and change in personality organization.

V. FURTHER THOUGHTS AND IMPLICATIONS

As the Mills longitudinal study has shown, not all people are responsive to opportunities for change. In Helson's terms, this has much to do with the quality of ego structure and ego defenses. In the Mills study, the women who changed in contrast to those who did not appeared to vary most in an aspect of personality that resembles the dimension of "openness to experience"—one of the five major dimensions of personality described by the Big Five Model (Costa & McCrae, chap. 20, this volume). We can also approach the issue of permeability to change from the perspective of affect theory.

Tomkins (1962, 1981) described personality as an ideoaffective organization or structure. This structure was conceived of as consisting of certain core affects and supporting cognitions. In affect terms then, the openness to experience of the Mills women who underwent change likely reflected an ideoaffective structure linked to trait interest. There are other trait emotions or dispositional emotions that may be more or less conducive to change as well. In our view, individuals whose ideoaffective structures predispose them to orient towards experiences of sadness and shame are more likely to absorb new experience rather than to defend against it because these emotions are quintessentially inclusive of and exquisitely responsive to the other within a relationship. In contrast, persons inclined to experience contempt and disgust in a dispositional way are more likely to resist change. Disgust and contempt involve sensory and interpersonal rejection, and a closing off of the self. The interpersonal aspect of the elements conducive to change is thus short-circuited.

This brings us to a fuller discussion of the role of emotion and interpersonal process. For this we turn back to the psychotherapy context. Indeed, the therapist's office is a potentially rich laboratory for the study of emotion process, and especially the processes involved in personality change.

The psychotherapy process has many significant emotional junctures, as noted by Greenberg (1993). Paying attention to these junctures appears to offer a fruitful way of focusing emotion work in therapy. However, there is much that the therapist and personality psychologist can learn about emotion dynamics and personality change process by (a) examining the process more closely, and (b) by bringing the therapist's emotions and personality structure more explicitly into the picture.

Using a typed transcript of a psychotherapy session and coding the presence of shame markers and other emotion cues, Scheff (1987) was able to illustrate how the moment-to-moment tracking of emotional reactions lets us understand the "small changes" that may lead to either productive personality work, ensnarement in cul de sacs, or even premature termination of therapy. In identifying shame markers and other emotional cues in the transcript of a psychotherapy session, Scheff (1987) was able to show how an ill-timed interpretation by the therapist provoked shame in the patient, which subsequently led to anger and a veering off into a long, frustrating, and nonproductive tangent. In such situations, which are probably more common than any of us would like to admit, the patient, instead of being led to a clarifying insight, followed by a new openness to experience, girds himself with defenses, which the therapist then may interpret as "resistence." In its wake, there is a shutting down, rather than an expansion of awareness in both the patient and therapist.

Like everyone else, therapists can err, but perhaps are less likely to do so if they attend to the momentary changes that take place in the patient's affect as well as their own, and less so if they have a good grip on the ideoaffective structure that the patient brings to the session. Training in affect theory is currently not a standard part of the curriculum in therapist training programs; one could argue that it should be.

Affect theory has implications as well for the "fit" between therapist and client, which may have a very direct bearing on the success of the change process. In an effort to clarify the change process and the elements of successful therapy, the psychotherapy process literature has identified *patient characteristics* and *therapist characteristics* that are associated with positive therapeutic outcomes, but has scarcely begun to consider how particular "pairings" affect the course and outcome of psychotherapy. We may find that therapeutic relationships work in ways that are similar to other dyadic relationships. The literature on affect and attachment indicates that different attachment styles are linked to different patterns of emotion regulation; moreover, the literature on adult romantic relationships and attachment styles indicates that certain attachment types are drawn to one another and that certain types have a greater capacity to endure over time than others (Magai & McFadden, 1995).

In psychotherapy research, focus on individual characteristics is a good beginning but it is still imbued with a linear systems perspective. And if we should know anything about psychotherapy, it is that it is a quintessential dynamic system. We should be looking at small changes and small perturbations within the larger system. And, as Greenberg has intuited, emotions may be the crucial pivots.

In conclusion, the study of the change process, whether in psychotherapy, in micronarrative research, or other creative approaches to the analysis of transformative life experiences, promises an exciting new opening for research on personality. In the physical world, the seemingly solid world of matter often undergoes radical transformation of state—for example, when solid changes to liquid. Similarly, the seeming solidity of personality can be caught up in transformation in response to certain mutative agents and experiences in ways that are not yet clearly understood. The mutative phenomena often appear to be small or even incidental to change. But as chaos theory indicates, minor perturbations can give rise to large systemwide changes. The kinds of transformative experience that people report in narrative accounts at least subjectively appear to be of this kind of magnitude, and the experiences are invariably couched in emotional terms. Indeed, emotions appear to constitute fractals in the stream of life experience.

REFERENCES

Aldwin, C. M., Levenson, M. R., & Spiro, A. (1994). Vulnerability and resilience to combat exposure: Can stress have lifelong effects? *Psychology and Aging, 9,* 34–44.

Anderson, J. W. (1988). Henry A. Murray's early career: A psychobiographical exploration. *Journal of Personality, 56,* 139–171.

Baumeister, R. F. (1994). Personality stability, personality change, and the question of process. In T. F. Heatherton & J. L. Weinberger (Eds.), *Can personality change?* (pp. 281–297). Washington, DC: American Psychological Association Emotion.

Camras, L. (1991). A dynamical system perspective on expressive development. In K. T. Strongman (Ed.), *International review of studies on emotion* (Volume 1, pp. 16–28). New York: John Wiley.

Caspi, A., & Moffitt, T. E. (1993). When do individual differences matter? A paradoxical theory of personality coherence. *Psychological Inquiry, 4,* 247–271.

Costa, P. T., & McCrae, R. R. (1994). Set in plaster? Evidence for the stability of adult personalty. In T. F. Heatherton & T. L. Weinberger (Eds.), *Can personality change?* (pp. 21–40). Washington, DC: American Psychological Association.

Diclemente, C. C. (1994). If behaviors change, can personality be far behind? In T. F. Heatherton & J. L. Weinberger (Eds.), *Can personality change?* (pp. 175–198). Washington, DC: American Psychological Association.

Fogel, A., & Thelen, E. (1987). Development of early expressive and communicative action: Reinterpreting the evidence from a dynamic systems perspective. *Developmental Psychology, 23,* 747–761.

Gould, R. L. (1980). Transformations during early and middle adult years. In N. J. Smelser & E. H. Erikson (Eds.), *Themes of work and love in adulthood* (pp. 213–237). Cambridge, MA: Harvard University Press.

Greenberg, L. S. (1993). Emotion and change processes in psychotherapy. In M. Lewis & J. Haviland (Eds.), *Handbook of emotions* (pp. 499–508). New York: Guilford.

Greenberg, L. S., & Safran, J. D. (1984). Integrating affect and cognition: A perspective on the process of therapeutic change. *Cognitive Therapy and Research, 8,* 559–578.

Haviland, J. M., & Walker-Andrews, A. S. (1992). Emotion socialization: A view from development and ethology. In V. B. Van Hasselt & M. Hersen (Eds.), *Handbook of social development* (pp. 29–50). New York: Plenum.

Heatherton, R. F., & Nichols, P. A. (1994). Conceptual issues in assessing whether personality can change. In T. F. Heatherton & J. L. Weinberger (Eds.), *Can personality change?* (pp. 3–18). Washington, DC: American Psychological Association.

Helson, R., Mitchell, V., & Moane, G. (1984). Personality and patterns of adherence and nonadherence to the social clock. *Journal of Personality and Social Psychology, 46,* 1019–1096.

Helson, R., & McCabe, L. (1994). The social clock project in middle age. In B. F. Turner & L. E. Troll (Eds.), *Women growing older* (pp. 68–93). Thousand Oaks, CA: Sage.

Helson, R., & Moane, G. (1987). Personality change in women from college to midlife. *Journal of Personality and Social Psychology, 52*(1), 176–186.

Helson, R., & Roberts, B. W. (1994). Ego development and personality change in adulthood. *Journal of Personality and Social Psychology, 66*(5), 911–920.

Helson, R., & Wink, P. (1992). Personality change in women from the early 40s to the early 50s. *Psychology and Aging, 7*(1), 46–55.

Heatherton, T. F., & Weinberger, J. H. (1994). *Can personality change?* Washington, DC: American Psychological Association.

Izard, C. E. (1991). *The psychology of emotions.* New York: Plenum Press.

James, W. (1961). *The varieties of religious experience.* New York: Collier Books. (Originally published 1902)

Levinson, D. J., Darrow, C. N., Klein, E. B., Levinson, M. H., & McKee, B. (1978). *The seasons of a man's life.* New York: Alfred A. Knopf.

Lewis, M. D. (in press). Personality self-organization: Cascading constraints on cognition-emotion interaction. In A. Fogel, M. C. Lyra, & J. Valsiner (Eds.), *Dynamics and indeterminism in developmental and social processes.* Hillsdale, NJ: Erlbaum.

Luborsky, L., & Spence, D. P. (1971). Quantitative research on psychoanalytic therapy. In A. E. Bergin & S. L. Garfield (Eds.), *Handbook of psychotherapy and behavior change* (pp. 408–438). New York: Wiley.

Magai, C., & McFadden, S. (1995). *The role of emotions in social and personality development: History, theory, and research.* New York: Plenum.

Malatesta, C. Z. (1990). The role of emotion in the development and organization of personality. In R. Thompson (Ed.), *Socioemotional development* Nebraska Symposium on Motivation (pp. 1–56). Lincoln: University of Nebraska Press.

McAdams, D. P. (1994). Can personality change? Levels of stability and growth in personality across the lifespan. In T. F. Heatherton & J. L. Weinberger (Eds.), *Can personality change?* (pp. 299–313). Washington, DC: American Psychological Association.

Miller, W. R., & C'deBaca, R. (1994). Quantum change: Toward a psychology of transformation. In T. F. Heatherton & J. L. Weinberger (Eds.), *Can personality change?* (pp. 253–280). Washington, DC: American Psychological Association.

Pervin, L. A. (1994). Personality stability, personality change, and the question of process. In T. F. Heatherton & J. L. Weinberger (Eds.), *Can personality change?* (pp. 315–330). Washington, DC: American Psychological Association.

Scheff, T. J. (1987). The shame–rage spiral: A case study of an interminable quarrel. In H. B. Lewis (Ed.), *The role of shame in symptom formation.* Hillsdale, NJ: Lawrence Erlbaum.

Tomkins, S. S. (1962). *Affect, imagery, consciousness. Vol. 1: The positive affects.* New York: Springer.

Tomkins, S. S. (1981). The quest for primary motives: Biography and autobiography of an idea. *Journal of Personality and Social Psychology, 41,* 306–329.

Ullman, C. (1989). The transformed self: *The psychology of religious conversion.* New York: Plenum Press.

Weiner, I. B. (1975). *Principles of psychotherapy.* New York: John Wiley & Sons.

CHAPTER 23

Emotional Episodes and Emotionality through the Life Span

Jennifer M. Jenkins *and* Keith Oatley

Institute of Child Study　　*Center for Applied Cognitive Science*
University of Toronto　　*Ontario Institute for Studies in Education*
Toronto, Canada　　*Toronto, Canada*

WHAT IS CHARACTER BUT THE DETERMINATION OF INCIDENT? WHAT IS
INCIDENT BUT THE ILLUSTRATION OF CHARACTER?
　　　　　　　　—*Henry James (1884)*, The Art of Fiction

I. INTRODUCTION

If development in childhood is about the process of maturation interacting with the accidents of family, what are we to say of development during adulthood? The emphasis changes. By the end of adolescence, a person no longer has mere temperament but a personality or, as it is called in
fiction, character. Throughout adulthood, the interaction of personality
or character with the accidents of life gives rise to the central themes and
meanings of life.

In this chapter our plan is to present evidence that episodes of emotion are the units by which we can understand important aspects of personality and psychopathology, and also how lives come to have personal
meaning. By episodes of emotion we mean emotions that last long enough

for the person experiencing the emotion, or some observer, to be aware that something has occurred that is significant to the person's goals. Here we propose that people develop relational goals in childhood, goals about what is most important to them in relationships and that such relational goals underlie a significant part of emotional experience across the life span. As people face the tasks of different phases of the life span, finding employment, choosing a mate, rearing children, what they want in relationships influences their actions and choices: does it feel comfortable to be intimate with others, do we need to get the better of other people in relationships, how threatening is the world to our sense of well-being?

First we need to make some distinctions among the different terms and concepts of emotions, for without such distinctions understanding emotional life can be confusing—understanding the academic literature on emotions, even more so.

II. EMOTION INCIDENTS ALONG THE SPECTRUM OF EMOTIONAL PHENOMENA

We propose the idea of an affective spectrum organized in terms of the time course of different kinds of emotional phenomena. This spectrum is sketched in Figure 1.

Facial expressions last between .5 sec and 4 sec, and autonomic events last not much longer (Ekman, 1984). Episodes of emotion that people become aware of in themselves and others typically last a few minutes to a few hours (Frijda, Mesquita, Sonnemans, & van Goozen, 1991). Moods last for hours or days. Most psychiatric syndromes are defined as lasting for at least 2 weeks and can last for years (American Psychiatric Association, 1994). Temperament and personality traits, by definition, extend over most of a lifetime.

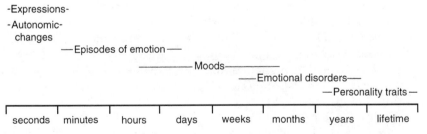

Figure 1 A time spectrum of different kinds of emotional phenomena, ranging from the shortest term changes of facial expression and autonomic response to traits of temperament and personality that can last a lifetime. (From Oatley & Jenkins, 1996. Reprinted with permission.)

The far left-hand side of the spectrum, facial expressions of emotion lasting for seconds, has been the primary focus for research endeavors in the psychology of the emotions for the last 20 years. Here we argue that patterns of emotionality such as those we see in personality and psychopathology are best understood by paying attention, not to these fleeting expressions, but to episodes of emotion that last for minutes, hours, or sometimes days. In an emotion episode the person knows that something of significance has happened. A woman's boss chastises her at work and she replays the discussion for hours. A toddler wants his mother to help him construct a building. She is busy. His disappointment colors their interactions for the rest of the day.

Emotions point to goals. As the earliest appraisal theorists (Arnold & Gasson, 1954) pointed out, emotions are relational—they relate events in the world with what is important to ourselves. So an appraisal is, in the first place, an evaluation of some event as good or bad, suitable or unsuitable, helping or hindering progress towards a goal. All emotions, both short and long term, point to goals, but only those episodes of emotion that last for minutes, hours, or days, and which sometimes have repercussions for years, point to the achievement or violation of *significant* goals.

Emotions that mark significant goals can monopolize attention. Empirically there is much evidence for the constraining effect of moods and emotions on attentional tasks (Mathews, 1993). But although the objects of emotions are usually obvious to us, neither these objects nor their implications are always fully understood (Oatley & Duncan, 1992). What emotions do, therefore, is to focus attention, sometimes ruminatively (Nolen-Hoeksema, Parker, & Larson, 1994), sometimes in such a way as to prompt important life decisions as when falling in love or deciding angrily to quit a job. When an episode of emotion occurs it organizes cognitive functioning in a particular way, with the implication that over longer periods of time we pay attention to certain aspects of our experience and not to other aspects. Dynamic systems theorists have argued that as emotional states become more coherent they act like attractors, pulling in similar emotional states and repelling dissimilar emotional states (Lewis, 1996).

III. EMOTION EPISODES COMPILED INTO EMOTION SCHEMA

Emotion episodes are compiled over time into emotion schema. We see emotion schema as enduring patterns of emotional response. They underlie the long-term patterns of emotionality that are evident on the right-hand side of the emotion spectrum: emotional disorders and personality states.

In childhood, we argue, as well as developing skills and knowledge, each individual develops emotion schema. Based at first on genetic biases of temperament in interaction with caregivers, children compile into a coherent structure significant emotional episodes of their lives. Like skills and habits, emotion schema are adaptations to environments, typically family environments in which they arise, given the temperamental constraints of the child.

Following Tomkins (see his collected writings, 1995) emotion schema can be characterized as a persisting modality of emotional response to certain kinds of situation and certain kinds of people, that carries across time and across contexts. Probably the most typical way in which such schema arise is through repeated experience of similar emotion episodes; for instance, when a parent repeatedly yells at a child, and the child frequently becomes angry and resists. Repeated experiences of this type of emotion episode will get compiled into a schema for the child in which the world is a threatening place, and threats are most effectively warded off by getting angry.

Some schema may also develop from a very traumatic single event that functions to orient the person towards the perception of similar threats. Later, small emotion episodes are integrated into the schema, broadening its applicability. In adult life, onsets of anxiety may take this form. For instance, in posttraumatic stress disorder one traumatic event such as being assaulted, will elicit a high level of anxiety. Subsequently, many events that were previously nonthreatening are perceived as threatening (McNally, Kaspi, Riemann, & Zeitlin, 1990). Tomkins (1979) elaborated this kind of process in his work on script theory.

We suggest that there are two parts to an emotion schema: the goals in relationship (we call this the goal orientation) and the emotion-related strategies that have developed to achieve goals in relationship.

Goal orientation in a relationship is a bias such that some goals are more important in our lives than others: so generally, we humans aim for interactions with others that feel familiar to us. This goal orientation is implicit in interaction rather than explicit and can be inferred from emotion episodes. Emotion episodes are markers that signal that important goals have been achieved or violated. These are not necessarily recognized consciously, but they are indicated by the kinds of events that upset or please us, as well as in the way that we behave emotionally with other people. For instance, for people who disparage close relationships in their speech, and prefer to spend time by themselves, or in a series of short-term relationships, we can infer that emotional distance feels more comfortable than proximity. Someone with a Type A behavior pattern is often hostile and combative with others. We can infer that dominance in the relationship is more important than a sense of reciprocity or warmth. People seek emotional states in relationships that feel optimal because of familiarity.

Here we describe a few of the goal orientations that become prominent in people's lives, and particularly those that might underlie the most common of the emotionally based psychopathological conditions such as externalizing disorders, depression, and anxiety. This description is not exhaustive.

One dimension of importance is the experiencing of relatedness or intimacy with other people. This dimension of personality development has been discussed at length by psychoanalysts (Horney, 1950) and more recently operationalized by attachment theorists (Ainsworth, Blehar, Walters, & Wall, 1978; Bowlby, 1971). Attachment theorists argue that sensitivity and parental responsiveness in early infancy lead to babies feeling that other people can be relied on as a source of comfort. Consequently babies with this experience will seek out their parent at times of threat, receive comfort and reassurance, leading to a recovery in their capacity to explore the environment. This sense of being able to move close to others and trust them is a goal orientation that is stable over time, as we discuss below.

A second dimension in relationships is about whether other people and the world are perceived as actively threatening to our sense of well-being. Psychopathology in childhood and adult life is associated with severe adversity or threat in childhood (Brewin, Andrews, & Gotlib, 1993; Rutter, Yule, Quinton, Rowlands, Yule, & Berger, 1975). Child abuse or neglect, interparental conflict, a parent suffering form a psychiatric disorder, all raise the risk for children and adults of developing a psychiatric disorder. The way that we understand these risks is that they encourage the development of schema in which the self is perceived as being under threat. Such beliefs are stronger in people with psychopathology than those without. For instance Quiggle, Garber, Panak, and Dodge (1992) found that children with psychopathology are more likely to think that other people have hostile intentions towards them, than children without psychopathology. Mathews (1993) has described how people suffering from anxiety perceive the world as threatening.

A third goal orientation has to do with valuing of the self in relationships. Central to depressive symptomatology is a view of the self as worthless. Experiences in childhood contribute to a view of the self as devalued in relationship, and may lead to the creation of an environment in adult life in which this expectation is confirmed. For example, it has been found that women who will subsequently become depressed often marry men who are vulnerable to psychiatric disorder (Coyne, Burchill, & Stiles,

1991). In time these marriages become problematic and conflictual. The argument that we are making is that these vulnerable women expect less for themselves in a relationship, marry people who are themselves more vulnerable and less able to support them, and consequently end up in circumstances in which they are less valued than their nondepressed counterparts.

A fourth goal orientation that is important in understanding long-term continuities in affect is power or dominance in relationships. In the primate literature on emotion this dimension has been important in understanding social structures and hierarchy (Goodall, 1992). Animals reach the top of the dominance hierarchy through displays or threats of aggression. During conflict, other animals' displays of fear signal their acceptance of a lower place in the hierarchy. Dominance has also been used widely to understand the dynamics of human social relationships (Kemper, 1990). In marriages people signal dominance through displays of anger and aggression. Sadness and fear function to signal submission (Biglan et al., 1985). For some people (e.g., those with Type A behavior patterns), establishing dominance in relationship may be more important than experiencing closeness.

Emotion schema involve people compiling strategies in the satisfaction of these goal orientations. People develop characteristic ways of eliciting care and protection from someone, as well as for keeping them at bay if distance feels more comfortable. People develop ways of negotiating dominance in relationship. For some if dominance is a top-level goal, this may be most appropriately satisfied by displays of anger and aggression. If however, such displays lead to escalating interchanges with someone physically more powerful, other means, such as whining and refusing, may be evident. As a means of warding off threat one person may remain in the house all day, refusing to answer the door and experiencing high levels of anxiety. Another may use anger and retaliation knowing that in their environment it functions to suppress aversive interactions (Patterson, 1982). We argue that such strategies have developed because they have functioned effectively in specific environments in the achievement of relational goals.

IV. EMOTION SCHEMA AS UNDERLYING CONTINUITIES IN EMOTIONALITY ACROSS THE LIFE SPAN

Why do we need to postulate something like an emotion schema? It is because across the life span there are strong continuities for some kinds of emotional behavior.

We postulate that emotions are primarily relational and that they function to structure interactions between people (Oatley & Jenkins, 1996). Consequently we see the schema that are responsible for continuities within people as primarily relational (Mead, 1913; Sullivan, 1952). Some of their structure arises from biological biases, some from certain kinds of experience, most, no doubt, from an interaction between these two kinds of influence. Here is some of the evidence of continuities.

Kagan and his colleagues (Kagan, Reznick, & Snidman, 1988) have identified some children who show extreme avoidance of new things, and they postulate a strong biological basis. Children who were very shy at age 2 were still very shy and inhibited at age 7. Caspi, Elder, and Bem (1988) found that shyness was stable over a 30-year period.

Aggressiveness too shows strong continuity: Caspi, Elder, and Bem (1987) found that children who were angry and ill-tempered when they were age 8 continued to be ill-tempered as adults, with accumulating effects. Males were less likely to stay in school. As adults their work life was more erratic, with lower occupational status and more downward mobility than their even-tempered counterparts. Ill-tempered females tended to marry below the expectations of their social class and to have less marital satisfaction, to show more ill temper in parenting, and to divorce more often than their even-tempered counterparts.

Other emotionally based aspects of personality show continuities: Costa and McCrae (1988) have reported stability coefficients of between 0.79 and 0.95 on the personality factors neuroticism, extraversion, and openness, over a 6-year period. It is not only the subjective element of these ratings that gives them their high levels of stability over time. Spouses' ratings of their partners' emotional functioning were also stable over time and agreed with self-reports (Costa & McCrae, 1988).

Some measures of psychopathology across the life span also show high levels of continuity. From a study by Harrington, Fudge, Rutter, Pickles, and Hill (1990), it was evident that people who suffered from depression as children were more likely to suffer depression than any other kind of psychiatric disorder in adulthood. The stability of aggression both during childhood and from childhood to adulthood is extremely high and of the same order as the stability of IQ (Olweus, 1979). Graham and Rutter (1973) found that 75% of children with an externalizing disorder at age 10 still had externalizing disorder at age 14. Robins (1978) found that about half of all children with an externalizing behavior disorder went on to have an antisocial personality disorder in adulthood; in both childhood and adulthood, such disorders are characterized by activities such as stealing, hostility, and lack of concern for others.

Disorders do not continue constantly throughout childhood. They come and go. Yet when stress returns, the person tends to show their own emotionally characteristic way of responding to it.

Another reason for postulating an emotion schema is that family relationship variables (including how emotions are expressed) are strong
predictors of psychopathology in children and adults. One needs some
way of thinking about how such emotion episodes in childhood can be
incorporated into a longer term structure that influences action across
time and situations.

Such continuities indicate that a style of emotional response is elaborated and maintained, and then moves to new contexts. It is easiest to understand these continuities in terms of persisting emotional schema;
early emotional experiences or temperamental biases are amplified by
learning and given content in further specific episodes of interaction
with others. The extent to which they are self-sustaining and resistant to
change then increases.

V. EPISODES OF EMOTION, EMOTION SCHEMA, AND STAGES OF THE LIFE SPAN

In terms of life span development, schemas from childhood and adolescence are expressed through the tasks of adult life. Erikson (1950)
suggested eight life stages—each with a characteristic life task, each with
a thoroughly emotional quality. If any remains unresolved it tends to cast
a shadow over the rest of life and to keep presenting the person with
repercussions of the issue. Erikson postulated that the sequence starts in
the first year with the question of trust versus mistrust. When this issue is
resolved it gives rise to hope, which can sustain one in life and in relationships with others. The sequence continues through childhood and
adolescence up to the stages of young adulthood (intimacy in love versus
self-absorption), maturity (generativity versus stagnation), and old age
(integrity versus despair).

As Magai and Hunziker (1993) argued, one of the problems with the
idea of life span development is the tension between nomothetic and
idiographic approaches. On the nomothetic side, researchers in development have sought general continuities and discontinuities over the life
span. With an idiographic perspective, as in biography and autobiography, we become interested in how an individual copes not just with the
general process of getting older, but with the particularities and accidents of a life.

Erikson's theory resonates with works of art—as Erikson (1978) himself shows in his analysis of Ingmar Bergman's 1957 film *Wild Strawberries*,
in which the aging Dr. Isak Borg takes a journey across Sweden to be

awarded an honorary doctorate. Simultaneously he travels back towards his own childhood, revisiting and reflecting on his life. In the film, and to some extent in Erikson's analysis of it, what characterizes the revisited stages is not periods of time, but specific episodes of emotion, and scenes of emotional significance, which form the turning points of the narrative. So, in a memory of the house in the country where Isak had spent his summers until the age of 20, he vividly remembers the young woman Sara, whom he was to marry, being made love to (in the Victorian sense) by his older brother. Isak's emotional response to this jealous scene is to withdraw. This withdrawal was not just a response to this event; it was paradigmatic of the way in which he created within himself a kind of fastidiousness, thereby placing himself more and more outside life, looking in. Such emotional episodes are not just typical, but formative, as Singer and Salovey (1993) have shown. In their occurrence they become part of our self, and in their remembering and recounting they become part of our self-definition. For Borg, this scene becomes another brick built into a structure whose form was already discernible early in life. As Erikson tells us in his commentary on the film, Borg means "fortress." Below we will elaborate more generally on how such episodes are built into emotion schema that can become very strong and represent important aspects of selfhood.

Conceiving the central elements of life as those brought into relief as episodes of emotion gives a satisfactory fit between empirical research and the characteristically literary way of regarding lives in terms of narrative. Emotional episodes, like the episodes of a story, are the fundamental parts of the structure. Narrative, moreover, which links such episodes of emotion, gives us perhaps our most clearly defined sense of integration of the self (Oatley, 1992).

VI. WAYS OF MEASURING EMOTION EPISODES ACROSS THE LIFE SPAN

Although we are still in the early stages of devising measures that capture the significance of emotions in individual lives and that have psychometrically acceptable properties, there are some useful examples. Emotion episodes are made up of eliciting events that are significant to individuals, the individual's appraisals of the events, and the emotional expressions or actions in response.

Brown and Harris pioneered a method of evaluating the significance of life events. Using their method respondents are interviewed at length about events that have happened to them over the previous year. Their narrative accounts are analyzed for the severity of life event based on the meaning of the event in the person's life. If they lost a job, was this a job that they needed in order to be able to feed their children, or a part-time job that contributed to nonessentials? This method of determining the severity of the event using knowledge of the context in which the event occurred has raised the levels of prediction of who becomes depressed (Brown & Harris, 1978).

Other emotion researchers have been working on ways to assess characteristic ways that individuals' appraise events. Stein, Folkman, Trabasso, and Christopher-Richards (1995) have analyzed narrative accounts of individuals who have lost their partners. They interviewed partners of AIDS patients (who were themselves HIV negative) directly after their bereavement and 1 year later. The proportion of positive appraisals to total appraisals at the time of the partners' death was a remarkably strong predictor of emotional functioning 1 year later.

Another innovative method of assessing how people appraise events comes from psychotherapy outcome research. Methods have been devised for assessing the transference relationship. During psychotherapy patients talk about the upsets, conflict, and achievements of their lives. From these narratives, "core conflictual relationship themes" are determined and three elements are coded: the patient's wishes, needs or intentions in relation to the other, responses from the other, and the response from the self. Core conflictual relationship themes are similar to our concept of emotion schema, and have proven useful in understanding changes in the transference relationship as a result of psychotherapeutic intervention (Luborsky & Crits-Christoph, 1990).

What methods do we have for examining characteristic ways of responding emotionally? Interview and questionnaire measures of personality and psychopathology provide such measures. Assessments of psychopathology and temperament in childhood are based on parents' and teachers' ratings of the frequency of shyness, withdrawn behavior, tearfulness, angry hitting of other children, stealing, lying, and so forth. Adult measures of personality and psychopathology rely on subjective reports by the self across a large number of different circumstances. They provide us with a way of assessing an amalgam of emotion episodes, across time and situations, that are significant to the person.

We see in these kinds of methods an attempt to combine the nomothetic and idiographic methods of assessment. Using these methods we are getting closer to the significance of emotions in people's lives, and how emotional experiences become pivotal in personality development.

VII. FROM EMOTION EPISODES TO SCHEMA: THE ROLE OF FAMILY RELATIONSHIPS, TEMPERAMENT, AND LIFE'S ACCIDENTS

Here we give some examples, through work on family relationships, emotion, and temperament, to show how emotion schema are formed (Baldwin, 1992). In the cloth of a life, these continuities form the warp; among them the woof of events is woven. In adulthood as well as being equipped with a personality, partly based on such emotion schema, our task may be taken to include becoming aware of these threads and structures, of the characteristic patterns that continue to be woven, seeking through experience, reflection, planning, to be able to affect the further structure of our lives. We also want to examine some of the turning points in our lives. Although there are continuities from early childhood to adult life, there are also considerable discontinuities—times when our early experience or behavior does not predict later behavior. What kinds of events provide opportunities for change?

A. Mistrust in Relationships

Erikson suggested that the first task for the human infant was the negotiation of issues around trust, which was resolved into a sense of hope in the possibilities of intimate relationships. This idea has been empirically investigated by attachment theorists with the use of Ainsworth et al.'s (1978) Strange Situation Test. In this test, trained observers diagnose not emotional expressions or autonomic responses, but episodes of emotional response, first to separation and then reunion, of a year-old infant and a parent. Behaviors and emotions shown during the strange situation are thought to be indicative of the child's sense of security in the relationship. On the basis of these responses three styles of attachment have been found: secure, avoidant, and ambivalent. Both temperamental characteristics of the baby and parenting behaviors towards the infant over the previous year are thought to contribute to patterns of attachment (Goldsmith & Alansky, 1987).

These styles of attachment have proven to be significant predictors of future social relationships. Insecurely attached babies are more likely to have negative social relationships with teachers when they enter school, to be less communicative and sociable, and to have less good relationships with other children (Sroufe & Fleeson, 1988). This concept of secure attachment was extended across the life span, and Main and colleagues developed the Adult Attachment Interview (AAI) (George, Kaplan, & Main,

1985). This is a semistructured interview, in which the person gives a nar-
ratively based, autobiographical account of earlier and current close relationships. The adult equivalent of secure status is assigned if the interviewee gives a coherent story of early life and current relationships. The
equivalent of avoidant status is assigned to those who give a very distanced
account. The equivalent of ambivalent status is assigned if the interviewee
is still overwhelmed by memories of childhood. This approach unites
nomothetic and idographic concerns, and has life span implications.
People for whom these styles were measured at age 1 using the strange
situation, were interviewed at age 20 (Waters, Merrick, Albersheim, & Treboux, 1995), using the AAI. Waters and colleagues found that of those babies who had been classified as secure or avoidant in the strange situation, two-thirds were still classified in the same way in the AAI, and of
those who were classified ambivalent as babies, slightly less than half continued with the same classification. Transgenerational links in attachment
status have also been reported. Women who were classified as insecure
before the birth of their baby, are more likely to have insecure babies,
than women classified as secure (Fonagy, Steele, & Steele, 1991).

Although there is considerable continuity over time and across adults
and children, there is also discontinuity. Emotion episodes later in life involving positive attachment experiences can provide the opportunity for
a positive relational trajectory with long-term beneficial consequences.
Quinton and Rutter (1988) followed up a group of girls into adult life
who were brought up in institutions as children. The institutionalized
girls had been deprived of a continuous attachment to a single person,
which had been thought by Erikson, Bowlby, and others, to be essential for any kind of successful emotional life in adulthood. These women
did show more psychiatric disturbance and more parenting difficulties
than women who had been brought up by their parents. Some of the ex-
institutionalized women, however, did manage well as parents. They were
sensitive, warm, and effective with their children. The main factor found
to differentiate these women who were managing well in spite of their
difficult background from those with major problems was the presence
in the home of a supportive spouse in their adult life. Women who had
married someone in whom they could confide, and on whom they could
count for help, functioned better as mothers, and were less likely to be
depressed. So, even after a gross lack of love in early life, young adults
who do find love later on show a remarkable ability to recover from early
deleterious experiences.

Attachment theorists have explained such continuities in terms of
children developing a model of intimate relationships in early childhood.

This model is based on the child's sense of security and trust in the relationship, and comes about through the parental responsiveness to children's signals of distress. The reason that we prefer to describe continuities over time in terms of emotion schema is that we think that adults and children compile schema that are much broader than trust and mistrust in relationship. Attachment categorizations have also not been found to be strong predictors of one of the main dimensions of long-term emotionality: psychopathology (Fagot & Kavanagh, 1990). We see attachment processes around protection and security as one of the important influences on the development of emotion schema, but other dimensions in relationship, to be discussed below, are important for understanding patterns in psychopathology.

B. Anger in Relationships

Studies in psychiatric epidemiology have demonstrated those factors in people's lives that contribute to the development of externalizing psychopathology. Being the recipient of parental hostility and anger (Dodge, Bates, & Pettit, 1990) and being exposed to interparental hostility or high levels of anger expression between parents are both important predictors of this pattern of behavior (Jenkins & Smith, 1991). Temperamental factors are also important in understanding the development of externalizing psychopathology (Olweus, 1980). Boys are more likely to react with aggression to family disharmony (Smith & Jenkins, 1991). Of particular interest are the studies by Patterson (1982) in which he shows that in families in which one child has an externalizing disorder, anger and aggression are reinforced by parents giving in and withdrawing to such displays. Children's goals are met through their expressions of anger.

We have hypothesized that on the basis of these experiences children develop an anger schema, a win–lose schema about relationships in which the need to be dominant is a top-level goal, with this dominance being expressed through anger displays. We see this as the basis of externalizing psychopathology. How do episodes of emotion in the home get compiled into generalized schema? Children living in the circumstances described above will often be the target of anger expression from parents. Constitutional differences of children, probably around distress to limitation (Goldsmith, 1993), will make some likely to react to aversive environments with anger rather than other emotions. Through watching parents fighting they may experience anger through emotion contagion, but also learn that problems are negotiated through the escalation of anger. These emotion episodes have in common displays of dominance in the relationship, as well as anger expression as a strategy for achieving goals. In an otherwise emotionally aversive environment, the value of dominance in a relationship may become paramount, hence the compilation of episodes of emotion into a meaningful schema.

Children exposed to such relationships in family life carry the anger schema into peer relationships, showing patterns of aggression with their peers (Dodge et al., 1990). Such patterns extend across the life span. Children who have been aggressively parented are more likely to parent aggressively themselves (Simons, Whitbeck, Conger, & Chyi-In, 1991).

Again it is apparent that positive relationships during the life span may be able to moderate such schema. Jenkins and Smith (1990) found that the presence of a grandparent to whom the child was close was associated with a much reduced risk of psychopathology in children experiencing high levels of interparental conflict. Presumably through such relationships children develop a sense that relationships other than those based on dominance can occur. The child learns that feeling valued and comforted may provide more satisfaction than being dominant.

C. Depression, Life Events, and Early Experience

We have sketched some of the ways in which conditions of family life—of trust, of hostility—translate into characteristic patterns of relating emotionally. Now we consider how early experiences interact in later life with life's accidents such that specific patterns of emotionality are formed.

Magai and Hunziker (1993) have argued that although there is a good deal of psychology about the continuities and stages of life, there is not much on life's accidents. But there is a psychology of the accidents of adult life; it is in a place where not all psychologists look—in the epidemiological study of psychiatric disorder.

Brown and Harris (1978) found that in 89% of cases of women, randomly sampled from the community, who had experienced a depressive breakdown, the breakdown had been preceded by a severe life event or difficulty. Those who became depressed had suffered someone in the family becoming seriously ill, an eviction from home, an adolescent son getting in serious trouble with the police, the family's breadwinner being fired without prospect of reemployment . . . serious life events in which the structure and fabric of a person's life is torn away. More poor people than rich people become depressed in part because these devastating events are more likely in their lives, in part because the less well-off have fewer resources with which to meet them.

What has been found in the research of Brown and Harris, and many others (Gotlib & Hammen, 1992; Oatley & Bolton, 1985), is that when such devastating "accidents" occur—let us call them adversities—if the person is vulnerable in certain possible ways, then he or she is very likely to suffer an episode of major depression. Again we argue that emotion schema are important in whether one succumbs to these adversities, or whether one manages to function in spite of them.

1. Vulnerability to Adversity

The vulnerabilities that make for depression when serious adversities occur were found (among women) by Brown and Harris to include lack of an intimate relationship with another person, and having lost one's own mother in childhood. Let us look a little more closely at these two kinds of vulnerability—lack of social support, and early loss of a mother.

a. Lack of Social Support. If a person suffers a severe adversity and has social support that provides a source of definition of the self apart from the role that has been lost or damaged by the event or difficulty, then this person is likely to experience episodes of strong negative emotion as he or she tries to make sense of what has happened, but will not become depressed. But if the person lacks social support then after a severe adversity, an episode of major depression is more likely to occur. If a person has become depressed, then the person will recover from depression if new sources of valuing the self can be built by means of new plans or relationships, alleviations of chronic difficulties (Oatley & Perring, 1991). Without such means, depression is likely to become chronic.

b. Effects of Early Failures of Parenting. Next let us look at the effects of early loss of a parent. Though such loss has long been suspected as making people vulnerable to later depression, only rather recently have the processes involved become clear.

It could be imagined, as implied both by Erikson and Bowlby, that failure of attachment at an early stage, not having established a sense of trust, leaves a person vulnerable. It seems now, however, that it is not the loss of a parent as such that makes the difference. It is the lack of parental care that typically follows loss of a mother that has the principal negative effects on the person and on the person's sense of self. Brewin et al. (1993) and Brown and Harris (1993) found that women who were neglected during childhood, and those who had been subjected to early physical or sexual abuse, were at increased risk of both depression and anxiety as adults.

The vulnerability of early neglect or abuse probably consists of damage to people's sense of themselves as being valuable and worthy of love.

Negative emotion schema in turn increase the likelihood of creating the kinds of situations that are likely to turn out badly. People who have experienced early neglect or abuse may have yearnings for love and protection. These seem to propel them into hasty sexual relationships. With choices that are not perhaps as considered as they might be, the risk of such relationships being punitive is increased. Early pregnancies, and single-parent status leads for most people in Western society to severe and intractable economic difficulties. All this can confirm expectations of loss and worthlessness, which become part of the self-deprecating pattern.

D. Personality and Emotion Bias

Although, as we have argued the reasons for onsets of depression are not mysterious, the etiological effects of severe life events and difficulties does not mean that constitutional effects, including those of temperament, are absent.

Recent evidence from twin studies (Kendler, Neale, Kessler, Heath, & Eaves, 1993b) indicates that there is some genetic predisposition towards depression. This could work in terms of bias, for instance of emotion schemas tipped towards feelings of sadness, worthlessness, and low confidence. Perhaps, too, as Kramer (1993) has suggested this might be mediated in part by mechanisms based on the transmitter substance serotonin. There is, for instance, suggestive evidence from monkeys that lack of serotonin gives rise to less social confidence and more withdrawal (Raleigh, McGuire, Brammer, Pollack, & Yuwiler, 1991).

Genetic influences do not only operate on the risk of depression *per se*. Plomin et al. (1990) examined life events in the last half of the life span in a twin population. They found that monozygotic twins (who share 100% of their genes) were much more similar to each other than dizygotic twins (who share on average only 50% of their genes) in the number of severe life events experienced during their lifetime, and Kendler, Neale, Kessler, Heath, and Eaves (1993a) also found that frequencies of life events were more strongly correlated in monozygotic than dizygotic twins. Plomin and Bergeman (1991) have reviewed a number of studies that have shown how variables thought to be environmental (like life events) are influenced by genetics. The inference is that some people, via personality traits or emotional biases, bring more severe events and difficulties upon themselves. Even so-called uncontrollable events show a modest association with genetics. Severe events in turn influence the incidence of depression. It is also easy to see that some people may have biases for or against forming long-lasting supportive relationships than others.

VIII. CONCLUSION

In adulthood, we confront the accidents of life equipped not just with resources which in Western society are based on money, but with the resources of supportive relationships, and social structures. Importantly, too, we have inner resources, of the kinds of emotion schema that we have built up since childhood. In memories, such as those of Dr. Borg in *Wild Strawberries,* particular episodes that seem especially redolent of characteristic patterns come to seem significant and serve as anchors in the narratives we tell about our lives, to define ourselves. The principal events of our autobiographies are episodes of emotion, and for some of us, very large and significant emotional episodes can become classified as depression or anxiety states. Such states give rise to the possibilities of tragedy in lives where the resources on which we depend are not universally available. But at the same time the emotional crises that we face, by way of the intense preoccupation that they create, give rise to the possibilities of self-reflection, and from such reflections arise the possibilities of self-understanding and change.

REFERENCES

Ainsworth, M. D. S., Blehar, M. C., Walters, E., & Wall, S. (1978). *Patterns of attachment: A psychological study of the strange situation.* Hillsdale, NJ: Erlbaum.

American Psychiatric Association (1994). *Diagnostic and statistical manual of mental disorders, Fourth edition: DSM-IV.* Washington, DC: American Psychiatric Association.

Arnold, M. B., & Gasson, J. A. (1954). Feelings and emotions as dynamic factors in personality integration. In M. B. Arnold & S. J. Gasson (Eds.), *The human person* (pp. 294–313). New York: Ronald.

Baldwin, M. (1992). Relational schemas and the processing of social information. *Psychological Bulletin, 112,* 461–484.

Bergman, I. (1957). *Wild strawberries.*

Biglan, A., Hops, H., Sherman, L., Friedman, L. S., Arthus J., & Osteen, V. (1985). Problem solving interactions of depressed women and their husbands. *Behavior Therapy, 16,* 431–451.

Bowlby, J. (1971). *Attachment and loss, Volume 1. Attachment.* London: Hogarth Press (reprinted by Penguin, 1978).

Brewin, C., Andrews, B., & Gotlib, I. H. (1993). Psychopathology and early experience: A reappraisal of retrospective reports. *Psychological Bulletin, 113,* 82–98.

Brown, G. W., & Harris, T. O. (1978). *Social origins of depression: A study of psychiatric disorder in women.* London: Tavistock.

Brown, G. W., & Harris, T. O. (1993). Aetiology of anxiety and depressive disorders in an inner-city population. 1. Early adversity. *Psychological Medicine, 23,* 143–154.

Caspi, A., Elder, G. H., & Bem, D. J. (1987). Moving against the world: life course patterns of explosive children. *Developmental Psychology, 23,* 308–313.

Caspi, A., Elder, G. H., & Bem, D. J. (1988). Moving away from the world: life-course patterns of shy children. *Developmental Psychology, 24, (no. 6),* 824–831.

Costa, P. T., & McCrae, R. R. (1988). Personality in adulthood: A six-year longitudinal study of self reports and spouse ratings on the NEO Personality Inventory. *Journal of Personality and Social Psychology, 54,* 853–863.

Coyne, J. C., Burchill, S. A., & Stiles, W. B. (1991). An interactional perspective on depression. In C. R. Snyder & D. O. Forsyth (Eds.), *Handbook of social and clinical psychology: The health perspective* (pp. 327–349). New York: Pergamon.

Dodge, K. A., Bates, J. E., & Pettit, G. S. (1990). Mechanisms in the cycle of violence. *Science, 250,* 1678–1683.

Ekman, P. (1984). Expression and the nature of emotion. In K. R. Scherer & P. Ekman (Eds.), *Approaches to emotion* (pp. 319–344). Hillsdale, NJ: Erlbaum.

Erikson, E. H. (1950). *Childhood and society.* London: Penguin (reissued 1965).

Erikson, E. H. (1978). Dr. Borg's life cycle. In E. H. Erikson (Ed.), *Adulthood* (pp. 1–31). New York: Norton.

Fagot, B. I., & Kavanagh, K. (1990). The prediction of antisocial behavior from avoidant attachment classifications. *Child Development, 61,* 864–873.

Fonagy, P., Steele, H., & Steele, M. (1991). Maternal representations of attachment during pregnancy predict the organization of infant-mother attachment at one year of age. *Child Development, 62,* 891–905.

Frijda, N. H., Mesquita, B., Sonnemans, J., & van Goozen, S. (1991). The duration of affective phenomena or emotions, sentiments and passions. In K. T. Strongman (Ed.), *International review of emotion, Vol. 1* (pp. 187–226). Chichester: Wiley.

George, C., Kaplan, N., & Main, M. (1985). *The Berkeley Adult Attachment Interview.* Unpublished protocol. Department of Psychology, University of California, Berkeley.

Goldsmith, H. H. (1993). Temperament: Variability in developing emotion systems. In M. Lewis & J. M. Haviland (Eds.), *Handbook of emotions* (pp. 353–364). New York: Guilford.

Goldsmith, H. H., & Alansky, J. A. (1987). Maternal and infant temperamental predictors of attachment. A meta-analytic review. *Journal of Consulting and Clinical Psychology, 55,* 805–816.

Goodall, J. (1992). Unusual violence in the overthrow of an alpha male chimpanzee at Gombe. In T. Nishida, W. C. McGrew, P. Marler, M. Pickford, & F. B. M. d. Waal (Eds.), *Topics in primatology, Vol. 1. Human origins* (pp. 131–142). Tokyo: University of Tokyo Press.

Gotlib, I. H., & Hammen, C. L. (1992). *Psychological aspects of depression: Toward a cognitive-interpersonal integration.* Chichester: Wiley and Sons.

Graham, P. J., & Rutter, M. (1973). Psychiatric disorder in the young adolescent: A follow-up study. *Proceedings of the Royal Society of Medicine, 66,* 1226–1229.

Harrington, R., Fudge, H., Rutter, M., Pickles, A., & Hill, J. (1990). Adult outcomes of childhood and adolescent depression. *Archives of General Psychiatry, 47*, 465–473.

Horney, K. (1950). *Neurosis and human growth.* New York: Norton.

James, H. (1884). The art of fiction. *Longmans Magazine*, Sept.

Jenkins, J. M., & Smith, M. A. (1990). Factors protecting children living in disharmonious homes: Maternal reports. *Journal of the American Academy of Child and Adolescent Psychiatry, 29*, 60–69.

Jenkins, J. M., & Smith, M. A. (1991). Marital disharmony and children's behaviour problems: Aspects of a poor marriage which affect children adversely. *Journal of Child Psychology and Psychiatry, 32*, 793–810.

Kagan, J., Reznick, J. S., & Snidman, N. (1988). Biological bases of childhood shyness. *Science, 240*, 167–171.

Kemper, T. D. (1990). Social relations and emotions: A structural approach. In T. D. Kemper (Ed.), *Research agendas in the sociology of emotions* (pp. 207–237). Albany, NY: State University of New York University Press.

Kendler, K. S., Neale, M., Kessler, R., Heath, A., & Eaves, L. (1993a). A twin study of recent life events. *Archives of General Psychiatry, 50*, 789–796.

Kendler, K. S., Neale, M. C., Kessler, R. C., Heath, A. C., & Eaves, L. J. (1993b). A longitudinal twin study of 1-year prevalence of major depression in women. *Archives of General Psychiatry, 50*, 843–852.

Kramer, P. D. (1993). *Listening to Prozac.* New York: Viking.

Lewis, M. (1996). Cognition-emotion feedback and the self-organization of developmental paths. *Human Development, 38*, 71–102.

Luborsky, L., & Crits-Christoph, P. (1990). *Understanding transference.* New York: Basic Books.

Magai, C., & Hunziker, J. (1993). Tolstoy and the riddle of developmental transformation: A lifespan analysis of the role of emotions in personality development. In M. Lewis & J. M. Haviland (Eds.), *Handbook of emotions* (pp. 247–259). New York: Guilford Press.

Mathews, A. (1993). Biases in emotional processing. *The Psychologist: Bulletin of the British Psychological Society, 6*, 493–499.

McNally, R. J., Kaspi, S. P., Riemann, B. C., & Zeitlin, S. B. (1990). Selective processing of threat cues in posttraumatic stress disorder. *Journal of Abnormal Psychology, 99*, 398–402.

Mead, G. H. (1913). The social self. *Journal of Philosophy, Psychology and Scientific Methods, 10*, 374–380.

Nolen-Hoeksema, S., Parker, L. E., & Larson, J. (1994). Ruminative coping with depressed mood following loss. *Journal of Personality and Social Psychology, 67* (92–104).

Oatley, K. (1992). Integrative action of narrative. In D. J. Stein & J. E. Young (Eds.), *Cognitive science and clinical disorders* (pp. 151–170). San Diego: Academic Press.

Oatley, K., & Bolton, W. (1985). A social-cognitive theory of depression in reaction to life events. *Psychological Review, 92*, 372–388.

Oatley, K., & Duncan, E. (1992). Incidents of emotion in daily life. In K. T. Strongman (Ed.), *International review of studies on emotion* (pp. 250–293). Chichester: Wiley.

Oatley, K., & Jenkins, J. M. (1996). *Understanding emotions: In psychology, psychiatry, and social science.* Cambridge, MA: Blackwell.

Oatley, K., & Perring, C. (1991). A longitudinal study of psychological and social factors affecting recovery from psychiatric breakdown. *British Journal of Psychiatry, 158,* 28–32.

Olweus, D. (1979). Stability of aggressive reaction patterns in males: A review. *Psychological Bulletin, 86,* 852–875.

Olweus, D. (1980). Familial and temperamental determinants of aggressive behavior in adolescent boys: A causal analysis. *Developmental Psychology, 16,* 644–660.

Patterson, G. R. (1982). *Coercive family process.* Eugene, OR: Castalia.

Plomin, R., & Bergeman, C. S. (1991). The nature of nurture: Genetic influence on environmental measures. *Behavioral and Brain Sciences, 14,* 373–427.

Plomin, R., Lichtenstein, P., Pedersen, N., McClearn, G. E., & Nesselroade, J. R. (1990). Genetic influences on life events during the last half of the life span. *Psychology of Aging, 5,* 25–30.

Quiggle, N. L., Garber, J., Panak, W. F., & Dodge, K. A. (1992). Social information processing in aggressive and depressed children: *Child Development, 63,* 1305–1320.

Quinton, D., & Rutter, M. (1988). *Parenting breakdown: The making and breaking of inter-generational links.* Aldershot: Avebury.

Raleigh, M. J., McGuire, M. T., Brammer, G. L., Pollack, D. B., & Yuwiler, A. (1991). Serotonergic mechanisms promote dominance acquisition in adult male vervet monkeys. *Brain Research, 559,* 181–190.

Robins, L. N. (1978). Sturdy childhood predictors of adult antisocial behavior: Replications from longitudinal studies. *Psychological Medicine, 8,* 611–622.

Rutter, M., Yule, B., Quinton, D., Rowlands, O., Yule, W., & Berger, M. (1975). Attainment and adjustment in two geographical areas: III. Some factors accounting for area differences. *British Journal of Psychiatry, 126,* 520–533.

Simons, R. L., Whitbeck, L. B., Conger, R. D., & Chyi-In, W. (1991). Intergenerational transmission of harsh parenting. *Developmental Psychology, 27 no. 1,* 159–171.

Singer, J. A., & Salovey, P. (1993). *The remembered self: Emotion and memory in personality.* New York: Free Press.

Smith, M. A., & Jenkins, J. M. (1991). The effects of marital disharmony on prepubertal children. *Journal of Abnormal Child Psychology, 19,* 625–644.

Sroufe, A. L., & Fleeson, J. (1988). The coherence of family relationships. In R. A. Hinde & J. Stevenson-Hinde (Eds.), *Relationships within families: Mutual influences* (pp. 27–47). Oxford: Clarendon Press.

Stein, N., Folkman, S., Trabasso, T., & Christopher-Richards, A. (1995). The role of appraisal processes in predicting psychological well-being. In *Roshomon Conference, Center for the Study of AIDS Prevention, January 3 & 4.*

Sullivan, H. S. (1952). *The interpersonal theory of psychiatry.* New York: Norton.

Tomkins, S. S. (1979). Script theory: Differential magnification of affects. In H. E. Howe & R. A. Dienstbier (Eds.), *Nebraska Symposium on Motivation, 1978* (pp. 201–236). Lincoln, NE: University of Nebraska Press.

Tomkins, S. S. (1995). *Exploring affect: The selected writings of Sylvan S. Tomkins (Ed. E. V. Demos).* New York: Cambridge University Press.

Waters, E., Merrick, S. K., Albersheim, L. J., & Treboux, D. (1995, March/April). *Attachment security from infancy to early adulthood: A 20-year longitudinal study of attachment security in infancy and early adulthood.* Paper presented at Biennial Meeting of the Society for Research in Child Development, Indianapolis, IN.

CHAPTER 24

The Story of Your Life

A Process Perspective on Narrative and Emotion in Adult Development

Jefferson A. Singer
Department of Psychology
Connecticut College
New London, Connecticut

I. INTRODUCTION

Adult development is one of the few fields in American psychology that has traditionally embraced the collection and analysis of individuals' narrative accounts of their lives. In this chapter, I discuss newer perspectives on the relationship of these narratives to adult development. In particular, I suggest that narratives can no longer be considered mere vessels that contain truths or insights about stages of the life course. Instead, individuals' narrative accounts (whether collected through interviews, autobiographies, letters, or diaries) play a major role in the very construction and understanding of these stages. By drawing on a personological theory of identity (McAdams, 1987, 1988, 1993) and social construction theories of both narrative and affect (Gergen, 1985, 1994; Singer & Sarbin, 1995), I describe different process approaches that demonstrate how the stories we tell of our lives reveal and define the developmental and affective challenges of adult life. Each of these approaches has generated a new body of empirical research that has broadened and deepened our understanding of the psychosocial "stages" of identity, intimacy, generativity, and ego integrity. To place these newer process perspectives in historical context, it is necessary to provide an account of how narratives have previously been used to study adult development.

II. EARLIER NARRATIVE APPROACHES TO ADULT DEVELOPMENT

The willingness to rely upon individuals' stories and life histories as valid sources of data may be traced to adult development's scientific roots in psychoanalytic and personological perspectives. Dating back to Freud's psychobiographical analysis of Leonardo da Vinci (Freud, 1910/1957) and Adler's (1927) emphasis on "individual psychology," there has been a broad tradition in psychoanalytic thinking that has valued theoretical interpretations of an individual's life through historical events, personal documents (letters, diaries, memos, etc.), and written works. Psychoanalytically oriented psychobiographies became a mainstay of scholars in both the social sciences and humanities for most of this century (Runyan, 1988) and have continued up to the present (Burlingame, 1994), despite criticism of their historical veridicality, idiographic focus, and their reductionist emphasis on childhood conflicts (Runyan, 1990).

American researchers in personality, Henry Murray and Gordon Allport, were impressed with the comprehensive concern for the individual life that psychoanalytic psychobiographies displayed. However, they were less enthusiastic about the Freudian preoccupation with sexual conflict in early childhood as the driving engine in personality (Anderson, 1990). Nevertheless, as they and their students went on to apply their own theoretical frameworks to investigations of personality, they continued to make analysis of life histories and personal documents central to their work (Allport, 1965; Murray, 1938, 1955/1981; White, 1975). This personological tradition of narrative perspectives on the life course was sustained through Robert White's *Lives in Progress* (1975) and is still vibrant in contemporary research (Franz, 1995; McAdams & Ochberg, 1988).

Given his psychoanalytic background (trained and psychoanalyzed by Anna Freud) and his role in the creation of Murray's (1938) *Explorations in personality* (he is listed among the co-authors as Erik Homburger), it should not be surprising that Erik Erikson, the founding father of contemporary adult development theory (Erikson, 1950), should have embraced narrative techniques. In telling the life stories of Martin Luther and Gandhi, he analyzed their autobiographical narratives, personal documents, and published writings to argue for the influence of psychosocial conflicts on their life choices. In proposing both an adult developmental theory and a narrative approach to its study, Erikson opened the way for the more recent and well-known interview studies of stages and transitions in the adult life course (Gould, 1980; Levinson, Darrow, Klein, Levinson, & McKee, 1978; Sheehy, 1984). Though none of these studies are as theoretically driven or psychoanalytically oriented as Erikson's work, they all draw upon the premise that individuals' accounts of their adult lives will reveal Eriksonian struggles with identity, intimacy, generativity, and ego integrity. In each case, the authors conducted lengthy and repeated interviews with their participants and then subjected these interviews to a qualitative interpretative analysis usually conducted by a research team that included the study's author. Other researchers have subsequently continued this approach with an emphasis on particular areas of adult development, such as women's transitions (Brown & Gilligan, 1992; Mercer, Nichols, & Doyle, 1989), generativity (Kotre, 1984), and life review (Sherman, 1991).

III. A NARRATIVE AND AFFECTIVE PROCESS APPROACH TO ADULT DEVELOPMENT

The traditional narrative perspectives outlined above all share a common assumption, one also held by sociologists and anthropologists who have engaged in life history techniques to study the lives and cultures of marginalized individuals. Peacock and Holland (1988, cited in Linde, 1993) described this "portal" assumption as a belief that the collected narrative will open the way to an understanding of an "actual world" that exists beyond the words of the narrative. In the case of sociologists and anthropologists, there was originally a hope that first-person accounts might give less stereotyped and more insightful visions of excluded members of the society (e.g., hobos—N. Anderson, 1923; dance hall girls—Cressey, 1932; delinquents—Shaw, 1930/1951). This perspective has persisted to the present day in social science and journalistic work (Coles, 1967; Kozol, 1991; Liebow, 1993; Howell, 1973; Terkel, 1974).

In contrast to this direct portal approach, George Herbert Mead and the Chicago school of symbolic interactionism elected to conduct life studies in order to understand how an individual's self-understanding shapes and is shaped by autobiographical events (see Polkinghorne, 1988, for a helpful account of this movement). Similarly, Murray and other personological researchers believed that the collection of narrative material through interviews, personal documents, and projective stories told to the ambiguous pictures of the T.A.T. (Thematic Apperception Test) would capture the unique ways in which individuals structured their experience of both their interior and exterior worlds. Peacock and Holland (1988, cited in Linde, 1993) call this second orientation the "subjectivist" portal approach. It seeks to depict not an external world of physical realities, but the internal reality of the participants narrating their stories. Through listening to or reading their stories, one gains entry to the universe of their feelings, thoughts, and motives.

Implicit in both the objective and subjectivist portal perspectives is a conviction that there is a "truth" beneath the narrative; the narrative serves only as a casing that may be discarded once the essential facts or meanings are extracted. The collection of narratives was meant to be a refinement, not a repudiation of positivist empiricism. Formal quantitative methods simply could not capture the complexity of human motive and thought available through the case study and narrative history. In recent decades, as Rosenwald and Ochberg (1992) detail, "a new conception of personal report (and of social science itself) has entered the scene. As a result, personal accounts are now read with an eye not just to the scenes they describe but to the process, product, and consequences of reportage itself" (p. 2). This hermeneutic perspective places its emphasis on the symbolic vocabulary, narrative structure, and cultural meanings of the stories themselves rather than on an independent objective or subjective reality the stories are putatively meant to depict (Bleicher, 1980). In contrast to the portal approach, Peacock and Holland define this newer concern with narrative qua narrative as a "process" approach and it is typified in psychology by the social constructionist work of K. Gergen (1985), Howard (1989), Sarbin (1986), and Spence (1982, 1987).

Rosenwald and Ochberg (1992) correctly pointed out that this new narrative emphasis owes a great debt to feminist and multicultural challenges to the domination of psychology by what Polkinghorne (1988) calls a "stringent formal science behaviorism" (p. 105), which has been associated over this century with a white male hierarchy. The excluded voices of women, ethnic/racial minorities, gays, and lesbians now summon competing narratives that highlight the necessity of listening to multiple stories (Garnets & Kimmel, 1991; Gilligan, 1982; Riger, 1992; Sue, 1991). When one no longer accepts an inherited single narrative as "truth," one is forced to acknowledge a given narrative's power to reveal as much about the group or culture to which individuals belong as it does about the individuals themselves. Rosenwald and Ochberg (1992) concluded, "The culture 'speaks itself' through each individual's story" (p. 7).

Just as the objective or "portal" perspective on narratives has been challenged by a more process-oriented perspective, so too have recent researchers questioned the depiction of emotional states as physiological "facts." In a recent special issue of the *Journal of Narrative and Life History* (J. A. Singer & Sarbin, 1995), a series of papers argue that emotions are first and foremost narrative constructions that express interpersonal transactions based in cultural rules and scenarios. Combining this position with the narrative process perspective on life stories leads to a very different view of the meaning of stories and emotions in the life course. In the sections that follow, I will review theoretical and research efforts that explore this new process perspective on narrative and emotion in adult development.

IV. McADAMS'S LIFE STORY THEORY OF IDENTITY: PERSONOLOGY AND PROCESS

In contrast to previous narrative research on the life course, Dan P. McAdams (1987, 1990, 1993) has not simply employed his participants' narratives to provide examples of how adults pass through the various psychosocial stages of adult development (identity, intimacy, generativity, and ego integrity). Rather, he has proposed that the life story individuals begin to construct in adolescence and continue to refine over the life course is in fact the core of their identity and affective experience.

> *Beginning in late adolescence, we become biographers of the self, mythologically rearranging the scattered elements of our lives—the different "selves," or what Erikson terms "identifications"—into a narrative whole providing unity and purpose. Thus,* identity is a life story *[italics in the original]. The identity configuration to which Erikson alludes is a configuration of plot, character, setting, scene, and theme. (McAdams, 1988, p. 29)*

McAdams believes that storytelling is a defining feature of human nature and that within our own Western individualistic culture, this storytelling capacity leads each person to fashion a unique life narrative. This life narrative follows a temporal course that is in accordance with the stages of adult development. It first comes to being during adolescence and struggles with dominant questions of "who am I?" and "who will I become?" (Identity vs. Role Confusion). As the "chapter" of adolescence comes to an end, young adults in their 20s and 30s turn their narrative powers more intensely to questions of intimacy and social integration; their story centers on questions of "how am I connected to others?" (Intimacy vs. Isolation). As adults enter the middle years of their 40s through their 60s, their narrative shift to acknowledgment of their mortality and limited reign upon the earth; they turn to consideration of their legacies and contributions to society, whether in the form of children, an intellectual or material product, or an act of service or distinction (Generativity vs. Stagnation). In the final chapters of advanced age, the 70s and beyond, individuals look back upon the story they have written, reviewing, critiquing, and in some cases attempting to add to it, as they approach its end (Ego Integrity vs. Despair).

As individuals move through these phases of story construction and revision, McAdams proposes that they rely upon elements common to all stories. There are four major components—*nuclear episodes, imagoes, ideological settings,* and *generativity scripts.* There are also two basic dimensions that link to each component, *thematic lines* and *narrative complexity.* Beginning with the thematic lines, McAdams proposes two major motivational themes run through our stories, sometimes in tandem and sometimes in conflict. The first is "agency" or the desire of human beings for independence, autonomy, and mastery. Agency encompasses our impulse to achieve self-definition through acts of creativity, individuation, and power. The second is "communion" or the desire to enter into relationship with others—to nurture or be nurtured, to give or receive love, to create bonds with or be bonded to a community. Communion involves the giving up of self to either another person, a community, or an idea. In this self-surrender, individuals merge with a transcendent whole and let go of their individual identity. The agency-communion distinction was coined by Bakan (1966) and is employed by many other contemporary researchers with similar wordings and dichotomies (Blatt, 1990; Fine, 1990; Gilligan, 1982; J. L. Singer, 1988; Smelser & Erikson, 1980).

According to McAdams, all of the four story elements will vary in the degree to which they express themes of agency and communion. At each stage of story construction, individuals confront the often-conflicting pulls in their lives toward greater engagement with others or greater separation and differentiation. Their stories shape themselves around the relative weight the narrative affords to each theme. For example, Mercer et al. (1989) in their study of women who were born in or before 1929, found their participants' life narratives to be dominated by interpersonal themes of spousal and maternal engagement. Reflecting a similar generational constraint in gender roles, Levinson et al.'s (1978) collection of men's narratives was organized around vocation and transitions within work life over time.

The other basic dimension of the life story is narrative complexity. In considering the structure of individuals' life histories, McAdams focuses squarely on "process" aspects of narratives. In other words, to understand individuals and their self-conceptions, we need to know how they construe the trajectory of their life stories. Some individuals tell an A to B to C kind of story—all events fall into a logical place; their life in their perception has followed a predictable and uncomplicated course. For example, consider a character in Heinrich Boll's novel, *Billiards at Half Past Nine*, who recounts the moment in his life at which he arrived in the city where he would find his livelihood and his wife:

> *From the moment I set foot in the city I had my moves all figured out, an exact*
> *daily routine, the steps of a complicated dance all down to a tee—myself soloist*
> *and ballet master all in one. Cast and decor were there for the asking, not costing*
> *a penny. (Boll, 1975, p. 62)*

Alternatively, other individuals depict their lives as filled with complicated twists and turns, ambiguity and conflict.

In addition to these two narrative dimensions of thematic lines and narrative structures, there are the four basic elements of the life story. The first element is ideological setting. Individuals craft their life stories with a eye toward a value system about right and wrong, "good" and "bad," what they should and not should do with their lives. This setting draws on individuals' convictions about the importance of agency and communion in their lives; do they value friendship over achievement or excellence over compromise? As individuals narrate their life stories, they reveal not just the circumstances of their lives, but the backdrop of values and commitments that make that life meaningful to them.

The second component of the life story is the nuclear episode. In each life story, there are particular critical events or incidents that individuals can describe with remarkable clarity and detail. Individuals often describe these scenes as turning points or benchmark moments of their lives. McAdams has suggested that nuclear episodes may contain crucial moments of change (where a reversal and new beginning occur) or of continuity (where the incident crystallizes a fundamental and defining aspect of the person). Nuclear episodes may be considered a particularly important subtype of a larger category of "self-defining memories" (Moffitt & Singer, 1994; J. A. Singer & Moffitt, 1991–92; J. A. Singer & Salovey, 1993). Self-defining memories are memories about a vivid and repeatedly recalled personal experience that reveals an ongoing concern or unresolved issue of the personality. They need not be as monumental or life changing as nuclear episodes, but they have the capacity to evoke strong emotion even years after the recollected events took place.

The affective power of nuclear episodes and self-defining memories highlights how a process perspective offers a different view of emotion from those held by traditional personality or emotion theorists. The story of individuals' lives is also a story of repeated affective patterns. Drawing on Silvan Tomkins's script theory (1979, 1987), McAdams recognizes that individuals tend to structure the major events of their lives according to sequences of affect. As Tomkins suggests, some individuals may alternately discover and impose a familiar affective pattern on the experiences of the lives. In Tomkins's terms, some of the most familiar patterns are *nuclear* and *commitment*. In the nuclear scene, individuals experience positive affect that changes abruptly to negative affect (e.g., an eager child happily awaiting the holiday, only to open the door to an angry dispute between her parents). This pattern—happy expectation betrayed by rancor—repeatedly surfaces in the individual's life, until it becomes a "scripted" set of affective rules that are often projected on to ambiguous experiences. At the other extreme, individuals may have "commitment scripts" (Tomkins, 1987) that depict sharp changes of affect from negative to positive. Commitment scenes are the positive turning points of McAdams's nuclear episodes, moments in which we overcome adversity and achieve a desired outcome (e.g., a child struggles with a frustrating dance step, but masters it and gives a successful recital). This process characterization of affect in adult lives moves us away from simple trait or physiological descriptions of affect. Rather, affect is embedded in the characteristic narrative episodes of an individual's life.

The next element in McAdams's life story perspective is the imago. Imagoes are the archetypal characters that populate individuals' narratives. They resurface throughout the narratives as friends or enemies, helpers or hindrances, sages or fools. Individuals will have their own particular set of character types. Even though the names may change as the narrative evolves, the types will tend to define and locate how the old and new characters are depicted. McAdams suggested that imagoes can be placed within the four possible combinations of high and low agency and communion. For example, a life story could contain a recurrent imago of a wise, but distant mentor (high agency, but low communion) and a charming, but ineffectual spouse (high communion, low agency). As individuals detail the story of their lives and the critical figures that have influenced them, it is possible not simply to note these influences, but to perceive the narrators' own internal concerns for agentic and communal figures in their lives.

The last element is the generativity script. Here McAdams means individuals' concern with the outcome of their life stories—their visions of life's ending and legacy. In assessing how individuals perceive or anticipate their stories' closings, we can once again determine their relative concerns with agency and communion. McAdams (1888, McAdams & de St. Aubin, 1992) suggested that generativity in the adult is a fusion of agency concerns for the perpetuation of the self and communion concerns for the welfare of descendants and society in general. By leaving a legacy, a mark on the world (whether in terms of the quality of one's off-spring or the excellence of one's material products), individuals achieve a kind of personal immortality at the same time that they make a contribution to the health of the society. Generativity scripts consist of individuals' own narrations of their efforts at fashioning a personal legacy. Within these life narratives, do individuals emphasize more agentic aspects of personal expression and triumph or communal aspects of nurturance and service?

McAdams and de St. Aubin (1992) have demonstrated that there is convergence among individuals' scores on a self-report inventory of generativity, their endorsement of behavioral acts of generativity, and their autobiographical accounts of important nuclear episodes in their lives (e.g., peak and nadir experiences). Kotre (1984) used life stories collected through intensive interviews to illustrate four different forms of generativity (biological, parental, technical, and cultural). Franz (1995) also found that narratives excerpted from letters and diaries can be content analyzed for agentic and communal themes in relationship to generativity. Examining the British writer Vera Brittain's personal documents, Franz found that themes of intimacy and generativity increased as she moved from her 20s into her early 30s. On the other hand, her certainty about her agentic identity as a writer also increased over this period, although other more general identity concerns tended to decline. This combination of increased intimacy and occupational confidence suggests that Britain's generativity script at the threshold of her 30s held the potential to balance both agentic and communal concerns. These kinds of personological and narrative approaches to the study of generativity and identity as a whole help to move researchers away from an overly simplistic and lock-step view of adult development; they also make clear that the process of identity formation proceeds throughout adult life rather than falling neatly into place at the beginning of young adulthood (Whitbourne, 1986).

From an affective perspective, the reconciliation of agentic and communal forces that accompanies generativity allows for a freeing up of affective experience that may have been previously restricted for both genders. For example, Gould (1980) detailed the case of Nicole, who after raising four children, made a decision to return to work and pursue her professional interests (a revival of her agentic needs). As she underwent the reverberations of this decision in all domains of her life, she experienced a surge of power that led to a freeing of sexual desire and increased excitement in her romantic life with her husband. In a parallel fashion, and more anecdotally, I have noted how many of my male colleagues have described to me a greater access to feelings of tenderness and to the ability to cry since the birth of their children. Once again, these examples locate affective experiences in the context of identity development over the life course, as opposed to viewing affect in a fixed or biological manner.

In summary, individuals' life stories, carried internally and narrated to others, contain the crucial components of identity. Our narrative understanding of ourselves is literally who we are and how we are known. As individuals grow and change over the life course, they waver between agentic and communal themes; they add and delete complexity from their life structures; they experience affectively intense moments of change and affirmation that become touchstones of their consciousness; they shape those around them into sagacious mentors, co-conspirators in their pleasures, or adversaries to be overcome. Individuals are constantly writing and revising their stories to create "unity" and coherence in their lives, as well as to define a generative "purpose" that moves them beyond themselves (McAdams, 1988, p. 3). Narratives are not windows through which researchers will glimpse the life course of adult development; narratives are the life course itself.

V. SOCIAL CONSTRUCTIONISM AND THE PROCESS PERSPECTIVE ON NARRATIVE AND AFFECT

By placing the emphasis in the life story of adult development on narrative and affective processes, McAdams's work encourages us to ask about the origins of individuals' stories. McAdams is always careful to acknowledge the sociocultural influences on any given life story; the content and style of the stories are very much constrained by the available tales extant in the culture. Yet as a personologically oriented psychologist, McAdams is primarily interested in the part of the story written by the individual. He wants to convey the most rich and comprehensive characterization of the individual life and the search for meaning within that life. Social construction theorists (Cushman, 1990; Gergen 1985; Greenberg, 1994; Sarbin, 1986) start from the other end of the continuum; they are interested in how culture writes the story of lives. Though individuals may construct their personal narratives and experience these stories as unique and spontaneously lived, social constructionists emphasize the cultural determinants that organize the narrative and affective elements of the self.

A chief proponent of this position, K. J. Gergen (1994) has attempted to recast the idea of a "remembered self" into a more contextual and interpersonal form; he suggested that memory is a shared transaction among members of a common culture. To remember an event and recount it to someone else, individuals rely upon certain rules of narration and familiar "relationship scenarios" (K. J. Gergen & Gergen, 1988). For example, most autobiographical narratives are organized around the following criteria (K. J. Gergen & Gergen, 1988, pp. 22–23): a valued end point or goal toward which the protagonist of the narrative is striving; a subset of events selected to be included in the narrative that are relevant to the major goal states emphasized in the narrative; a recognizable order, most often temporal, for the events in the narrative; a causal linkage of these same events in a culturally accepted sequence such that later ones seem logically to be the outcome of earlier ones; and a demarcation of the narrative's beginning or end by well-understood signs (e.g., "let me tell you a story" or "so now you know the story of my first . . .").

Just as these criteria govern the form that our personal stories may take, our adherence to the norms of emotional experience may strongly guide the content of the story. K. J. Gergen and Gergen (1988) described individuals' emotional interactions as dependent on cultural norms. For example, if I feel angry and express this anger through a furrowed brow and clenched fist, a co-worker may sense my strong emotion and either avoid me or ask very gingerly what is bothering me. Since I am in a workplace, I cannot show my anger by yelling or throwing things, so I must reply in strong but measured tones about the source of my anger. Once I have articulated my anger and its object, there is a strong pull on a friendly co-worker to share in my indignation and to make statements that indicate support and a fellow outrage. It is easy to see how all of us play out this emotional exchange; however, if individuals change the object of anger from a reasonable one (an unfair boss) to a highly trivial one (a broken shoelace), it becomes clear that there are clear constraints over what is and is not a socially sanctioned emotional response. The emotion is given its meaning and semantic value through this interchange and acknowledgment of it by others with whom we are engaging in relationships (Sarbin, 1986).

Further influences on the narratives individuals tell about themselves can be found by considering the recipients of the narratives and the purposes behind the telling of the narratives to the recipients. Gergen (1994) suggested that many personal remembrances serve rhetorical purposes and are responses to interactions in which individuals' identities have been doubted or subject to inquiry. In order to answer the individual who has pushed us to clarify who we are (such challenges could take place in the course of a beginning courtship, a workplace collaboration, a justification of an unexpected or embarrassing action, a psychotherapy intake, an admissions or job interview, a class reunion, etc.), we offer a self-narrative in the form of a personal remembrance. The recipient becomes part of this narrative by engaging in questions about the events described and ultimately by greeting the narrative with acceptance (e.g., "now I understood you a bit better" or "that explains to me why you are this way") or continued challenge (e.g., "I'm not sure I buy this story" or "what am I supposed make of all this?"). Obviously, the degree that the recipient will be inclined to accept a personal narrative as "authentic" will vary on the perceived purpose behind the narrative. In the case of psychotherapy, the listening therapist tends to see the client's personal remembrances as sincerely intended if not always historically accurate (Spence, 1982). On the other hand, a job interviewer has some reason to believe that stronger forces of self-presentation may be in action during the recounting of an applicant's past experiences. The consideration of all these influences—narrative and affective rules, relationship scenarios, identities of the narrative recipients, and the rhetorical purposes served by narratives—combine to change the telling of one's life story from an individual's revelation of a given life's unity and purpose to an interpersonal transaction located within a set of cultural rituals.

If we take this argument a step further, we are forced to question the original stage theory approach to adult development. Though Erikson's original proposal of the adult moving through stages of identity, intimacy, generativity, and ego integrity was highly sensitive to both cross-cultural and idiographic influences regarding the timing and full manifestation of these stages, there was still an ontological commitment to these stages as part of the human life cycle. For example, as Smelser (1980, pp. 19–20) pointed out, Erikson conceived of the psychosocial stages as "epigenetic," a new stage could not emerge until the preceding stage's developmental tasks had been engaged. Although the life stages were heavily dependent upon interaction with culture, they were perceived in quasi-biological terms and as part of the evolutionary inheritance of what it meant to be human.

K. J. Gergen (1977) suggested that the existence of these stages and the narratives that have been collected to verify their existence (e.g., Gould, 1980; Levinson et al., 1978) are evidence of emergent Western cultural themes and scenarios as opposed to essential components of a "human nature." Their linear structure reflects our cultural preoccupation with progress and product, with life as an accumulation of accomplishment and commodities. Similarly, their presentation of a dichotomy between selfness (agency) and selflessness (communion) expresses our own culture's absorption in the concept of the individual. In a society that prizes individuality above all, we find it hard to imagine a social life in which this endless trade-off between caring for others or caring for ourselves would no longer seem a relevant or sensible dilemma (Greenberg, 1994). In addition, the original ordering of the psychosocial stages, in particular the location of identity achievement before intimacy has been questioned for its male-centered perspective. As more contemporary re-

searchers have made clear (Franz & Stewart, 1994; Josselson, 1973; Whitbourne & Tesch, 1985), the original location of identity formation before
the creation of intimacy says much more about the traditional weight
given to self-actualization through vocation by males than it does about
the psychological necessities of identity formation.

In the wake of these critiques, does this mean that social constructionists or researchers informed by social construction theory should
cease to study life stages in adult development or at the very least eschew
the use of narrative techniques to study them? No at all. What these critiques encourage researchers to do is to see these different tasks within
the life course as rich sources of information for the investigation of how
culture structures our choices and affective responses as individuals mature and age. As Smelser (1980, p. 23) suggested, we need not see the
psychosocial stages as "stages" at all; rather we might consider them life
"challenges" that will likely confront adults at different junctures in the
course of a lifetime (see also Mishler, 1992, pp. 36–37). Their particular
temporal order and their relationship to each other may be dictated
strongly by individuals' particular cultural contexts. Similarly, individuals'
responses to these challenges—how they choose to conceptualize them
and incorporate them into their life narratives—would be susceptible to
cultural influence as well. What follows are examples of how social constructionist research reexamines adult developmental stages through the
lens of a process analysis of narrative and emotion.

VI. PROCESS ANALYSIS OF INTIMACY

Social constructionist research has been applied to issues of intimacy
and romantic love (M. M. Gergen & Gergen, 1995), as well as failed intimacy or "unrequited love" (Baumeister, Wotman & Stillwell, 1993). The
Gergens have suggested that conceptions of relationships and affective
expressions of love are highly prone to historic and societal context. To be
in love in the period of 19th-century romanticism is extremely different
than the rational contractual emphasis of the subsequent modernist period or the self-reflexiveness of our current postmodern era. The affective
scenarios of love in the romantic period required "an intensity of expression—for example, tears, profound sadness, the swoon, joyous laughter"
(M. M. Gergen & Gergen, 1995, p. 226). In contrast, affective scenarios
of love in our postmodern period highlight the self-consciousness and
reflexivity of our time; we may engage in signs of sentiment, but we are
more likely to do so with a playful, ironic air.

In their study of unrequited love, Baumeister et al. (1993) asked participants to generate autobiographical accounts of episodes in which they

had assumed the role of either a "would-be lover" or a "rejector" of a potential lover. The participants' narratives were then analyzed for differences in emotion, self-esteem, guilt, key events, and perceptions of the other. The results showed clearly that cultural demands strongly influenced the roles and responses adopted by individuals who find themselves caught in the "drama" of unrequited love. In particular, would-be lovers drew upon the mass culture's depiction of the pining and brokenhearted lover. The easy availability of this cultural "script" for the would-be lover may in fact help to mitigate the pain of the experience and allow the would-be lover to draw consolation from joining the ranks of misunderstood romantics. On the other hand, rejectors often depicted their experience in more negative terms, clearly wishing the episode had never occurred. Rejectors also were less able to draw upon a familiar or sympathetic script for their part in not reciprocating the relationship. This "scriptlessness," as Baumeister et al. (1993, p. 385) depicted it, is an additional source of tension and distress for the reluctant recipients of the would-be lovers' advances. This study demonstrates that individuals have potential access to a variety of interpersonal and affective scripts already stored in consciousness and that these scripts may guide their affective responses in actual situations.

VII. PROCESS ANALYSIS OF MIDLIFE CAREER CHOICES

Recent analyses of individuals' narratives of their paths of career choice and advancement have again supported the need to treat these narratives as meaningful and symbolic in their own right (Mishler, 1992; Ochberg, 1988; Wiersma, 1988). Mishler (1992) presented a life story of an artist-craftsman and demonstrated how the narrative follows a structure of "origins," "detours," "craft skills," and "turning points," that is idiographically meaningful, but also reveals a cultural path that craftspeople tend to travel in our society. In order to make his narrative sensible to himself and to his interviewer, the craftsman profiled by Mishler began to "craft" his own story to fit a comprehensible and recognizable cultural form. Mishler emphasized that this process of identity formation through the construction of a socially recognizable narrative provides meaning and direction to the craftsman's conception of his life.

Extending this perspective, Ochberg (1988) and Wiersma (1988) provided life histories of other individuals' career choices; however, their emphasis is on more nonconscious meanings and ambivalent affect accrued by these narratives. Similar to Mishler, Ochberg demonstrated with two case histories of men at midcareer transitions, that their narratives reflect cultural narrative structures and themes—in this case the need for advancement and aggressive accomplishment in the workplace. Their stories rely upon narrative conventions of besting the competition, impressing the boss, accumulating capital, and the accompanying affects of pride, joy, and contempt. On the other hand, through a careful analysis of their biographical information, Ochberg also demonstrated that their narratives are equally revealing for what they leave out or cannot say about their intrapersonal dynamics. In each case, unarticulated needs for tenderness and connection with their fathers influence how they proceed and at times stumble in their career paths. The unspoken aspects of their narratives contain affects of sadness, guilt, and anger. Ochberg offered a synthesis of a social constructionist perspective with a continuing attention to the symbolic and analysis familiar to depth psychology.

Wiersma (1988) applied the same synthetic technique to her examination of women's narratives of their midlife transitions from domestic work to a career outside the home. She pointed out that narrative accounts cannot be taken on face value as valid windows into the meanings or needs of the narrators. The women in her study initially provided what Wiersma dubbed "press releases" that explained their transitions in socially sanctioned ways. In particular, the women's initial narratives conformed to certain cultural and social class expectations held by their peer group that this transition should offer liberation and rebirth for women trapped in domestic routines. The dominant affective expression of these press release narratives is upbeat, confident, and triumphant. However, after more careful analysis of the symbolic import of their actual narrative statements and further interviewing over a 2-year period, subtexts behind these press releases become more apparent. Wiersma was able to detect a more concealed narrative text that expressed their own ambivalence that this new course was acceptable and an unwillingness to acknowledge that their new roles were actively chosen and pursued by them. Behind these press releases, she was able to detect less "acceptable" affective themes of guilt, regret, and anxiety. Wiersma's hermeneutic "decoding" of these narratives suggested again that great caution must be exercised in accepting the narrative validity of individual's life histories on the basis of an initial account.

VIII. NARRATIVE PROCESS ANALYSIS OF THE LIFE COURSE TRAJECTORY

Having looked at different challenges within the life course, it is worthwhile to consider a process perspective on the life course as a whole. Within the more personological framework, McAdams might ask about the ideological setting or "narrative tone" (McAdams, 1993) a particular participant assigns to the overall flow of his or her life story. Is the story's basic affective orientation optimistic or pessimistic, filled with the belief in possibilities or obstacles? McAdams might examine this question by considering the early upbringing of participants and how effectively they developed a capacity for trust from parental–infant transactions. Alternatively, social constructionists would avoid consideration of a given individual's psychogenic history and instead look at the narrative palettes available to a cohort of individuals at a given time in the culture.

K. J. Gergen and Gergen (1988) described their study of 29 college-aged participants who were asked to chart the trajectory of the general affective tone of their lives up to the time of the study. The overall pattern suggested a happy childhood moving in an upward direction, followed by a stormy and downward sloping adolescent period, but finishing for the present in a upward slope, predicting happiness ahead in the early adult years. Though the particular circumstances varied widely from participant to participant, the emergent pattern reveals the adolescents share a common narrative and affective structure for understanding the general flow of their lives. The Gergens suggested that this particular pattern may actually rely upon the conventions of television drama, which often follows the same formula of calm beginning, dramatic disruption, and happy resolution. Similarly, the portrayal of "stormy adolescence" has become an encompassing myth in our culture and may exert a certain self-fulfilling influence on our perception of that period of life.

In contrast, M. Gergen (1980) looked at the overall pattern for 72 participants ranging from 63 to 93 years of age. This group generated a narrative and affective pattern that looked more like a rainbow with a slowly rising positive slope from childhood through the early adult years, peaking at the "golden years" of the 50s and 60s and then declining with advanced age from the 70s on. Once again, the Gergens proposed the possibility that media and social science foster this pattern by describing earlier phases of life in "developmental" terms and later life as a period of "declining years." A recent *New York Times* article (Angier, June 11, 1995) actually points to the surprisingly robust health and hardiness of individuals who have survived into their 80s and beyond. Perhaps, these kinds of revisionist accounts will begin to influence the cultural perceptions of life's trajectory and of "adult development" in general.

IX. CONCLUSION

The process perspective on narrative and emotion has engendered a great deal of empirical research, both quantitative and purely interpretive. By turning the focus on to the narrative and affective patterns themselves, it has allowed the units of analysis (recurrent plot structures, affective sequences, thematic motives, prototypical characters, dominant metaphors or symbols) to become more measurable and manageable than the full vista of a life. The result has been rich studies that allow for a greater reconciliation of idiographic and nomothetic techniques, creating more cross-talk and convergence in personality and social psychological perspectives than ever before. At the same time, these studies have a phenomenological feel that brings us closer to what students call "the real world." With the movement in psychotherapy to embrace narrative analysis (Spence, 1982, 1987; Schafer, 1992), there is an emerging convergence between more pure and applied branches of psychology. How the introduction of social constructionist ideas about narrative and affect will influence the process of psychotherapy and the story-creating function of that enterprise is indeed a challenging question. If culture writes itself through our stories, treating individuals for their particular incomplete or troubling stories may be focusing energies in a misleading direction (Greenberg, 1995). At the very least, whether in the course of studying adult development or treating a client in psychotherapy, the simple request to "tell me about yourself" no longer seems so simple or straightforward. The narrative and affective processes that ensue in answer to that question will be a source of study as much as the "facts" that are reported. For psychologists who have too often been "paradigmatic thinkers" and researchers (Bruner, 1986), it may be time to develop our narrative sides and attend more closely both to the stories people tell and the way that they are telling them.

REFERENCES

Adler, A. (1927). *Understanding human nature.* New York: Greenberg.

Alexander, I. E. (1988). Personality, psychological assessment, and psychobiography. *Journal of Personality, 56,* 265–294.

Allport, G. W. (Ed.) (1965). *Letters from Jenny.* New York: Harcourt, Brace, & World.

Anderson, J. W. (1990). The life of Henry A. Murray: 1893–1988. In A. I. Rabin, R. A. Zucker, R. A. Emmons, & S. Frank (Eds.), *Studying persons and lives* (pp. 304–334). New York: Springer.

Anderson, N. (1923). *The hobo.* Chicago: University of Chicago Press.

Angier, N. (June 11, 1995). If you're really ancient, you may be better off. *Sunday New York Times, 4,* 1, cont. on p. 5.

Bakan, D. (1966). *The duality of human existence: Isolation and communion in western man.* Boston: Beacon Press.

Baumeister, R. F., Wotman, S. R., & Stillwell, A. M. (1993). Unrequited love: On heartbreak, anger, guilt, scriptlessness, and humiliation. *Journal of Personality and Social Psychology, 64,* 377–394.

Blatt, S. J. (1990). Interpersonal relatedness and self-definition: Two personality configurations and their implications for psychopathology and psychotherapy. In J. L. Singer (Ed.), *Repression and dissociation* (pp. 299–335). Chicago: University of Chicago Press.

Bleicher, J. (1980). *Contemporary hermeneutics.* London: Routledge & Kegan Paul.

Boll, H. (1975). *Billiards at half past nine.* New York: Avon.

Brown, L. M., & Gilligan, C. (1992). *Meeting at the crossroads: Women's psychology and girls' development.* Cambridge, MA: Harvard University Press.

Bruner, J. S. (1986). *Actual minds, possible worlds.* Cambridge, MA: Harvard University Press.

Burlingame, M. A. (1994). *The inner world of Abraham Lincoln.* Urbana: University of Illinois Press.

Coles, R. (1967). *Children in crisis.* Boston: Little Brown.

Cressey, P. G. (1932) *The taxi-dance hall.* Chicago: University of Chicago Press.

Cushman, P. (1990). Why the self is empty: Toward a historically situated psychology. *American Psychologist, 45,* 599–611.

Erikson, E. H. (1950). *Childhood and society* (1st ed.). New York: Norton.

Fine, R. (1990). *Love and work.* New York: Continuum.

Franz, C. E. (1995). A quantitative case study of longitudinal changes in identity, intimacy, and generativity. *Journal of Personality, 63,* 27–46.

Franz, C. E., & Stewart, A. J. (1994). *Women creating lives: Identities, resilience, and resistance.* Boulder, CO: Westview.

Freud, S. (1910/1957). Leonardo da Vinci and a memory of his childhood. In J. Strachey (Ed.), *The standard edition of the complete psychological works of Sigmund Freud* (Vol. 11, pp. 63–137). London: Hogarth.

Garnets, L., & Kimmel, D. (1991). Lesbian and gay male dimensions in the psychological study of human diversity. In J. D. Goodchilds (Ed.), *Psychological perspectives on human diversity in America* (pp. 143–192). Washington DC: American Psychological Association.

Gergen, K. J. (1977). Stability, change, and chance in human development. In N. Datan & H. W. Reese (Eds.), *Lifespan developmental psychology* (pp. 136–158). New York: Academic Press.

Gergen, K. J. (1985). The social constructionist movement in modern psychology. *American Psychologist, 40,* 266–275.

Gergen, K. J. (1994). Mind, text, and society: Self-memory in social context. In U. Neisser & R. Fivush (Eds.), *The remembering self* (pp. 78–104). New York: Cambridge University Press.

Gergen, K. J., & Gergen, M. M. (1988). Narratives and the self as relationship. In L. Berkowitz (Ed.), *Advances in experimental social psychology* (Vol. 21, pp. 17–56). New York: Academic Press.

Gergen, M. M. (1980). *Antecedents and consequences of self-attributional preferences in later life.* Unpublished doctoral dissertation, Temple University, Philadelphia, PA.

Gergen, M. M., & Gergen, K. J. (1995). What is this thing called love? Emotional scenarios in historical perspective. *Journal of Narrative and Life History, 5,* 221–237.

Gilligan, C. (1982). *In a different voice.* Cambridge, MA: Harvard University Press.

Gould, R. L. (1980). Transformations during early and middle adult years. In N. J. Smelser & E. H. Erikson (Eds.), *Themes of work and love in adulthood* (pp. 213–237). Cambridge, MA: Harvard University Press.

Greenberg, G. (1994). *The self on the shelf: Recovery books and the good life.* Albany: State University of New York Press.

Greenberg, G. (1995). If the self is a narrative: Social construction in the clinic. *Journal of Narrative and Life History, 5,* 269–283.

Howard, G., (1989). *A tale of two stories: Excursions into a narrative approach to psychology.* Notre Dame, IN: Academic Publications.

Howell, J. T. (1973). *Hard living on clay street.* Garden City, NY: Anchor Press.

Josselson, R. (1973). Psychodynamic aspects of identity formation in college women. *Journal of Youth and Adolescence, 9,* 117–126.

Kotre, J. (1984). *Outliving the self: Generativity and the interpretation of lives.* Baltimore: Johns Hopkins University Press.

Kozol, J. (1991). *Savage inequalities.* New York: Crown.

Levinson, D. J., Darrow, C. N., Klein, E. B., Levinson, M. H., & McKee, B. (1978). *The seasons of a man's life.* New York: Alfred A. Knopf.

Liebow, E. (1993). *Tell them who I am.* New York: Free Press.

Linde, C. (1993). *Life stories: The creation of coherence.* New York: Oxford University Press.

McAdams, D. P. (1987). A life-story model of identity. In R. Hogan & W. H. Jones (Eds.), *Perspectives in personality* (Vol. 2, pp. 15–50). Greenwich, CT: JAI Press.

McAdams, D. P. (1988). *Power, intimacy, and the life story: Personological inquiries into identity.* New York: Guilford Press.

McAdams, D. P. (1990). Unity and purpose in human lives: The emergence of identity as a life story. In A. I. Rabin, R. A. Zucker, R. A. Emmons, & S. Frank (Eds.), *Studying persons and lives* (pp. 148–200). New York: Springer.

McAdams, D. P. (1993). *Stories we live by: Personal myths and the making of the self.* New York: William Morrow.

McAdams, D. P., & de St. Aubin (1992). A theory of generativity and its assessment through self-report, behavioral acts, and narrative themes in autobiography. *Journal of Personality and Social Psychology, 62,* 1003–1015.

McAdams, D. P., & Ochberg, R. L. (Eds.). (1988). *Psychobiography and life narratives.* Durham, NC: Duke University Press.

Mercer, R. T., Nichols, E. G., & Doyle, G. C. (1989). *Transitions in a woman's life: Major life events in developmental context.* New York: Springer.

Mishler, E. G. (1992). Work, identity, and narrative: An artist-craftsman's story. In G. C. Rosenwald & R. L. Ochberg (Eds.), *Storied lives* (pp. 21–40). New Haven: Yale University Press.

Moffitt, K. H., & Singer, J. A. (1994). Continuity in the life story: Self-defining memories, affect and approach/avoidance strivings. *Journal of Personality, 62,* 21–43.

Murray, H. A. (1938). *Explorations in personality.* New York: Oxford University Press.

Murray, H. A. (1955/1981). American Icarus. In E. S. Schneidman (Ed), *Endeavors in psychology: Selections from the personology of Henry A. Murray* (pp. 312–330). New York: Harper & Row.

Ochberg, R. L. (1987). *Middle-aged sons and the meaning of work.* Ann Arbor, MI: Mi Research Press.

Ochberg, R. L., (1988). Life stories and the psychosocial construction of careers. *Journal of Personality, 56,* 173–204.

Polkinghorne, D. E. (1988). *Narrative knowing and the human sciences.* Albany: State University of New York Press.

Riger, S. (1992). Epistemological debates, feminist voices: Science, social values, and the study of women. *American Psychologist, 47,* 730–740.

Rosenwald, G. C., & Ochberg, R. L. (Eds.) (1992). Introduction: Life stories, cultural politics, and self-understanding. In G. C. Rosenwald, & R. L. Ochberg (Eds.), *Storied lives* (pp. 1–18). New Haven: Yale University Press.

Rosenwald, G. C., & Ochberg, R. L. (Eds.). (1992). *Storied lives: The cultural politics of self-understanding.* New Haven: Yale University Press.

Runyan, W. M. (1984). *Life histories and psychobiography: Explorations in theory and method.* New York: Oxford University Press.

Runyan, W. M. (1988). Progress in psychobiography. *Journal of Personality, 56,* 295–326.

Runyan, W. M. (1990). Individual lives and the structure of personality psychology. In A. I. Rabin, R. A. Zucker, R. A. Emmons, & S. Frank (Eds.), *Studying persons and lives* (pp. 10–40). New York: Springer.

Sarbin, T. R. (Ed.), (1986). *Narrative psychology: The storied nature of human conduct.* New York: Praeger.

Schafer, R. (1992). *Retelling a life: Narration and dialogue in psychoanalysis.* New York: Basic Books.

Shaw, C. R. (1930/1951). *The jack-roller: A delinquent boy's own story.* Philadelphia: Albert Saifer.

Sheehy, G. (1984). *Passages.* New York: Bantam.

Sherman, E. (1991). *Reminiscence and the self in old age.* New York: Springer.

Singer, J. A., & Moffitt, K. H. (1991–92). An experimental investigation of specificity and generality in memory narratives. *Imagination, Cognition, and Personality, 11,* 233–257.

Singer, J. A., & Salovey, P. (1993). *The remembered self: Emotion and memory in personality.* New York: The Free Press.

Singer, J. A., & Sarbin, T. R. (Eds.). (1995). Narrative construction of emotional life. *Journal of Narrative and Life History* [Special issue], 5, 203–283.

Singer, J. L. (1988). Psychoanalytic theory in the context of contemporary psychology: The Helen Block Lewis memorial address. *Psychoanalytic Psychology, 5,* 95–125.

Smelser, N. J. (1980). Issues in the study of work and love in adulthood. In N. J. Smelser & E. H. Erikson (Eds.), *Themes of love and work in adulthood* (pp. 1–26). Cambridge, MA: Harvard University Press.

Smelser, N. J., & Erikson, E. H. (1980). *Themes of love and work in adulthood.* Cambridge, MA: Harvard University Press.

Spence, D. P. (1982). *Narrative truth and historical truth: Meaning and interpretation in psychoanalysis.* New York: Norton.

Spence, D. P. (1987). *The Freudian metaphor.* New York: Norton.

Sue, S. (1991). Ethnicity and culture in psychological research and practice. In J. D. Goodchilds (Ed.), *Psychological perspectives on human diversity in America* (pp. 143–192). Washington, DC: American Psychological Association.

Taylor, S. J., & Bogan, R. (1984). *Introduction to qualitative research methods: The search for meanings* (2nd ed.). New York: Wiley & Sons.

Terkel, S. (1974). *Working.* New York: Pantheon.

Tomkins, S. S. (1979). Script theory: Differential magnification of affects. In H. E. Howe & R. A. Dienstbier (Eds.), *Nebraska symposium on motivation,* (vol. 26, pp. 201–236). Lincoln: University of Nebraska Press.

Tomkins, S. S. (1987). Script theory. In J. Aranoff, A. I. Rabin, & R. A. Zucker (Eds.), *The emergence of personality* (pp. 147–216). New York: Springer.

Whitbourne, S. K. (1986). *The me I know: A study of adult identity.* New York: Spring-Verlag.

Whitbourne, S. K., & Tesch, S. A. (1985). A comparison of identity and intimacy statuses in college students and alumni. *Developmental Psychology, 21,* 1039–1044.

White, R. W. (1975). *Lives in progress.* New York: Holt, Rinehart, & Winston.

Wiersma, J. (1988). The press release: Symbolic communication in life history interviewing. *Journal of Personality, 56,* 205–238.

Index